Most Likely Diagnosis
USMLE Step 2 CK
Clinical Knowledge

Amninder S. Dhesi, MD

Note to Reader

Although the information, ideas, management, in this book is carefully reviewed for correctness, neither authors or editors nor the publisher can accept the legal responsibility for any errors or omissions that maybe made. Neither the publisher nor editor makes any warranty, expressed or implied, with respect to the material contained herein.

DEDICATION

Completing this book required a lot of patience and love for teaching. I would like to thank my parents for teaching me the value of perseverance and always believing in me. I am very thankful to my brother and sister for always supporting me. Lastly, I would like to thank my wife for her endless love and encouragement.

TABLE OF CONTENTS

Cardiology
- o   Internal medicine --- 1
- o   Infectious diseases --- 24
- o   Surgery --- 26

Hypertension -- 29

Hematology --- 33

Pulmonology
- o   Internal medicine --- 59
- o   Infectious diseases --- 73
- o   Surgery --- 79

Endocrinology - --- 81

Electrolytes --- 99

Acid-base disorders -- 107

Nephrology
- o   Internal medicine --- 109
- o   Infectious diseases --- 127
- o   Surgery --- 131

Gastroenterology
- o   Internal medicine --- 133
- o   Surgery --- 159

Rheumatology
- o   Internal medicine --- 165
- o   Infectious diseases --- 177
- o   Surgery --- 179

Neurology
- o   Internal medicine --- 187
- o   Infectious diseases --- 207
- o   Surgery --- 213

Postoperative fever -- 215

Psychiatry
- o   Adults -- 217
- o   Pediatrics -- 235

Pediatrics -- 239

Gynecology --- 285

Obstetrics -- 309

Human Immunodeficiency Virus (HIV) ----------------------------- 335

TABLE OF CONTENTS

Bites --- 339

Adult immunization --- 341

Biostatistics -- 343

Ethics --- 347

Dermatology -- 353

Ophthalmology -- 365

Toxicology --- 371

Vitamins -- 375

CARDIOLOGY

CHEST PAIN

CHEST PAIN DIFFERENTIAL DIAGNOSIS

- **Pericarditis:** Chest pain in pericarditis is characterized by sharp chest pain, which is worst when patient is supine and relives with leaning forward. EKG shows **ST elevation in all leads**
- **Costochondritis:** Chest pain is characterized by localized, and stabbing chest pain, which can be reproduced by physical motion. Physical exam shows chest wall tenderness. EKG is usually normal
- **GERD:** Chest pain in GERD is felt after eating certain foods and it gets better with antacids
- **Esophageal spasm:** Chest pain that starts after drinking cold water or beverage
- **Aortic dissection:** Chest pain is characterized by sharp, tearing chest pain, **radiating to the back.** It is mostly seen after trauma, motor vehicle accident at the speed > 45mph or collagen vascular disease, such as Marfan syndrome, Ehlers–Danlos syndrome. Physical exam shows different blood pressure in each arm. Chest X-ray shows widened mediastinum
- **Pneumothorax:** It is mostly seen in young patients. Patient usually presents with **sudden onset of chest pain and shortness of breath.** Physical exam shows JVD, and auscultation of lungs shows absent breath sounds on the affected side of the lungs
- **Cocaine abuse:** Cocaine abuse may cause angina. Look for other clues such as history of drug abuse, nosebleed, or pupillary dilation.
  Panic attacks: Chest pain in panic attacks is felt suddenly after feeling overwhelming sense of fear

CHARACTERISTIC OF CHEST PAIN IN A MI

Three main characteristics of chest pain in a MI are:

- Substernal chest pain that may radiate to left arm, shoulder, or jaw
- Chest tightness or pressure sensation
- Chest pain that is not reproducible by body motion

Note: Diabetics, postmenopausal women, elderly and heart transplant patients likely to have silent MI or atypical symptoms such as nausea, dyspnea, weakness or confusion

RISK FACTORS FOR CORONARY ARTERY DISEASE (CAD)

- Cigarettes smoking
- Diabetes mellitus
- BP > 140/90 or on BP medications
- HDL < 40
- Male > 45 years, or female > 55 years of age
- First-degree male relative < 55 years of age with CAD , or first-degree female relative < 65 years of age with CAD

Note: Diabetes mellitus is the **greatest risk factor** for CAD, and cigarettes' smoking cessation is the **most preventable** CAD risk factor.

Cardiac enzymes

Enzyme	Detectable after infarction
Myoglobin	• Is detectable within 1-4 hours
CK-MB	• Is detectable within 4-6 hours, peaks in 12-24 hours and normalizes within 2-3 days • Is also used to detect MI **re-infraction**
Troponin	• Is detectable within 3-4 hours, peaks in 12-16 hours and remains elevated for up to 2 weeks

TYPES AND MANAGEMENT OF ANGINA

1. STABLE ANGINA

Stable angina occurs due to poor blood flow through the coronary arteries, which are either blocked or narrowed

Mechanism: Blocked or narrowed coronary arteries may supply enough blood to the heart when the oxygen demand is less such as while sitting, walking or working at normal pace. However, during physical exertion or stress blocked arteries are unable to meet heart's oxygen demand, and that leads to stable angina.

Si/Sx: chest pain or discomfort with **predictable amount of exertion and relieves by rest or nitroglycerin**

Diagnosis: EKG shows ST depression and inversion or flattening of T-wave.

Note: EKG may be normal when patient's heart is not stressed anymore. In that case, patient's heart is stressed with a stress test, and EKG is monitored for any changes. Stress test is discussed in details below

Stress test

In a stress test patient's heart rate is raised to his heart rate (maximum heart rate= 220 – patient's age) via treadmill stress test or chemical stress test, and heart activity is monitored. Which stress test is appropriate for a patient is determined based on the followings:

- If patient can walk and has no pre-existing baseline EKG changes, then do **treadmill stress**
- If patient cannot walk or has pre-existing baseline EKG changes, then do **one of following chemical test:**

Types of stress test and indications

Type of stress test	Indications
Dipyridamole, or adenosine thallium	• If patient is deconditioned, cannot walk due to lower extremity defect, amputations, peripheral vascular diseases (PVD), weakness
Dobutamine stress echo	• If patient has COPD, asthma, 2nd or 3rd degree heart block
Do **nuclear stress test** (Exercise thallium)	• If patient has preexisting **baseline EKG changes,** such as: Left bundle block, left ventricular hypertrophy, taking digoxin, pacemakers implanted

Stress test interpretation:

- Treadmill stress test is considered positive, if a patient shows ≥ 2mm ST-segment depression and/or a drop in systolic BP > 10mmHG
- Dobutamine stress echo test shows **abnormal wall motion** in ischemic area
- Exercise thallium and adenosine thallium tests show **decreased isotope uptake** in ischemic area

Angiography is performed after a positive EKG or stress test for unstable angina. It shows the extent of coronary artery occlusion, and number of coronary arteries occluded, which helps in deciding whether or not a patient needs coronary artery bypass grafts (CABG)

Treatment for stable angina is as follow:
Acute treatment: If a patient presents with anginal chest pain, then give **morphine, oxygen, sublingual nitroglycerin, aspirin and beta-blockers**, even before doing EKG or other tests. As this management lowers the mortality by preventing further blood from clotting, opening the arteries and lowering the oxygen demand. Further management may include PCI or CABG, which is as follow:

Percutaneous coronary intervention (PCI), commonly known as coronary angioplasty, is a standard care

Coronary artery bypass graft (CABG) is indicated when any of these are present:
    1. Angiography shows any of the followings:
    1a. Significant stenosis of the left main coronary artery
    1b. >70% stenosis of proximal LAD and left circumflex
    1c. 3- vessels occluded in a patient with CAD or 2-vessels occluded in a patient with DM
    2. Ejection fraction <25%
    3. Medicine failure

Internal mammary **artery** grafts are preferred because they lasts 10 years, whereas saphenous **vein** grafts lasts only 5 years

---

Long-term treatment is focused towards lowering the future MI risk such as diet modification, lower diabetes, lower cholesterol levels, lower the risk of clot formation
- Aspirin (if a patient is allergic to aspirin, then give clopidogrel)
- Statins
- Long-acting nitroglycerin
- Beta-blockers (metoprolol or carvedilol)
- Life style modification such as stop smoking, exercise
- Diet modification

2. ACUTE CORONARY SYNDROME (ACS)

Acute coronary syndrome refers to a group of heart conditions that are caused by obstruction (atherosclerosis or clot) of the coronary artery. ACS should be distinguished from stable angina, which occurs predictable amount of exertion and relieves by rest or nitroglycerin

ACS is classified into two main groups according to the ST-segment on EKG

1. **ST-segment elevation MI (STMI)**
2. Non-ST-segment elevation coronary syndrome, which is further sub-divided into two, based on cardiac enzymes
2a. **Non-ST-segment elevation MI (NSTMI)** in which **cardiac enzymes are elevated**
2b. **Unstable angina** in which **cardiac enzymes are absent**

In a nutshell: ACS refers to three types of MI: ST-segment elevation MI (STMI), Non-ST-segment elevation MI (NSTMI), and unstable angina, which are **diagnosed based on EKG and cardiac enzymes**

Important: NSTMI and unstable angina are caused by obstruction of coronary arteries by **atherosclerosis**, and **STMI** is caused by obstruction of coronary arteries by a **clot**.

Si/Sx: Chest pain, heaviness, tightness, pressure, pain radiating to left arm, shoulder or jaw, which is **not relieved by rest or nitroglycerin**

STMI area of infarction & blood supply

ST elevation, T wave inversion on EKG	Heart infarction area	Blood supply
II, III, aVF	Inferior	Right coronary
I, V4, V5, V6, aVL	Lateral	Left anterior descending
V1, V2	**Posterior**	**Posterior** descending
V1, V3	Anteroseptal	Left anterior descending
V2, V4	Anterior	Left anterior descending

Treatment: all patients before EKG gets morphine, oxygen, aspirin and beta-blockers. Rest of the treatment is as follow:

Note: do not wait for the cardiac enzymes results because they may take hours to be detectable

Acute treatment of for **NSTMI and unstable angina** is heparin and /or PCI and adjuvant treatment

Acute treatment for **STMI** is PCI or thrombolytics and adjuvant therapy
- PCI is proven to be superior to thrombolytics. The standard care is to perform PCI within 90 minutes, " door-to-ballon time. However, if PCI is delayed for some reasons, then give thrombolytics. Furthermore, make sure that the patient does not have any contraindications for thrombolytics. (Discussed below)

Contra-indications for thrombolytics (tPAs)

Absolute contraindications	Relative contraindications
- Intracranial hemorrhage - Ischemic stroke within last 6 months - Aortic dissection - Active bleeding - Surgery within last 2 weeks	- BP> 180/110 mmHg at the time of presentation - Prolong CPR (>10 minutes) within 2-4 weeks - Active peptic ulcer disease - Major surgery within 3 weeks - INR> 2.0 - Pregnancy

Important: tPAs are beneficial only in **STMI** because a clot in coronary arteries causes STMI, and tPAs **restore the perfusion by lysing the clot.** (A summary of acute treatment of ACS is on the next page)

- **Adjuvant treatment** with **aspirin, ACE-inhibitors and GIIa/IIIb inhibitors, are given to all patients with ACS. Clopidogrel and heparin are added only if PCI is planned.**

Long-term treatment of ACS:
- Aspirin
- Clopidogrel for 9-12 months
- Statins
- Short-acting nitrates
- Beta-blockers (metoprolol or carvedilol)
- Life style and diet modification

Summary of acute treatment of different types of angina

Medication	Stable angina	NSTMI and Unstable angina	STMI
Aspirin	Yes	Yes	Yes
Nitroglycerin	Yes	Yes	Yes
Beta-blocker	Yes	Yes	Yes
Morphine	Yes	Yes	Yes
ACEIs*	Yes	Yes	Yes
Clopidogrel	No	Yes, if PCI is planned	Yes if PCI is planned
Low-molecular weight heparin	No	Yes, if PCI is not planned	Yes, if PCI is planned
IV heparin	No	Yes, if PCI is planned	Yes, but only after tPA
GP IIb/IIIa	No	Yes (Tirofiban or eptifibatide)	Yes, abciximab if PCI is planned
Thrombolytics (tPAs)*	**No**	**No**	Yes (only if PCI is delayed or cannot be performed)

*ACEIs prevent cardiac remodeling. They also lower the mortality in patients with ejection fraction (EF) < 45%. ACEIs are given to a patient with stable angina if patient has CHF, systolic dysfunction or EF< 45%.

* tPAs can be given up to 12 hours of onset of symptoms of STMI or new LBBB

LIPIDS GOAL IN A POST-MI PATIENT
1. LDLs goals are as follow:
   1a. LDLs goal in a patient with **CAD or CAD equivalents alone** is < 100 mg/dl
   1b. LDLs goal is a patient with **CAD plus diabetes** is <70 mg/dl
2. Triglycerides goal is <150 mg/dl
3. HDLs goal is > 40 mg/dl

CORONARY ARTERY DISEASE (CAD) EQUIVALENTS:
- Diabetes
- Peripheral artery disease
- Aortic artery disease
- Carotid disease

LDLs goals and management

Risk factors	Lifestyle modification	Initiate drug treatment
0-1 risk factor for CAD	≥ 160 mg/dl	>190 mg/dl
≥ 2 risk factor for CAD	≥ 130 mg/dl	≥160 mg/dl
CAD or CAD equivalents	≥ 100 mg/dl	≥130 mg/dl

NOTE: A patient with **CAD and diabetes** should be started on medication to keep LDLs <70 mg/dl.

Lipid lowering medications

Medication	Effects	Side effects
Statins	Lowers LDL & triglyceride	Increases liver enzymes (AST, ALT), myositis
Fibric acid derivatives	Lowers triglyceride & increases HDL	Myositis, GI upset
Ezetimibe	Lowers LDL	Diarrhea, abdominal pain
Bile acid resins	Lowers LDL	Flatus & abdominal cramping, myalgia
Niacin	Lowers LDL & Increase HDL	Skin flushing, pruritus

Drugs that lower the mortality in ACS are:
- Metoprolol
- Clopidogrel
- Aspirin
- Thrombolytic
- Statins
- ACE-Inhibitors (ACEIs)
- Angiotensin receptor blockers (ARBs)

POST-MI COMPLICATIONS
- Most common cause of death after MI is ventricular arrhythmias
- Other complications of post-MI are third-degree heart block, pericarditis, papillary muscle rupture, cardiac tamponade, left ventricular wall rupture
- Late complication of MI is Dressler's syndrome

3. PRINZMETAL ANGINA

Prinzmetal angina, which is also known as variant angina, is characterized by episodes of angina that usually occurs **at rest**. It is caused by a **spasm in the coronary arteries**.

Diagnosis: EKG shows **transient ST elevation** and cardiac enzymes are negative

Treatment: nitroglycerin or calcium channel blockers, and cardiac catheterization should be performed because vasospasm usually occurs at the site of an atherosclerosis

CARDIAC ARRHYTHMIAS AND CONDUCTION ABNORMALITIES

A normal heart rate is 60-100 beats per minute (bpm)
- Bradycardia: heart rate < 60 bpm
- Tachycardia: heart rate > 100 bpm

Note: some people have arrhythmia that occurs only during a particular activity. Moreover, EKG does not detect heart rhythm abnormalities that do not occur during the test. In that case, patient may need a **Holter** (stable, outpatient) **or telemetry monitor** (unstable or hospitalized patients). These are medical deceives that continuously monitor the heart rate and rhythm. Please note that these are not used to detect stable angina.

1. SINUS BRADYCARDIA

Sinus bradycardia is referred to a heart rate that originates from the sinus node and has a **heart rate < 60 bpm**

Cause: Medicines (beta-blockers, calcium channel blockers, digitalis and antiarrhythmics), sinus node dysfunction, increased vagal tone, hypothyroidism

Si/Sx: some patients may be asymptomatic, but symptoms may include lightheadedness, shortness of breath, dizziness, hypotension

Diagnosis:
- **EKG shows heart rate < 60 bpm, with normal P wave, PR interval and QRS complexes**

Treatment: treatment depends on symptoms
- No treatment is required for a asymptomatic patient
- Atropine or pacemakers for symptomatic patient

Note Beta-blockers, and calcium channel blockers medicines should be avoided in sinus bradycardia because both of these slow the heart conduction and worsen the symptoms

2.   FIRST-DEGREE HEART BLOCK
In a first-degree heart block, electric impulse moves slower than normal trough the AV node.

Cause: it can occur in normal individual, but risk factors include increased vagal tone, drugs (beta-blockers, calcium channel blockers digoxin, amiodarone), acute myocardial infarction, myocarditis

Si/Sx: Asymptomatic

Diagnosis:
*   EKG shows normal sinus rhythm with prolong **PR interval (>. 02ms)**

Treatment:
    *   No treatment required

Note: Beta-blockers, calcium channel blockers medicines should be avoided in first-degree heart block because both of these slow the heart conduction and can worsen the symptoms

3.   SECOND-DEGREE HEART BLOCK
Second-degree heart block is sub-classified into two types:
*   Second-degree type I heart block
*   Second-degree type II heart block

3a. SECOND-DEGREE TYPE I HEART BLOCK
In a second-degree type I heart block (also known as Mobitz Type I or Wenckebach's block), the electric signals moves slower and slower with each heartbeat until the heart skips a heartbeat.

Cause: increased vagal tone, medicine (beta-blockers, calcium channel blockers, digoxin)

Si/Sx: some patients may be asymptomatic, but symptoms may include lightheadedness, dizziness, syncope

Diagnosis:
    *   EKG shows progressive prolonged PR intervals until a noncaonducted P wave

Treatment:
    *   Stop the offending drug
    *   Atropine or pacemaker is only for symptomatic patients

3b. SECOND-DEGREE TYPE II HEART BLOCK

In a second-degree type II heart block (also known as Mobitz Type II), some electrical signals move normally between atria and ventricles, while other signals are blocked.

Cause: Anterior septal MI, fibrosis of conducting system, inflammatory conditions (rheumatic fever, Lyme disease), autoimmune (SLE, systemic sclerosis), infiltrative myocardial disease (amyloidosis, sarcoidosis)

Si/Sx: light-headedness, dizziness syncope

Diagnosis:

- EKG shows normal PR intervals with unexpected non-conducted P wave

Treatment: Pacemaker

Complication: second-degree type II heart block can progress to 3rd degree heart block

4. THIRD-DEGREE HEART BLOCK

In a third-degree heart block (also known as complete heart block) all electric signals are blocked from atria to ventricles. As a result, both **atria** and **ventricles** are contracting at **their own rate**.

Cause: acute MI, inferior MI, second-degree type II heart block, Lyme disease

Si/Sx: Syncope, dizziness, hypotension, acute heart failure

Diagnosis:

- EKG shows uncoordinated P waves and QRS complexes

Treatment: Pacemaker

5. VENTRICULAR FIBRILLATION (VF)

Ventricular fibrillation is uncoordinated contractions of ventricle muscles of the heart

Cause: CAD, MI, heart surgery, heart muscle disease

Si/Sx: Syncope, hypotension, pulselessness, sudden death

Diagnosis: EKG shows disorganized heart rhythm

Treatment: VF is a life threatening condition; it can lead to death within few minutes if the patient is not treated quickly. **Unsynchronized** defibrillation (200-300-360 J) is the primary standard care

6. VENTRICULAR TACHYCARDIA

Ventricular tachycardia is defined as rapid high heartbeat (>100 bpm) that starts in the ventricles, and has least 3 consecutive premature ventricular contractions (PVCs)

Cause: CAD, MI, myocarditis, cardiomyopathy, valvular heart disease, anti-arrhythmic medicines

Si/Sx: Most of the patients are asymptomatic, but symptoms may include palpitations, angina, syncope, shortness of breath, light-headedness

Diagnosis:
- EKG shows wide QRS complex with ventricular rate > 100 bpm, 3 or more consecutive PVCs

Treatment: Treatment depends on symptoms
- If a patient is **unstable, hypotensive or has no pulses**, then do **synchronized defibrillation**
- If a patient is **stable**, then treat the patient with **amiodarone or lidocaine**

7. ATRIAL FIBRILLATION

Atrial fibrillation is uncoordinated contractions of atrial muscles of the heart

Cause: pulmonary disease, ischemia, rheumatic heart disease, anemia, atrial myxoma, thyrotoxicosis, ethanol, sepsis

Si/Sx: most of patients are asymptomatic, but symptoms may include hypotension, tachycardia, chest pain, palpitations, irregularly irregular pulses

Diagnosis:
- EKG shows absent P wave, variable and irregular QRS complex

Treatment: depends on the symptoms
- If a patient is **hemodynamic unstable** (lightheadedness, confusion, CHF, hypertension, or chest pain), then do **synchronize electrical cardioversion**.
- If a patient is **stable,** then slow the heart rate with **calcium channel blockers** (diltiazem, verapamil), **beta- blocker** (metoprolol, esmolol), or digoxin

Complication: Patients with atrial fibrillation are at increased risk of embolic stroke. To prevent that, the patient should be kept on anticoagulant **(warfarin or aspirin) to maintain INR 2-3 indefinitely.** Anticoagulation is given **based on total risk,** also known as **CHADS2** score, is discussed below

Risk factor	Relative risk
CHF	1
HTN	1
Age > 65	1
Diabetes	1
Previous stroke	2

- **For score** 0 or lone A-fib, give **aspirin**
- **For** scores **1-2**, give **aspirin or warfarin**
- **For** score **3 or higher**, give **warfarin**

For example:
- A patient with CHF and HTN has a CHADS2 score: 1+1= 2
- A patient with CHF, HTN and previous stroke has a CHADS2 score: 1+1+2 =4

8. ATRIAL FLUTTER
Atrial flutter is uncoordinated contractions of atrial muscles of the heart. Atrial rate is usually 250-300 bpm in atrial flutter
Cause: COPD, CHF, ASD, surgically repaired congenital heart disease
Si/Sx: most of patients are asymptomatic, but symptoms may include hypotension, tachycardia, chest pain or palpitations
Diagnosis: EKG shows regular rhythm with **"saw tooth appearance"** of P wave
Treatment: same as A-fib

9. SUPRAVENTRICULAR TACHYCARDIA (SVT)
Supraventricular tachycardia is a fast heart rhythm that originates at or above the atrioventricular node
Si/Sx: palpitation, **tachycardia,** syncope
Diagnosis: EKG shows narrow QRS complex with ventricular rate 160- 180 bpm

Treatment: depends on patient's symptoms:
- **A stable patient** can be treated with **carotid massage, Valsalva maneuver, or ice water face immersion**. If this is ineffective, then use **IV adenosine**
- **Synchronized** cardioversion is done in a **unstable patient**

10. MULTIFOCAL ATRIAL TACHYCARDIA
Multifocal atrial tachycardia is a rapid heart rate that occurs when multiple electric signals are sent from atria to ventricles
Cause: COPD, hypoxemia, reentrant pathway
Si/Sx: most of patients are asymptomatic, but symptoms may include hypotension, tachycardia, chest pain, palpitations
Diagnosis:
- EKG shows **multiple P waves** with heart **rate > 100 bpm**

Treatment: Slow the heart rate with calcium channel blockers (verapamil, diltiazem) or beta-blockers, and treat the underlying cause

11. WANDERING PACEMAKER
Wandering pacemaker (also known as atrial arrhythmia) occurs when heart pacemaker site shifts from SA node to atria, and or AV node
Diagnosis:
- EKG shows **multiple P waves** with heart **rate of < 100 bpm**

Treatment: None

12. WOLFF–PARKINSON–WHITE SYNDROME (WPW)
Wolff–Parkinson–white syndrome is a heart condition caused by an abnormal extra electrical pathway in the heart that allows the electrical signal to bypass the AV node.
Cause: " short-circuit" conducting system that bypasses the AV node and allow reentrant
Diagnosis: EKG shows **delta wave** (slurred upstroke of QRS complex)
Treatment: Procainamide

HEART VALVE LESIONS

Valvular lesions and effects of maneuvers

Valvular lesions	Squatting/ leg Raise	Standing/ Valsalva
AS, AR, **MS**, MR, VSD	Murmur increases	Murmur decreases
MVP, HOCM	Murmur decreases	Murmur increases

Valvular lesions and effects of maneuvers

Valvular Lesion	Hand grip	Amyl Nitrate
AR, MR, VSD	Murmur increase	Murmur decrease
AS, MVP, HOCM	Murmur decreases	Murmur increases
MS	Minimal effect	Minimal effect

AS= Aortic stenosis, AR= Aortic regurgitation, MS=Mitral stenosis, MR= Mitral regurgitation, VSD= Ventricular septal defect, HOCM=Hypertrophic subaortic stenosis

SYSTOLIC MURMUR GRADES:
- I/VI is barely audible
- II/VI is faint, but audible
- III/VI is loud, but without a palpable thrill
- IV/VI is loud with palpable thrill
- V/VI is loud that it can be heard with the stethoscope lightly placed on the chest
- VI/VI is so loud that it can be heard even without a stethoscope.

Innocent murmurs are systolic murmur, I/VI or II/VI grade murmur.

SUMMARY OF HEART MURMUR LOCATIONS
- Aortic stenosis: 2nd right intercostal space radiating to the carotid arteries
- Aortic regurgitation, tricuspid murmur: let lower sternal border
- Mitral regurgitation: 5th intercostal space, below the left nipple
- Pulmonic valve: 2nd left intercostal space

1. AORTIC STENOSIS (AS)

Aortic stenosis is characterized by abnormally narrowed opening of aortic valve. This leads to lower blood flow from heart to the body

Cause: most common cause in a young patient is **congenital bicuspid valve**, and in an old patient is **calcification of normal aortic valves**

Si/Sx: angina-type chest pain, syncope, exertional dyspnea, palpitation

Diagnosis:

- Physical exam shows peripheral pulses that are weak and late compare to heat sounds (pulsus parvus et tardus)
- Auscultation of heart usually shows midsystolic **crescendo-decrescendo systolic** murmur heard at **second right intercostal space radiating to the carotid arteries and apex,** paradoxically split S2
- ECG shows **left ventricular hypertrophy**
- Diagnosis is confirmed with **echocardiography**

Treatment:

- Valves are replaced in all symptomatic patients or when valve area is < .8cm2. If a patient cannot tolerate valve replacement, then do balloon valvuloplasty

Note: Beta-blockers or afterload reducers should be avoided

2. AORTIC REGURGITATIONA (AR)

Aortic regurgitation is caused by improper closure of aortic valves. This leads to backward flow of blood from aorta to ventricle during ventricular diastole

Cause: Most common cause is hypertension; other causes may include endocarditis, **Marfan syndrome,** syphilis, ankylosing spondylitis, aortic dissection

Si/Sx: Patients often are asymptomatic, but symptoms may include shortness of breath, bounding pulses, fatigue, fatigue, shortening of breath

Diagnosis:

- Physical exam may show:
  1. Corrigan pulse: **rapid rise** and **fall of pulse**
  2. Duroziez sign: **diastolic murmur** heard over **femoral artery**
  3. De Musset sign: **head-bobbing** with each pulse
  4. Hill sign: **systolic blood pressure > 30 mmHg** higher in **lower extremities**
  5. Quincke pulse: **pulsation in fingernails**

- Chest auscultation shows **diastolic murmur** over left lower sternal border
- **EKG** shows **left ventricular hypertrophy**
- Diagnosis is **confirmed** with **echocardiography**

Treatment:
- Decrease the afterload with ACE-inhibitors, ARBs, or vasodilators such as Nifedipine, hydralazine
- Aortic valve are replaced in symptomatic patients or, when echocardiograph shows **ejection fraction (EF) <50% or left ventricular end systolic diameter > 5.0 cm**

3. MITRAL REGURGITATION (MR)

Mitral regurgitation is caused by improper closure of mitral valve. This lead to backward flow of blood from ventricle to atrium during ventricular systole

Cause: Mitral valve prolapse, ischemic heart disease, collagen vascular disease, papillary muscle dysfunction

Symptoms: dyspnea on exertion, orthopnea, paroxysmal nocturnal dyspnea, pulmonary edema

Diagnosis:
- Chest auscultation shows **holosystolic murmur heard** at 5th intercostal space **below left nipple radiating to axilla**
- **EKG** shows left atrial enlargement
- Diagnosis is confirmed with echocardiography

Treatment:
- ACE-inhibitors, ARBs, or vasodilators such as Nifedipine, hydralazine
- Diuretic and digoxin
- **Mitral Valve are replaced** when echocardiograph shows ejection fraction (EF) <60% or left ventricular **end systolic** diameter > 4.0 cm

4. MITRAL STENOSIS

Mitral stenosis is characterized by abnormally narrowed opening of mitral valve. This leads to lower blood flow from ventricle to atrium

Cause: rheumatic fever disease is the most common cause

Si/Sx: most of the patients' stay asymptomatic until A-fib develops or woman becomes pregnant. Symptoms may include **dysphagia, hoarseness,** hemoptysis

Diagnosis:

- Chest auscultation shows **opening snap** followed by **mid diastolic rumble,** loud S1
- Chest X-ray shows **elevation of left main bronchus & straightening of left heart border**
- **EKG** shows left atrial enlargement
- Diagnosis is confirmed with echocardiography

Treatment:

- Beta-blockers and digitalis to control heart rate
- Fluid overload is managed with diuretics and fluid reduction
- Anticoagulants (warfarin) is given for embolus prophylaxis, (maintain INR 2-3)
- Most effective therapy is **balloon valvuloplasty; it is well tolerated even in pregnancy**
- Surgical valve are replaced in refractory cases

Complication of mitral stenosis is stroke

5. MITRAL VALVE PROLAPSE (MVP)

Mitral valve prolapse is caused by improper closure of mitral valve. This lead to backward flow of blood from ventricle to atrium during ventricular systole

Risk factor: MVP is seen in 7 % of the population, mainly in young women

Cause: connective tissue disorder especially Marfan syndrome, and in rare genetic disorders

Si/Sx: most of the patients are asymptomatic, but symptoms may include lightheadedness, palpitations, syncope, chest pain

Diagnosis:

- Chest auscultation shows **late systolic murmur with midsystolic click**
- **Echocardiography can be used to confirm diagnosis**

Treatment:

- Usually no treatment is required
- Beta-blockers or valve replacement is for symptomatic patients

CONGESTIVE HEART FAILURE (CHF)

Congestive heart failure is a heart condition in which heart is unable to pump enough blood to the rest of the body.

Types: CHF can be right-side heart failure, left-side heart failure, both sided heart failure, systolic dysfunction, or diastolic dysfunction

Causes: CAD, MI, HTN, faulty heart valves, arrhythmias, hypo/hyperthyroidism, cardiomyopathy, myocarditis, congenital heart defects, pulmonary HTN

Si/Sx: discussed in the table below

Right and left-sided heart failure symptoms

Right-sided heart failure symptoms	Left-sided heart failure symptoms
<ul><li>JVD</li><li>Hepatomegaly</li><li>Hepatojugular reflex</li><li>Bipedal edema</li><li>Cyanosis</li><li>Weight loss</li></ul>	<ul><li>Bilateral rales</li><li>S3 Gallops</li><li>Pleural effusion</li><li>Pulmonary edema</li><li>Orthopnea</li><li>Exertional dyspnea</li><li>Paroxysmal nocturnal dyspnea</li></ul>

New York Heart Association (NYHA) Functional Classification Of CHF

NYHA class	Symptoms
I	CHF, but no symptoms and no limitation with normal physical activity
II	Mild symptoms and slight limitation with normal physical activity
III	Marked limitation in activity due to symptoms, even with mild activity. Comfortable only at rest
IV	Severe limitations, symptoms, experienced even while resting. Patient are mostly bedbound

Diagnosis:

- Chest x-ray shows cardiomegaly, effusion, cephalization of pulmonary vessels, pulmonary vascular congestion
- EKG: Arrhythmias, sinus tachycardia

- **Echocardiograph** is the only test which helps differentiate systolic from diastolic dysfunction; ejection fraction is **< 45 % in systolic dysfunction**, and **> 45 % in disystolic dysfunction**
- **BNP**
- **Most accurate test is MUGA scan** (nuclear ventriculography)

Treatment: as follow

- **Acute treatment** for a patient with **pulmonary edema** is oxygen, furosemide, nitrate, and morphine
- **Chronic treatment** for a stable CHF patient depends on the type of dysfunction, discussed below:

Chronic CHF treatment

Systolic dysfunction	**Disystolic** dysfunction
- ACE-inhibitor or ARBS (lowers the mortality) - Beta-blockers such as metoprolol or carvedilol (Lowers the mortality) - Spironolactone (lowers the mortality in class III and IV CHF) - Digoxin (reduces the hospitalization) - Furosemide	- Beat-blockers (metoprolol or carvedilol) - Diuretics

Note: If a patient cannot tolerate ACE inhibitor, then use hydralazine and isosorbide

PULMONARY EDEMA

Pulmonary edema is characterized by abnormal fluid buildup in the air sacs of the lungs

Cause: CHF is the most common cause; other less common causes include kidney failure, lung damage, high altitude exposure

Si/Sx: SOB, pink frothy sputum, nocturnal dyspnea, orthopnea

Diagnosis:

- Clinical diagnosis
- Physical exam shows rales or crackles on lung exam, JVD
- Chest X-ray shows Kerley B lines, effusion, dilated pulmonary vessels

Treatment: Oxygen, furosemide, nitrate and morphine (morphine mobilizes the fluid, reduced pain and anxiety)

CARDIOMYOPATHY

1. DILATED CARDIOMYOPATHY
Dilated cardiomyopathy is a condition in which heart muscles become weakened and enlarged; mainly the left ventricle. As a result, heart cannot pump enough blood to the body.
Cause: ischemia is the most common cause; other causes include Infection (Chagas' disease, HIV, Coxsackie virus), medicines (Adriamycin doxorubicin), alcohol, beriberi,
Si/Sx: same as CHF
Diagnosis:
- Echocardiography shows decreased ejection fraction (systolic dysfunction)
- **Most accurate test is MUGA scan** (nuclear ventriculography)

Treatment: stop the offending agent or treat the underlying condition. And, treat the patient as per systolic dysfunction CHF

2. HYPERTROPHIC OBSTRUCTIVE CARDIOMYOPATHY (HOCM)
Autosomal dominant trait causes the thickening of the interventricular septum. Thickened septum bulges into the ventricle and blocks the blood outflow from ventricle. It is the most common cause of death in young athletes.
Si/Sx: Chest pain, palpitation, dyspnea
Diagnosis:
- Physical exam shows systolic murmur, which increases with Valsalva & amyl nitrite, and decreases with handgrip, leg raise & squatting
- EKG shows left ventricular hypertrophy
- Echocardiograph shows decreased diastolic function

Treatment:
- Best initial treatment is beta-blockers or verapamil. If drug therapy is ineffective, then give pure alcohol injection in septal arteries. Myomectomy is a last resort
- AICD should be placed in patients with family history of sudden death at young age or unexplained syncope
- Patients should be advise against intense training or exercise

3.   RESTRICTIVE CARDIOMYOPATHY

Restrictive cardiomyopathy is a condition in which heart size is normal or slightly enlarged, but heart muscles are stiff and cannot relax during diastole. As result, heart does not fill and pump enough blood to the body

Cause: amyloidosis, hemochromatosis, radiation, sarcoidosis, scleroderma, glycogen storage disease

Si/Sx: Combination of right and left-sided heart failure

Diagnosis:

- Physical exam shows rise in jugular venous pressure (JVP) on inspiration (**Kussmaul's sign**)
- Chest X-ray shows cardiomegaly
- EKG shows low-voltage QRS complex
- Most accurate test is **endomyocardial biopsy**

Treatment: salt restriction, diuretic for fluid overload and treat the underlying cause

PERICARDIAL DISEASE

1.   CONSTRICTIVE PERICARDITIS

Constrictive pericarditis is a chronic inflammation of the pericardium that leads to calcification, fibrosis and stiffening of the heart muscles

Causes: tuberculosis, radiation therapy of chest, heart surgery, mesothelioma

Si/Sx: similar to right-sided heart failure (JVD, lower extremity edema, hepatomegaly)

Diagnosis:

- Physical exam shows rise in jugular venous pressure (JVP) on inspiration (**Kussmaul's sign**), and **pericardial knock**, an extra diastolic apical sound due to thickened pericardium
- Chest X-ray shows **pericardium calcification**
- CT or MRI of chest show thickened pericardium

Treatment: low sodium diet and diuretic and pericardiectomy

2. PERICARDITIS

Pericarditis is an inflammation of the pericardium

Causes: viral infection is the most common cause; other causes include fungal, bacterial, rheumatoid arthritis, MI, trauma, drugs

Si/Sx: retrosternal pain, which is **worst when patient is supine** and **relieves** with **leaning forward and sitting up.** Pain is not affected by activity or food.

Diagnosis:
- Physical exam shows **pericardial friction rub**
- EKG shows **ST elevation in all leads and PR depression** (PR depression very specific, but is not always present)

Treatment: Treat the underlying cause. NSAIDs for viral pericarditis, if NSAIDs is ineffective, then give prednisone

3. PERICARDIAL TAMPONADE

Pericardial tamponade is pressure on the heart due to blood or fluid buildup in pericardial sac (space between the heart muscles and pericardium)

Cause: infections (viral, bacterial), metastatic cancer, trauma, dissecting thoracic aorta aneurysm, heart surgery, SLE

Si/Sx: chest pain, palpitations, rapid breathing, difficulty breathing, light-headedness

Diagnosis:
- Physical exam shows blood pressure decreases > 10 mmHg during inspiration (**Pulsus paradoxus**), **Beck's triad** (distance heart sounds, JVD, and hypotension)
- EKG shows **low voltage QRS and electrical alternans** (beat-to-beat height difference of QRS complex axis)
- Diagnosis is confirmed with echocardiography, which shows right atrial and right ventricular **diastolic collapse**

Treatment:
- Give IV fluids to maintain blood pressure, and then immediate pericardiocentesis; needle drainage of the fluid from the pericardial sac
- Pericardial window or pericardiectomy may be done in a recurrent case

CARDIOLOGY INFECTIOUS DISEASES

ENDOCARDITIS

Endocarditis is an inflammation of the inner lining of the heart (endocardium). It usually involves the heart valves, but it may also involve other structures inside of the heart such as interventricular septum, chordae tendineae

Causes: most common cause is infection from bacteria, virus or fungus. Which most likely entered the bloodstream during central venous line access, injection drug use (IV drug abuse) or dental surgery. Other causes include SLE, cancer

Types:

1. **Acute bacterial** endocarditis affects the healthy heart valves. It is common in IV **drug abusers. Patient usually** develops symptoms **within days to weeks** after the exposure of infection. **S. Aureus and Strep. Pneumonia** is the most common causes.

2. **Subacute bacterial** endocarditis affects previously damaged heart valve. It is caused by **Strep. Viridian.**

3. **Culture negative endocarditis** is caused organisms that are hard to culture known as the **HACEK** group: **H.** Parainfluenzae, Actinobacillus, Cardiobacterium, Eikenella, Kingella kingae

4. Systemic lupus erythematosus (SLE) also causes endocarditis known as Libman-sacks endocarditis, which is probably due to autoantibody mediated damage of heart valves

5. Marantic endocarditis (also known as non-bacterial thrombotic endocarditis) is causes by metastatic cancer

Si/Sx: fever and new murmur are the most common symptoms, but other symptoms may include **splinter hemorrhage** (red brown streak in nail beds), **Osler nodes** (painful nodules on fingers and toes), **Roth spots** (retinal hemorrhage with clear central area), **Janeway lesions** (dark spots on palms and soles)

Diagnosis: based on Duke criteria: 2 major or 1 major + 3 minors or 5 minor

Major Criteria	Minor Criteria
• 2 positive blood cultures growing same organism • Positive echocardiogram or onset of new murmur	• Presence of predisposing valve abnormality • Fever >38 C or 100.4 F • Embolic disease • Immunologic phenomena (e.g., Roth spot) • 1 positive blood culture

Treatment:
- IV vancomycin and gentamicin, until the culture and sensitivity results are available
- Surgical valve replacement when there is abscess is on the valves, prosthetic valves are involved, AV block or recurrent emboli

ENDOCARDITIS PROPHYLAXIS
Endocarditis prophylaxis is give to patients to prevent endocarditis
Criteria to give prophylaxis is as follow:
- If a patient is going to have dental procedures, respiratory tract procedures, surgery of infected skin.
- Heart defects such as prosthetic valves, previous endocarditis Unrepaired cyanotic heart disease, heart transplant recipient who develops valve disease

Treatment: Amoxicillin prior to the procedure. Penicillin allergic patient can get clindamycin, macrolide or cephalosporin

CARDIOVASCULAR SURGERY

THORACIC AORTA DISSECTION
Thoracic aorta dissection is a transverse tear in the intima of the aorta in the chest region
Risk factors: Most Common risk factor is hypertension
Types: Two types of thoracic aorta dissections are:
- Type A, which affects the ascending aorta
- Type B, which affects the descending aorta

Si/Sx: chest pain radiating thorough the back between **scapula's**
Diagnosis:
- Physical exam shows **different high blood pressure** in **each arm**
- Best initial test is **chest X-ray, which** shows **widening of mediastinum**
- Most accurate test is **chest CT angiography**

Treatment: treatment depends on the type of dissecting aorta, which is a follow:
- Descending aortic dissection: control the blood pressures with **beta blockers** (IV labetalol or esmolol) or nitroprusside
- Ascending aortic dissection is a surgical emergency, it is managed by controlling the blood pressure and immediate surgical intervention

ABDOMINAL AORTA ANEURYSM (AAA)
Abdominal aorta aneurysm is characterized by aneurysm of aorta in abdomen region
Cause: there is no known cause, but risk factors includes smoking, male gender, obesity, high blood pressure, high cholesterol
Si/Sx: most of the patients are asymptomatic, but symptoms may include pain in the abdomen or back, clammy skin, dizziness, shock
Diagnosis:
- Physical exam usually shows show pulsatile abdominal mass or abdominal bruits.
- Diagnosis is confirmed with ultrasound
- CT to determine the size

Treatment: as follow:

- AAA < 4 cm: annual imaging
- AAA> 5 cm: surgically repair
- AAA 4-5 cm: follow-up every 6 months
- Ruptured AAA requires immediate surgical intervention

Screening for AAA: USPSTF recommended one-time ultrasound screening for men between 65- 75 years of age who have smoked at least 100 cigarettes in their lifetime

PERIPHERAL VASCULAR DISEASE
Peripheral vascular disease is characterized by narrowing of arteries by atherosclerotic plaque of arteries outside of the heart and brain

Risk factors: hypertension, diabetes, smoking, elevated blood cholesterol, obesity

Si/Sx: Depends on the location and extent of the blocked artery (discussed below), but common symptoms includes Intermittent claudication, smooth shiny skin,

Disease specific Si/Sx are

- **Aortoiliac disease:** Buttock claudication, loss of femoral pulses, impotence
- **Femoropopliteal disease**: calf claudication and loss of pulses below

Diagnosis:

- Complete physical exam, palpitations of pluses & auscultation for bruits
- **Ankle-brachial index (ABI)**: normal ABI is >1.0.
- **Doppler ultrasounds of legs** to find the pressure gradient
- **Angiography** to find the location of occlusion

Treatment:

- Smoking cessation
- Exercise, as tolerated
- Aspirin
- ACE to decrease the blood pressure
- Cilostazol
- Statins to keep LDL <100
- Angioplasty is done when medical therapy is ineffective

SUBCLAVIAN STEAL SYNDROME
Subclavian steal syndrome is characterized by occlusion of subclavian artery proximal to the origin of the vertebral artery. In this syndrome blood is reversed from the vertebrobasilar artery to supply arm during arm exercise
Si/Sx: **Arm claudication, confusion,** nausea, syncope, and supraclavicular bruits
Diagnosis: Angiography
Treatment: Bypass graft

ARTERIAL ULCERS
Arterial ulcers occurs because of inadequate perfusion of skin and subcutaneous tissue, they are usually found on **lower leg and lateral ankle**
Cause: secondary to atherosclerotic plaque it the arteries
Risk factors: Smoking, diabetes with poor glycemic control, inadequate footwear
Si/Sx: Painful ulcers on lower leg and lateral ankle, absent pulses, claudication
Diagnosis: same as PVD
Treatment: same as PVD

VENOUS ULCERS
Venous ulcer are usually found **above the medial ankle and below knees**
Risk factors: DVT, varicose veins, incompetent valves, obesity,
Si/Sx: Painless ulcers usually located above medical ankle and below knees, contain bleeding granulation tissues
Diagnosis: Doppler of legs
Treatment: elevation of affected leg to reduce the swelling, Unna's boot, compression stocking to increase the blood flow

HYPERTENSION

HYPERTENSION (HTN)

Hypertension is defined as systolic BP> 140 mmHg and diastolic BP >90 mm Hg

Cause:

- **Primary hypertension** or essential hypertension, accounts for 90-95 % of the cases of hypertension. There is no known cause for primary hypertension, but risk factors may include obesity, high sodium diet, alcohol, smoking, advanced age, family history of HTN or heart disease and race (African-Americans)
- **Secondary hypertension** accounts for remaining 5-10 % of the cases of hypertension (discussed below)

Causes of secondary HTN and specific findings

Cardiology	• Coarctation of aorta: BP is higher in upper extremity compare to lower extremity
Renal	• Renal artery stenosis: **abdominal bruits** • PCKD
Endocrine	• Pheochromocytoma: **episodic HTN** • Conn syndrome and Cushing syndrome: HTN with **hypokalemia** • Hyperthyroidism: **isolated systolic HTN** • Acromegaly
Drugs	• NSAIDs, OCPs, glucocorticosteroids

Si/Sx: most of the patient may have no symptoms and HTN is usually diagnosed incidentally during routine screening. But, even silent HTN can slowly lead to heart diseases, kidney diseases, or visual problems

Diagnosis: Diagnosis of HTN is based on:

- 3 separate measurement, taken at 4-weeks intervals
- Resting quietly for 5 minutes, before measuring BP
- Seated with arm at heart level
- Blood pressure cuff should encircle 80% of the arm

As discussed on the previous page that silent HTN can cause other problems. Therefore, a patient diagnosed with HTN should have following tests:

- Urinalysis (UA)
- Eye exam
- Cardiac exam & EKG
- Serum potassium & BUN/Cr
- Blood glucose and plasma lipids
-

Treatment: treatment **depends on the cause** of HTN (discussed below)

1. Treatment of **Primary hypertension** is as follow:

HTN stage	BP range	Treatment
Normal BP	<120/80	None
Pre-HTN	120/80 –139/89	**Lifestyle modification** for 3-6 months, if this fails, then start HTN medicine*
HTN stage 1	140/90 –159/99	**Lifestyle modification** for 3-6 months, if this fails, then start HTN medicine*
HTN Stage 2	>160/100	**Life style modification and combination of 2 HTN medicines***

* Best initial treatment is thiazide diuretics. If thiazide is ineffective, then add ACEIs, ARBs, beta-blockers or calcium channel blockers.

** 2-medicines combination usually includes thiazide + ACEIs, ARBs, beta-blockers or calcium channel blockers.

Lifestyle modifications and BP lowering benefits are, as follow:
- **Weight reduction** lowers systolic BP by **5-20 mmHg**
- **Healthy diet** lowers systolic BP **up to 14** mmHg
- **Exercise** lowers systolic BP by **4- 9** mmHg
- **Reduced sodium** lowers systolic BP **by 2-8** mm Hg
- **Limit alcohol** lowers systolic BP by **2-4** mmHg

Note: If a patient has comorbid disease(s), then start the medical treatment at the first visit, rather than waiting 3-6 months to check effect of lifestyle modifications

Compelling indications and contraindications for HTN medicines

Medicine	Indications	Contraindications	Side effects
Thiazide diuretics	• No comorbid disease • Osteoporosis	• Gout, • Diabetes	• Hyperglycemia • Hyperlipidemia • Hyperuricemia
β-blockers	• MI • CHF • Migraine • Hyperthyroidism	• COPD • Diabetes • Hyperkalemia	• Asthma • Hypertriglyceridemia • Bradycardia
Calcium channel blockers	• Systolic HTN • Angina • Depression • Migraine	• Heart block	• Peripheral edema • Constipation
ACEIs	• Diabetes • CHF • HTN in scleroderma	• Pregnancy • Renal artery stenosis • Renal failure	• Cough • Angioedema
α− blocker (Prazosin, terazosin	• BPH	• Orthostatic-hypotension	• Postural hypotension • Headaches

2. **Treatment for secondary HTN:** treat the underlying cause

HYPERTENSIVE URGENCY
Hypertensive urgency is defined as BP> 220/110 mm Hg **without the evidence of end-organ damage**
Treatment: oral blood pressure medicine such beta-blockers (labetalol), clonidine or ACEI, with the goal of slowly lowering the BP over several days

HYPERTENSIVE EMERGENCY

Hypertensive emergency is defined as BP> 220/110 mm HG with the **evidence of end-organ damage** such as acute renal failure, CHF, ischemia, encephalopathy

Treatment: hypertensive emergency is a medical emergency. Start the patient on IV nitroprusside, nitroglycerin, labetalol, or nocardin, but do not lower the BP more than 25 % within first 1-2 hour, otherwise patient may develop cerebral hypoperfusion or coronary insufficiency

HEMATOLOGY

ANEMIA

Anemia is a condition in which the body does not have enough red blood cells (RCBs) to carry oxygen to body tissues. It may also be diagnosed when **hemoglobin < 14 mg/dl or hematocrit < 41 % in men, and hemoglobin < 12 mg/dl or hematocrit <36 % in women**

Cause: There are many causes of anemia, which can be divided into three main groups.

1) Decreased red blood cell production in conditions such as Iron – deficiency anemia, Sickle cell anemia, Vitamin deficiency and bone marrow problem.

2) Blood loss from conditions such as ulcer, hemorrhoids, menstruation and NSAIDs.

3) Destruction of red blood cells in conditions such as infection, autoimmune hemolytic diseases and prosthetic heart valves.

Si/Sx: Signs and symptoms depend on the severity of anemia. Patents with **mild anemia may not have any symptoms**. As **anemia progress** patient may feel weak, tired even with usual activity, and problem with concentration. In **severe anemia** patient may experience shortness of breath, brittle nail, pale skin, chest pain and even MI in some cases.

Diagnosis:

- Complete blood count with peripheral smear is the best initial test for all forms of anemia
- Reticulocytes count
- Iron study
- LDH and indirect bilirubin
- Haptoglobin
- Urinalysis

Treatment: Treat the underlying cause

Blood transfusion is required in a young patient with hematocrit level < 20 %, an elderly with hematocrit is < 30%, or a patient with heart disease has hematocrit level < 30%.

Mean Corpuscular Volume (MCV) and Anemia Differential Diagnosis

MCV < 80 (Microcytic anemia)	MCV 80 -100 (Normocytic anemia)	MCV > 100 (Macrocytic anemia)
• Iron deficiency anemia • Anemia of chronic disease • Thalassemia • Sideroblastic anemia • Lead poisoning	• Acute blood loss • Sickle cell anemia • Hereditary spherocytosis • Autoimmune hemolysis • Drug Induced hemolysis • Glucose-6-phosphate dehydrogenase • Paroxysmal nocturnal hemoglobinuria • Aplastic anemia • Renal failure	• Vitamin B 12 deficiency • Folate deficiency • Alcoholism • Liver disease • Hypothyroidism • Medicine (Metformin, methotrexate, phenytoin, zidovudine, and Bactrim) • Myelodysplastic syndrome

Reticulocyte count: it measures the percentage of immature red blood cells in the blood.

Differential diagnosis of reticulocyte count

Low reticulocytes count	High reticulocytes count
• All types of macrocytic anemia • All types iron deficiency except thalassemia • Bone marrow failure • Radiation therapy	• Acute bleeding • Hemolytic anemia • Thalassemia

SPECIFIC CAUSES OF ANEMIA

MICROCYTIC ANEMIA (MCV <80)

1. IRON DEFICIENCY ANEMIA

Iron deficiency anemia is an anemia that is caused by inadequate iron in the body. Iron helps make red blood cells. Insufficient iron in the body will result in reduced RBCs production or reduced RBCs size

Cause: Many things can cause iron deficiency anemia. Some major causes include:
1. Body is not absorbing enough iron due to medical conditions such as celiac disease, Crohn's disease **or** gastric bypass surgery
2. Lot of blood is lost such as during heavy menstrual period, colon cancer, or peptic ulcer
3. More iron is required than normal such as during pregnancy or breastfeeding

Si/Sx: symptoms of anemia dependence on the severity of anemia
Diagnosis:
- CBC with peripheral smear is the **best initial test**
- Iron study shows **low ferritin,** iron & iron saturation and **increased** red cell distribution (RDW) and total iron binding capacity (TIBC)
- Bone marrow biopsy is the **most accurate test**, which shows decreased stainable iron

Treatment: Treat the underlying cause. Oral ferrous sulfate is often needed to replenish the iron body stores

Note: In the older patient (> 60 years of age) iron deficiency anemia is caused by colon cancer until otherwise proven. Make sure to rule out colon cancer with fecal occult blood test and colonoscopy.

2. ANEMIA OF CHRONIC DISEASE
Anemia of chronic disease is caused by certain chronic medical conditions
Risk factors: end-stage renal disease, cancers, liver cirrhosis, and autoimmune disease such as Crohn's disease, ulcerative colitis, rheumatoid arthritis or systemic lupus erythematosus.
Si/Sx: symptoms of anemia dependence on the severity of anemia.
Diagnosis:
- Iron study shows **increased ferritin**, and **decreased** iron, iron saturation and Total iron binding capacity (TIBC)

Treatment: Treat the underlying cause. However, anemia of chronic disease associated with end-stage renal disease is treated with erythropoietin.

3. SIDEROBALSTIC ANEMIA

Sideroblastic anemia is a condition in which **bone marrow** produces **ringed sideroblasts** (erythroblast with ferritin granules) rather than normal red blood cells. It results from **ineffective erythropoiesis** caused by a **defect in porphyrin pathway**

Cause: Two main causes of sideroblast are:

- Hereditary ALA synthase deficiency
- Acquired cause such as alcohol abuse, lead poisoning or Isoniazid

Si/Sx: symptoms of anemia dependence on the severity of anemia.

Diagnosis:

- Iron study shows **increased** Iron & ferritin, and **normal or low TIBC**
- Most accurate test is bone marrow biopsy with **Prussian blue stain**, which shows ringed sideroblasts

Treatment: depends on the cause

- ALA synthase deficiency is treated with pyridoxine (vitamin B 6).
- Acquired sideroblastic anemia is treated by treating the underlying cause

4. THALASSEMIA

Thalassemia is an inherited blood disorder in which abnormal hemoglobin is produced

Types: Hemoglobin is made up of alpha and beta chains. 4 genes are involved in the synthesis of alpha-hemoglobin chain and 2 genes are involved in the synthesis of beta-hemoglobin chain. Mutation in any gene(s) can lead to different symptoms.

Risk factors:

- Alpha-thalassemia is more common in Asian, African and Mediterranean
- Beat-thalassemia is more common in Mediterranean and African descent

Diagnosis:

- **Gel electrophoresis** is the only way to identify that if alpha or beta chain is affected
- HgF and HbA are **increased in beta thalassemia** and **normal in alpha thalassemia**

Si/Sx: See table on the next page

Treatment: See table below

Alpha –thalassemias, symptoms and treatment

Number of alpha genes mutated	Diagnosis	Symptoms	Treatment
1	Silent carrier	No signs or symptoms	No treatment
2	α-Thalassemia minor	Mild anemia symptoms	No treatment, may need iron pills
3	HbH disease	Mild to moderate anemia, Hemoglobin H, splenomegaly	Periodic transfusion
4	Hydrops fetalis	Fetus dies before delivery	No treatment

Beta-thalassemia symptoms and treatment

Number of beta genes mutated	Diagnosis	Symptoms	Treatment
1	Thalassemia-minor	Mild symptoms	No treatment
2	Thalassemia-major	**Newborn is asymptomatic for first 6 months of life.** They develop symptoms after that time due to **switch from γ- Hb to adult β -Hb**	Aggressive transfusion and splenectomy to enhance RBC survival. Deferoxamine to prevent iron overload

MACROCYTIC ANEMIA (MCV > 100)

Vitamin B- 12 deficiency and folate deficiency are the leading cause of macrocytic anemia

1.   VITAMIN B 12 DEFICIENCY

Vitamin B 12 plays an important role in red blood cell production. Deficiency of vitamin B 12 leads to megaloblastic anemia. Megaloblastic anemia is characterized by **large red blood cells (RBCs)**

Cause: malabsorption, autoimmune disease, pernicious anemia, atrophic gastritis

Si/Sx: Fatigue, peripheral neuropathy, loss of position and vibration sense, smooth tongue, diarrhea, psychosis and dementia

Diagnosis:

- Best **initial test** is **CBC with peripheral smear**, which shows MCV > 100, **macroovalocytes with hypersegmented neutrophils**
- Most **accurate test** is **Vitamin B 12 level**. However, not all cases show a low level of Vitamin B- 12 level, its level can be normal in acute phase reactant and elevated in stress, infection or cancer. In that case, **methylmalonic acid** may help.
- **Anti-parietal cell antibodies** and **anti-intrinsic factor** are used to **confirm the diagnosis**

Treatment: Vitamin B 12 replacement

2.   FOLATE DEFICIENCY ANEMIA

Folate plays an important role in red blood cell production. Folate deficiency can also lead to megaloblastic anemia

Cause: Causes of folate deficiency include inadequate folic acid intake (diet, during pregnancy, sickle cell anemia), reduced absorption, medicines such as phenytoin, methotrexate

Si/Sx: fatigues, lightheaded, forgetful, trouble concentrating.

Diagnosis:

- Best initial test is CBC with peripheral smear, which shows MCV > 100, macroovalocytes with hypersegmented neutrophils
- Folic acid levels

Treatment: Folic acid replacement

Note: Neurologic abnormalities are seen in vitamin B 12 deficiency, whereas, no neurologic abnormalities seen in folate deficiency anemia.

NORMOCYTIC ANEMIA (MCV 80- 100)

1. SICKLE CELL ANEMIA

Sickle cell is an autosomal recessive trait, caused by point mutation, which results in glutamic acid being substituted for valine at position 6 of the beta chain.

Si/Sx:

- Dehydration, hypoxia, infection, or acidosis, cause sickling of deoxygenated RBCs. These sickle **shaped cells obstructs the blood vessels and restricts the blood flow to organs**, which leads to ischemia, pain, necrosis and other conditions such as stroke, retinal infarctions, priapism and pulmonary infarction
- Autosplenectomy
- Aplastic crisis
- Intravascular hemolysis
- Avascular necrosis of the femoral head
- Osteomyelitis

Diagnosis:

- Best **initial test** is CBC with peripheral smear. Peripheral smear shows sickling of RBCs and Howell-jolly bodies
- Reticulocytes are usually increased by 10- 20 % from baseline
- Most **accurate test** is hemoglobin electrophoresis

Treatment:

- **Acute painful crisis** is managed with Oxygen, IV hydration and analgesia. IV ceftriaxone or levofloxacin is added to the treatment if the patient has a fever
- Exchange transfusion, if the patient has acute chest syndrome, eye infarction, lung infarction or stroke.
- Folic acid replacement to prevent aplastic crisis
- **Hydroxyurea** is given to prevent **recurrent vaso-occlusive painful crisis**
- Patients with autosplenectomy should receive H. Influenza and pneumococcal vaccine to prevent infections from encapsulated organisms

2.   HEREDITARY SPHEROCYTOSIS

Hereditary spherocytosis is characterized by the formation of RBCs that are sphere-shaped rather than bi-concave disk shaped. Sphere-shaped RBCs become trapped in the spleen, and spleen destroys them (hemolysis)

Cause: Autosomal dominant defect in spectrin gene

Si/Sx: Recurrent episodes of hemolysis, jaundice, pigmented gallstones, splenomegaly

Diagnosis:

- CBC shows low MCV and increased mean corpuscular hemoglobin concentration (MCHC)
- Peripheral blood smear shows spherocytes with **no central pallor** of normal RBCs
- Coombs' test is negative
- Most accurate test is **osmotic fragility test**. When patient's RBCs are placed in a hypotonic solution, RBCs absorb all the solution until the RBCs cell membrane bursts (cell lysis)

Treatment: There is no cure for hereditary spherocytosis,

- Mild spherocytosis is treated with **folic replacement**, which support the RBCs production
- Severe spherocytosis is treated by surgical removal of spleen (**Splenectomy),** which stops further hemolysis

3.   COLD-AGGLUTININ HEMOLYSIS

Cold-agglutinin hemolysis is a rare form of autoimmune hemolytic anemia caused by cold-reacting autoantibodies, usually **IgM.** Cold-reacting autoantibodies bind to the cell membrane of RBCs and cause premature lysis of RBCs.

Cause: For most of the cases there is no known cause (idiopathic). Some known causes are Mycoplasma pneumonia, mononucleosis, Epstein-Barr virus, cytomegalovirus or Waldenströn macroglobulinemia.

Si/Sx: anemia occurs after body exposed by cold temperature or following upper respiratory tract infection (URI). **Pain and purple discoloration** of body parts **exposed to cold temperature** such as the nose, ears, and fingers, which **resolves in warm temperature**.

Diagnosis:

- Direct coombs' test shows positive Anti-C3d, negative anti-IgG
- Most accurate test is **cold agglutinins titer**

Treatment:
- **Supportive treatment**, avoid cold weather, treat the underlying cause
- Rituximab (anti-CD 20 monoclonal antibody)
- In a case of **severe hemolysis** adjunct treatment with **plasmapheresis** can be done to **remove IgM antibody**
- **Immunosuppressive** agents such as cyclophosphamide, azathioprine, interferon and fludarabine to **stop IgM synthesis**

Note: Prednisone and splenectomy are not useful for cold-agglutinin disease. However, these can be used if IgG co-antibodies are present.

4. WARM AUTOIMMUNE HEMOLYSIS

Warm autoimmune hemolysis occurs when body immune system directs antibodies against its own RBCs. It is usually **IgG mediated**

Cause: most of the cases are idiopathic. Some known causes include lymphoproliferative disorders (CLL, lymphoma), autoimmune disorders (Lupus, scleroderma, rheumatoid arthritis), and drugs (alpha-methyldopa, penicillin, rifampin)

Si/Sx: dark urine, fatigue, jaundice, shortness of breath

Diagnosis:
- Peripheral blood smear shows spherocytosis
- Positive direct coombs' test

Treatment:
- **Prednisone** is the **best initial treatment**
- **Intravenous immunoglobulin** (IVIG) is used if acute hemolysis not responding to prednisone. IVIG reduces hemolysis by **reducing the interaction between spleen macrophage and antibody coated RBCs**
- If the patient has recurrent episodes of hemolysis, then do splenectomy
- Rituximab, azathioprine, cyclophosphamide, or cyclosporine are used in refractory cases

5. GLUCOSE-6-PHOSPHATE DEHYDROGENASE (G6PD) DEFICIENCY

G6PD deficiency is X-linked recessive hereditary disease

Precipitating factors: Fava beans and drugs such as sulfa drugs, primaquine, dapsone, nitrofurantoin, quinidine, quinine, and NSAIDs

Si/Sx: dark urine, fatigue, pallor, jaundice, and shortness of breath **after exposure of precipitating factor**

Diagnosis:

- Best initial test is peripheral blood smear, which show **Heinz body** (hemoglobin precipitates) and **bite cells** (damaged RBCs are removed by macrophages in the spleen)
- Most accurate test is G6PD level, measured 2-3 months after an acute episode

Treatment: There is no cure for G6PD deficiency. Mild hemolysis is treated with supportive care (IV fluids) and removing the precipitating factor. Severe hemolysis is treated with blood transfusion

6. PAROXYSMAL NOCTURNAL HEMOGLOBINURIA (PNH)

Paroxysmal nocturnal hemoglobinuria (PNH) is an acquired RBCs membrane **defect in phosphatidylinositol glycan A (PIG-A)** that allows RBCs to bind to complements and cause intravascular hemolysis.

Complement lysis mostly happens in an acidic environment. Every one is mildly acidotic while sleeping because a relative hypoventilation; as a result, most of the patient present with nocturnal or early morning hemoglobinuria.

Si/Sx: nocturnal or early morning hemoglobinuria, shortness of breath, headaches

Diagnosis: Most accurate test is CD 55 and CD 59 levels or flow cytometry for CD 55 and CD 59.

Treatment:

- Prednisone is the best initial treatment.
- Eculizumab is used for long-term treatment. It protects RBCs from immune destruction by inhibiting the complement pathway (inactivating C5 complement pathway).

Complications: PNH is an acquired RBCs stem cell defect it may cause ALL, aplastic anemia, blood clots, or myelodysplasia. **Large venous thrombosis is the most common cause of death**

7.   MICROANGIOPATHIC HEMOLYTIC ANEMIA

Microangiopathic hemolytic anemia is a subgroup of hemolytic anemia in which **RBCs are destroyed by coagulation factors** in the small capillaries. It is seen in conditions such as hemolytic uremic syndrome (HUS), disseminated intravascular coagulation (DIC), thrombotic thrombocytopenia purpura (TTP) and malignant hypertension.

Differential diagnosis of hemolytic anemia

Condition	HUS	TTP	DIC
Cause	E. Coli 157: H7, Shigella, salmonella	HIV infection, SLE and drugs such as OCP, ticlopidine, or clopidogrel	Sepsis, trauma, septic abortion, trauma
Si/Sx	Anemia, thrombocytopenia , acute renal failure	Anemia, thrombocytopenia , acute renal failure, **fever and neurological abnormalities**	**Bleeding from any site of the body**, acute renal failure, jaundice and confusion
Diagnosis	Normal PT/PTT	Normal PT/PTT and **increased bleeding time**	Increased PT/PTT and increased bleeding time. **Increased D-Dimer and fibrin split product. Decreased fibrinogen**
Treatment	IV fluids for mild symptoms, Plasmapheresis for severe symptoms. Dialysis, if needed	Same as HUS	Treat the underlying cause. Fresh frozen plasma and platelet transfusion, as needed

Note: Antibiotics are not given to a patient with HUS because they can worsen the HUS

MYELOPROLIFERATIVE DISORDERS

1. POLYCTHEMIA VERA
Polycythemia Vera is a disorder of the bone marrow in which production of RBCs, WBCs and platelets are increased, but RBCs are produced more than WBC s and platelets

Types and Causes:
- Primary polycythemia vera is caused by mutation in JAK protein
- Secondary polycythemia is caused by hypoxia (COPD, smoking, high altitude)

Si/Sx: headache, dizziness, vision problem, shortness of breath, **itchiness after warm showers**, fatigue, and splenomegaly

Diagnosis:
- CBC shows low MCV, increased RBC, increased hematocrit and increased hemoglobin
- Erythropoietin (EPO) levels, which is **low in primary** polycythemia, and **high in secondary** polycythemia

Treatment:
- Best initial treatment is Phlebotomy, it lower the blood volume, and reduces the risk of thrombotic events
- Aspirin is also added to treatment to reduce the risk of thrombotic events
- If a patient cannot tolerate phlebotomy, then give hydroxyurea
- Allopurinol if the patient develops gout

Complication: AML, Myelofibrosis, Gout, stroke

2. ESSENTIAL THROMBOCYTHEMIA
Essential thrombocythemia is characterized by overproduction of platelets in the absence of any other cause, such as cancer, infection, or iron deficiency.

Si/Sx: headache, vision disturbance, tingling of the hands and feet, weakness, chest pain, nosebleeds, bruising

Diagnose: platelet count > 450,000

Treatment: Hydroxyurea and aspirin. However, these are given only if the patient is > 60 years of age, history of thrombosis or platelet count more than 1.5 million

3.   MYELOFIBROSIS

Myelofibrosis is a disorder of the bone marrow, in which bone marrow is replaced by **fibrosis tissue**. This results in decreased production of RBCs, WBCs and platelets. Hematopoiesis shifts to the liver and spleen, and cause them to become markedly enlarged.

Si/Sx: fatigue, shortness of breath, pallor, bruising, easy bleeding, hepatosplenomegaly

Diagnosis:

- CBC with peripheral blood smear shows **pancytopenia** (low RBCs, WBCs, and platelets) and teardrop cell
- Most accurate test is bone marrow biopsy, which shows fibrosis

Treatment: Bone marrow transplant (BMT) is the best treatment for patients **< 60 years of age and healthy enough to have BMT. Thalidomide** or **lenalidomide** is best option for patients **> 60 years of age or are not healthy to have BMT.**

APLASTIC ANEMIA

Aplastic anemia is a condition in which bone marrow **does not produce** enough **RBCs, WBCs, and platelets**

Cause: idiopathic, chemotherapy, radiation, parvovirus B 19, lupus, and drugs (Sulfa drugs, chloramphenicol, phenytoin)

Si/Sx: fatigue, shortness of breath, pallor, bruising, easy bleeding due to low platelets, infections due to low WBCs

Diagnosis:

- Best initial test is CBC, which shows pancytopenia (low RBCs, WBCs, and platelets count)
- Most accurate test is bone marrow biopsy, which shows fewer-than-normal blood cells and an **increased amount of fat**

Treatment:

- Supportive treatment (IV fluids, antibiotics, blood transfusion and platelets), and treat the underlying causes.
- Bone marrow transplant (BMT) is recommended; if the patient is **< 45 years of age, has matched done and is in good health**. However, if the patient **does not meet** any of the criteria, then give **Antithymocyte globulin, cyclosporine and prednisone.**

LEUKEMIA

Leukemia is a cancer of white blood cells (WBCs), in which white blood cells are overproduced. WBCs grow faster and bigger and do not work as normal WBCs.

Over time, leukemia cell overcrowds the bone marrow that interferes with normal blood cell production, which can lead to other problems, such as anemia, infection and bleeding.

Types: four main types of leukemia are:

- Acute lymphoblastic leukemia (ALL)
- Acute myelogenous leukemia (AML)
- Chronic lymphoblastic leukemia (CLL)
- Chronic myelogenous leukemia (CML)

1. ACUTE LYMPHOBLASTIC LEUKEMIA (ALL)

ALL is the most common leukemia in children between 2-5 years of age.

Si/Sx: fever, fatigue, weight loss, bruising, petechia, bone pain, infection, lymphadenopathy and hepatosplenomegaly

Diagnosis:

- CBC shows anemia, thrombocytopenia, and leukocytosis
- **Best initial test is the peripheral smear**, which shows leukemic blast
- Bone marrow biopsy shows leukemic blast (WBC >20%)
- Immunochemistry may reveal **PAS +, TdT +, CALLA +**
- Some patients may have cytogenic translocation t(9;22) or t(4;11)
- Leukemic blast (WBC >20 %) on peripheral smear and bone marrow biopsy **confirms the diagnosis**

Treatment:

Best initial treatment for ALL is induction chemotherapy with daunorubicin, asparaginase, vincristine and steroids. Chemotherapy in ALL consists of three phases: induction, consolidation and maintenance therapy

- Induction therapy: Purpose is to kill tumor cells rapidly
- **Consolidation therapy**: purpose is to further kill any cancer cells that may be left in the body. It important to give **intrathecal chemotherapy** (methotrexate) during this phase to prevent CNS relapse of ALL

- Maintenance therapy - to kill any residual tumor cells.

Bone marrow transplant (**BMT**) is performed, if the patient **relapses after chemotherapy** or has a bad prognosis.

Bad prognosis defined as;
- Patient is less than 1 year of age at the time of diagnosis
- Patient is more than 10 years of age at the time of diagnosis
- Has cytogenic translocation such as t (9; 22)
- WBCs more than 100,000 at the time of diagnosis

2. ACUTE MYELOGENOUS LEUKEMIA (AML)

AML is the most common leukemia in adults 15-39 years of age. AML is divided into eight types, M0 – M7

Si/Sx: fever, fatigue, weight loss, bruising, petechia, bone pain, infection, lymphadenopathy and hepatosplenomegaly

Diagnosis:
- CBC shows anemia, thrombocytopenia, and leukocytosis
- Bone marrow biopsy shows myeloblasts that are **Auer rods, myeloperoxidase and sudan black**

Treatment:
- Best initial treatment for AML is chemotherapy with daunorubicin, cytosine and arabinoside. Chemotherapy in AML consists of two phases: induction, and consolidation
- If the patient has AML type M3 (promyelocytic leukemia), then add **all trans retinoic acid (ATRA) to the chemotherapy**

Note: M3, promyelocytic leukemia can cause disseminated intravascular coagulation (DIC).

3. CHRONIC LYMPHOBLASTIC LEUKEMIA (CLL)

CLL is the most common leukemia in adults 40-59 years of age. It affects B cell lymphocytes

Si/Sx: Most of the patients with CLL are asymptomatic, but some patients may have fatigue, lymphadenopathy and splenomegaly

Diagnosis:
- CBC shows isolated lymphocytosis (lymphocyte count > 5000/μL)
- Peripheral blood smear shows **smudge cell** (leukocytes that are partially lysed during the blood smear preparation)

Stages:

- Stage 0: Isolated lymphocytosis
- Stage 1: Enlarged lymph nodes
- Stage 2: Splenomegaly
- Stage 3: Anemia
- Stage 4: Thrombocytopenia

Treatment:

- **Supportive treatment** for patients with **stage 0** and **stage 1** CLL
- **Fludarabine plus rituximab** for patient with **stage 2, stage 3 or stage 4** CLL
- Cyclophosphamide is for treat refractory cases

4. CHRONIC MYELOGENOUS LEUKEMIA (CML)

CML is characterized by clonal bone marrow stem cell disorder in which proliferation of granulocytes (neutrophils, eosinophils, basophils), is seen
Cause: 90 % of the cases are associated with Philadelphia chromosome
t (9; 22), fusion **of BCR-ABL protein** with strong **tyrosine kinase activity**
Si/Sx: fatigue, night sweats, low-grade fever, abdominal fullness and splenomegaly
Diagnosis:

- CBC with peripheral smear shows elevated WBCs, predominantly neutrophils
- Most accurate test is chromosomal translocation (9; 22), which can be done by PCR or FISH

Treatment:
Best initial treatment is a **tyrosine kinase inhibitor** such as imatinib, dasatinib, or nilotinib. If tyrosine kinase inhibitors are ineffective, then do bone marrow transplant (BMT)

MYELODYSPLASTIC SYNDROME

Myelodysplastic syndrome is a cancer in which bone marrow does not make enough new blood cells and cells that are made are abnormal cells. It is most common in adults 60 -75 years of age.
Cause: there is no known specific cause, but risk factors are 5q- syndrome (deletion in the long arm of chromosome 5), radiation, benzene, acquired aplastic anemia, Fanconi anemia

Si/Sx: fever, fatigue, weight loss, bruising, petechia, bone pain, infection, lymphadenopathy and hepatosplenomegaly

Diagnosis:
- CBC shows low RBCs, WBCs, and platelet counts, MCV> 100
- Peripheral smear shows hypogranular neutrophil with pseudo-Pelger-Huet nucleus (**2 lobes neutrophils**)
- Blood chemistry shows **normal vitamin B 12 and folate level**
- Most **accurate test is bone marrow biopsy** that shows hypercellular to normocellular marrow. In 10% of the patients, marrow may be hypocellular
- Karyotyping to check for 5q- syndrome

Treatment:
- Blood products transfusion, as needed
- Erythropoietin injection, as needed
- **Bone marrow transplant** for patients **younger than 60 years of age**
- Azacitidine is a specific treatment for myelodysplasia; it **reduces the need for blood transfusion**
- **Lenalidomide** is effective in reducing blood transfusion requirement in patients with the **5q- syndrome**

HAIRY CELL LEUKEMIA

Hairy cell leukemia is a cancer of B lymphocyte. It mostly affects the men over 55 years of age.

Cause: There is no known cause

Si/Sx: Fatigue, night sweat, low-grade fever, abdominal fullness, recurrent infection, easy bruising or bleeding, splenomegaly

Diagnosis:
- CBC shows low RBCs, WBCs, and platelets
- Blood smear and a bone marrow biopsy show **hairy cell** (hair-like projection of cytoplasm of B-lymphocytes)
- Most accurate test is tartrate-resistant acid phosphatase (TRAP)

Treatment: Best initial therapy is cladribine or pentostatin. Splenectomy is reserved for refractory cases.

LYMPHOMA

Lymphoma is cancer of the lymphatic system (lymph nodes, lymphatic channels and lymph nodes such as spleen and thymus)

Types: Hodgkin's lymphoma and **Non-Hodgkin's lymphoma.**

1.   HODGKIN'S LYMPHOMA

Hodgkin's lymphoma is cancer of the lymphatic system. It has bi-modal distribution, seen between 15-35 years of age and over 55 years old.

Risk factors: Epstein-Barr virus, family history, HIV,

Si/Sx: painless, enlarged, nonerythematous, nontender lymph nodes (cervical, supraclavicular and axillary). Some patients may have "B" symptoms (fever, soaking night sweats, and unexplained weight loss)

Diagnosis:

- CBC
- Chest X-ray, CT head, chest, abdomen and pelvic
- Bone marrow biopsy
- Best initial test is **excisional lymph node biopsy**

Variants of Hodgkin Lymphoma

Type	Characteristics
Lymphocytes predominance	**Predominant lymphocytes**, few RS cells, variable number of histiocytes, little fibrosis
Lymphocytes depletion	**Few lymphocytes**, many RS cells, diffuse fibrosis may be seen
Mixed cellularity	**Mixture** of neutrophils, lymphocytes, plasma cells, eosinophil, histiocytes and a **large number of RS cells**
Nodular sclerosis	**Collagen bands create nodular pattern**; RS cells are lacunar cells. Mixture of neutrophils, lymphocytes, plasma cells, eosinophils and histiocytes. Mediastinal, supraclavicular and cervical lymph nodes

Treatment: depends on the following:

Characteristics	Treatment
• If "B" symptoms are present (fever, weight loss and night sweats) • Stage 3 lymphoma (lymph node affected on **both sides** of the diaphragm) • Stage 4 lymphoma (**disseminated disease)**	**Mnemonic: ABVD** Adriamycin, Bleomycin, Vinblastine, and Dacarbazine
• B symptoms are absent • Stage 1 lymphoma (Single lymph node affected) • Stage 2 lymphoma (2 more lymph node affected on the **same side of the diaphragm)**	**Radiation**

2. NON-HODGKIN'S LYMPHOMA

Signs and symptoms are same as Hodgkin's lymphoma, but Non-Hodgkin's lymphoma more likely to involve extralymphatic sites and it looks similar to CLL.

Diagnosis:

- CBC
- Chest X-ray, CT head, chest, abdomen and pelvic
- Bone marrow biopsy
- Best initial test is excisional lymph node biopsy

Treatment: depends on the following:

Characteristics	Treatment
• If "B" symptoms are present (fever, weight loss, and night sweats) • Stage 3 lymphoma (Lymph node affected on **both sides** of the diaphragm) • Stage 4 lymphoma (**disseminated disease)**	**Mnemonic: CHOP** Chemotherapy, Hydroxy-Adriamycin, Oncovin and **Prednisone**
• B symptoms are absent • Stage 1 lymphoma (Single lymph node affected) • Stage 2 lymphoma (2 more lymph node affected on the **same side of the diaphragm)**	**Radiation**

MULTIPLE MYELOMA

Multiple myeloma is a cancer of plasma cell in the bone marrow. It is characterized by **overproduction of IgG antibodies**. As the cancer grows it affects the production of normal blood cells, and causes bone pain, bone lesions,

Si/Sx: bone pain, multiple fractures, repeated infections, weight loss, weakness

Diagnosis:

- Labs: **hypercalcemia**, decreased anion-gap channel, elevated BUN and creatinine
- Peripheral smear shows **blood rouleaux formation**
- X-ray of affected bone shows punched out lytic lesion
- **Serum protein** electrophoresis shows **IgG or IgA spike**
- **Urine protein** electrophoresis shows **Bence-Jones protein**
- Bone marrow biopsy shows >10 % plasma cell

Treatment:

- **Best initial treatment** for patients **< 70 years age** is thalidomide and dexamethasone.
- Most effective therapy is **bone marrow transplant (BMT)**
- **Melphalan and prednisone** are for patients **> 70 years of age** or those who **cannot tolerate thalidomide and dexamethasone**

WALDENSTROM'S MACROGLOBULINEMIA

Waldenstrom's macroglobulinemia is cancer of B-lymphocytes. It is characterized by **overproduction of IgM antibodies** from B-lymphocytes. Uncontrolled production of IgM leads to hyperviscosity and interferes with RBCs and platelet production.

Si/Sx: Blurred vision, fatigue, headache, change in mental status, bleeding gums

Diagnosis:
- CBC shows increased lymphocytes and decreased RBCs and platelets
- **Best initial test** is serum viscosity
- Serum protein electrophoresis shows IgM spike

Treatment: Plasmapheresis

BLEEDING DISORDERS

1. IDIOPATHIC THROMBOCYTOPENIC PURPURA (ITP)

Idiopathic thrombocytopenic purpura is characterized by isolated low platelet count (thrombocytopenia)

Cause: there is no specific known cause. Some known causes include viral illness (such as mumps, measles or flu), leukemia, lymphoma, anti-platelet antibody

Si/Sx: petechiae, purpura, prolong bleeding from cuts, epistaxis, bleeding gums, heavy menstrual flow in women and **normal size spleen**

Note: enlarged spleen size suggests possible other causes of thrombocytopenia

Diagnosis:
- Idiopathic thrombocytopenic purpura is a diagnosis of exclusion. It is important to rule out other cause of thrombocytopenia
- CBC shows low platelet count, and normal RBCs and WBCs
- **Normal clotting factors with prolong bleeding time**

Treatment:

- **No treatment is required** if the patient have no active bleeding and platelet count> 50,000. Check **platelets count at regular interval**
- If platelet count is <30,000, start treatment with corticosteroids. Stop NSAIDs to improve platelet count, if applicable
- If platelet count is < 10,000, treat patient with IVIG or Anti-Rho
- If platelet count remains low after 4-6 weeks of treatment or recurrent bleeding, then do splenectomy
- Thrombopoietin receptor agonist (Romiplostim, eltrombopag) may be used if steroids or splenectomy is ineffective. These **stimulate platelet production in the bone marrow.**

Note: If splenectomy is planned, make sure to vaccinate patient against encapsulated bacteria (N. meningitides, H. influenza and pneumococcus) 2 weeks prior to the procedure

2. VON WILLEBRAND DISEASE (VWD)

Von Willebrand disease is the most common heredity bleeding disorder. It is an autosomal dominant disorder caused by a deficiency of von Willebrand factor (vWF). vWF is required for platelet adhesion
Si/Sx: Platelet type bleeding -petechia, purpura, epistaxis, bleeding form gums, and heavy menstrual flow in women
Diagnosis:

- CBC shows normal platelet count
- Bleeding time shows **increased aPTT**
- Factor VIII level
- Most accurate is VWF level and ristocetin cofactor test (detects VWF function)

Treatment: Best initial treatment is desmopressin (DDAVP), which releases the vWF from endothelial cells. If it is ineffective, then give factor VIII replacement.

3. HEMOPHILIA

Hemophilia is a rare **X-linked recessive disorder**, in which blood does not clot properly. It is more common in males and female are asymptomatic carriers

Types: Hemophilia A (Factor VIII deficiency), Hemophilia B (Factor IX deficiency)

Si/Sx: signs and symptoms depend on the level of the deficient factor. Patient with very low level of factor may experience spontaneous bleeding, whereas, patients with slight deficiency may only bleed after trauma or surgery.

Diagnosis:
- Normal bleeding time and PT, **increased PTT**
- **Most accurate** test is **specific factor assay**

Treatment: discussed below

Condition	Treatment
Hemophilia A	• Vasopressin for mild bleeding • Factor VIII replacement for severe bleeding
Hemophilia B	• Factor IX replacement

4. VITAMIN K DEFICIENCY

Vitamin K plays an important role in the synthesis of coagulation factor. Its deficiency can leads to **decreased production of factors 2,7,9 and 10**

Si/Sx: oozing at venipuncture site. Bleeding is similar to the bleeding of hemophilia and may occur at any site

Diagnosis:
- **Both PT and PTT are elevated**
- PT and PTT **normalizes after vitamin K infusion**

Treatment:
- Mild bleeding is treated with vitamin K
- Severe bleeding is treated with fresh frozen plasma and vitamin K

5. LIVER DISEASE

Almost all clotting factors are made in the liver, except for factor VIII and vWF

Si/Sx: similar to vitamin K deficiency

Diagnosis:

- Both PT and PTT are elevated
- PT and PTT **does not normalize** after Vitamin K infusion

Treatment: Fresh frozen plasma and vitamin K replacement

TRANSFUSION REACTION

1. ACUTE HEMOLYTIC REACTION

Acute hemolytic reaction occurs due to destruction of RBCs by preformed recipient antibodies

Cause: clerical error is the most common cause

Si/Sx: fever, chill chest pain, back pain, hemorrhage, shortness of breath, hypotension

Treatment: Stop transfusion, IV fluids and mannitol to prevent renal failure

2. FEBRILE NONHEMOLYTIC REACTION

Si/Sx: Fever, chills temperature rises 1.0 c- 1.8 F from the baseline

Cause: recipient's antibodies to donor WBCs

Treatment: Leukoreduction – filtration of donor white cell from red blood cells products

3. TRANSFUSION-ASSOCIATED ACUTE LUNG INJURY

Si/Sx: Abrupt onset of fever, hypotension, non-cardiogenic pulmonary edema

Cause: donor's plasma contains antibodies

Treatment: most cases resolve within 72 hours

4. ALLERGIC REACTION

Occurs when the recipient has preformed antibodies in donor blood

Si/Sx: urticaria, pruritus, may lead to anaphylactic shock

Cause: antibody in donor blood

Treatment: antihistamines such as diphenhydramine

5. ALLERGIC ANAPHYLAXIS
Si/Sx: hypotension, tachycardia, loss of consciousness, shock, cardiac arrhythmia, cardiac arrest
Cause: IgA deficiency
Treatment: stop transfusion, maintain ABCs and give IgA washed blood products

TRANSPLANT REJECTION

1. HYPERACUTE REJECTION
Hyperacute rejection occurs within minutes of transplant. It occurs due to antibodies in organ recipient's blood that reacts to a transplanted organ
Cause: ABO incompatibility
Treatment: Remove the organ
Prevention: check ABO compatibility prior to transplantation

2. ACUTE REJECTION
Acute rejection occurs between 5 days to 3 months after transplant. It occurs due to cytotoxic T lymphocytes against foreign MHCs
Diagnosis: biopsy of organ shows T lymphocytes and antibody induced graft tissue injury
Treatment: Steroids and immunosuppressive drugs

3. CHRONIC REJECTION
Chronic rejection takes place over months to years after transplant
Diagnosis: biopsy of organ shows anti-body mediated vascular damage (fibrosis of blood vessels)
Treatment: chronic rejection is considered irreversible. There is no effective treatment

Notes:

PULMONOLOGY

ACUTE PHARYNGITIS

Pharyngitis is a sore throat caused by inflammation of pharynx (throat)

Cause: it can be caused by bacterial or viral infection

- **Bacterial**: Group A beta-hemolytic streptococcus (GABHS) is the most common cause, other causes may include, streptococcus pneumonia, H. influenza, N. gonorrhea, C. pneumonia, Mycoplasma pneumonia
- **Viral:** Adenovirus, EBV, HSV, measles, rhinovirus, RSV, parainfluenza virus

Si/Sx: Symptoms of sore throat vary, depending on the cause, which is as follow:

- A symptomatic criterion that is used to diagnose Group A beta-hemolytic streptococcus (**GABHS**) is **fever, tonsillar exudate, cervical adenopathy, absence of cough**
- Symptoms for **non-GABHS includes** fever, body ache, enlarged lymph node in armpits, rhinorrhea, conjunctivitis,

Diagnosis:

- Best initial test is **rapid GAS antigen test**
- Most accurate test is throat culture

Treatment: depends on the cause of infection

- If **GABHS** is suspected, start empiric treatment with **penicillin.** But, if the patient is allergic to penicillin, then give azithromycin or clindamycin
- **Viral** pharyngitis is treated with **conservative management** such as fluids, rest, gargling with warm water, or antipyretics

Note: Penicillin or other antibiotics used during GABH reduces the risk of rheumatic fever.

SINUSITIS

Sinusitis is an inflammation of the tissue lining the sinuses

Types and causes:

- **Acute sinusitis**: when symptoms of sinusitis present for < **4 weeks**. It is commonly associated with bacteria (S. pneumonia, H. influenza non-type b, and M. catarrhalis) and viral (rhinoviruses, coronaviruses, and H. influenza)
- **Chronic sinusitis**: when symptoms of sinusitis lasts **> 12 weeks or 3 months**. It is associated with anaerobic bacteria or fungus (Diabetic patients are at increased of getting sinusitis from mucormycosis).

Si/Sx:

- **Acute sinusitis** symptoms include fever, headache, pain behind the eyes, facial tenderness, maxillary tooth pain, bad breath, nasal discharge.
- **Chronic sinusitis** symptoms include high fever, darkened nasal discharge, and respiratory illness that was getting better and then begins to get worse

Diagnosis:

- Clinical diagnosis
- Transillumination test
- X-ray or CT is not recommend for acute sinusitis, unless complication develops such as purulent discharge
- CT is recommended for chronic sinusitis

Treatment;

- Majority of the cases of acute and chronic sinusitis needs symptomatic treatment such as **fluids, humidifier, nasal saline, inhale steam 2-4 times per day**. However, if symptoms do not resolve after 7 days of symptomatic treatment, then give **amoxicillin**
- Surgery and antibiotics are recommended for chronic and fungal sinusitis

INFLUENZA
Influenza, which is commonly known as flu
Cause: RNA virus of the family orthomyxovirus
Si/Sx: Fever, chills, runny nose, body ache, cough, headache, watering eyes
Treatment: treatment depends on the onset of symptoms and time of presentation.

- If the patient presents **< 48 hours** of onset of symptoms, then treat the patient with **neuraminidase inhibitors** such as oseltamivir, or zanamivir. Neuraminidase inhibitors help by shortening the duration of symptoms
- If the patient presents **>48 hours of onset of symptoms**, then give **symptomatic treatment** such as acetaminophen for fever and pain, fluids, and the rest.

ALLERGIC RHINITIS
Allergic rhinitis is an allergic inflammation of the nasal cavity
Cause: pollen, dust, animal dander
Si/Sx: itching, sneezing, wheezing, boggy and **bluish turbinate**
Diagnosis: history, skin testing to identify allergen or IgE RAST tests
Treatment: **Avoid the** known allergen and **intranasal corticosteroids**

VASOMOTOR RHINITIS
Vasomotor rhinitis is a condition that causes constant runny nose, sneezing, and nasal congestion
Cause: there is no exact known cause, but risk factors may include air pollution, spicy food, strong emotions, alcohol
Diagnosis: diagnosis of exclusion
Treatment: depends on symptoms

- If the patient has **clogged nasal cavity,** then give **topical corticosteroids**
- If the patient has **postnasal drip,** then give **intranasal antihistamine (azelastine)**
- If the patient has pure **rhinorrhea, then** give **Ipratropium bromide**

LOWER RESPIRATORY TRACT INFECTION

OBSTRUCTIVE LUNG DIEASE

Obstructive lung disease is characterized by narrowing of lungs or damage to lungs, which results in obstruction of the airway, and difficulty with exhaling.

Cause: the most common causes of obstructive lung disease are:
- Asthma
- Bronchiectasis
- Chronic obstructive pulmonary disease (COPD), which includes chronic bronchitis and emphysema

Diagnosis: Diagnosis depends on the specific cause. However, all obstructive lung diseases show:
- **Increased** total lung capacity **(TLC)**, functional residual capacity **(FRC)**, and residual volume **(RV)**
- **Decreased FEV1/FVC ratio**

Treatment: treatment depends on specific cause (discussed below)

1. ASTHMA

Asthma is a chronic lung disease, characterized by inflammation and narrowing of airway

Cause: common triggers include pollen, pet dander, dust mites, tobacco smoking, respiratory infection, and medicines such as NSAIDs

Si/Sx: recurring episodes of expiratory wheezing, shortness of breath, chest tightness, and cough. Symptoms often are worse at night or early morning

Diagnosis:
- ABG shows mild hypoxia and respiratory ankylosis
- Pulmonary function test: increased TLC, FRC and RV, and decreased FEV1, FEV and FEV1/FEV ratio.
- CBC may show eosinophilia
- Chest X-ray may show hyperinflation

Bronchodilator test

Bronchodilator test can be used to diagnose asthma, when a patient experiences symptoms of asthma, but diagnostic tests are inconclusive. FEV1 is measured before and after administering nebulized albuterol. Asthmatic patient shows >20 % **increase** in FEV1 after receiving nebulized albuterol

Methacholine stimulation test

Methacholine stimulation test can be used to diagnose asthma, when a patient complains of asthma like symptoms, but symptoms are not clear. Methacholine is an artificial form of acetylcholine, which provokes bronchoconstriction. FEV1 is measured before and after administering nebulized methacholine. Asthmatic patient shows >20 % **decrease** in FEV1 after receiving nebulized methacholine

Note: Everyone shows decreased FEV1 after methacholine stimulation test, but asthmatic patient shows FEV1 decreased more than 20%.

Treatment: avoid trigger. Treatment for stable asthma is as follow

Type	Daytime symptoms	Night time symptoms	PFTs	Treatment
Intermittent	2 times a week	2 times a month	FEV1 >80%	Inhaled albuterol, as needed
Mild persistent	>2 times a week	>2 times a month	FEV1 >80%	**Add inhaled** corticosteroids
Moderate persistent	Everyday	>2 per week	FEV1 60 – 80%	**Add** inhaled salmeterol and oral montelukast
Severe	Continuous	Frequent	FEV1 <60%	**Add oral** corticosteroids

2. ASTHMA EXACERBATION

Asthma exacerbation is characterized by acute episode of progressive worsening wheezing, shortness of breath, chest tightness
Treatment: oxygen, albuterol, ipratropium bromide, and prednisone. Intubate as needed.

3. BRONCHIETASIS

Bronchiectasis is characterized by destruction of smooth muscles and elastic tissues of the bronchial tree. This damage leads to abnormal dilation of the large airway.
Cause: cystic fibrosis, Kartagener syndrome, infection (Tuberculosis, whooping cough), IBD, rheumatoid arthritis
Si/Sx: foul smelling sputum production, recurrent lung infection, and hemoptysis
Diagnosis:

- Best initial test is chest x-ray, which shows **"tram-tracks sign"** caused by thickened, dilated airway
- Most accurate test is High resolution CT
- Sputum culture to find the bacteria responsible for infection

Treatment: There is no specific cure for bronchiectasis. Supportive care includes:

- Postural drainage, chest physiotherapy, cupping and clapping of secretion,
- Bronchodilator, expectorants and hydration
- Antibiosis based on sputum culture, but keep rotating antibiotics to prevent development of drug resistance
- Surgical resection for localized bronchiectasis

4. CHRONIC OBSTRUCTIVE PULMONARY DISEASE (COPD)

Chronic obstructive pulmonary disease includes **emphysema** and **chronic bronchitis**

4a. CHRONIC BRONCHITIS

Chronic bronchitis is characterized by inflammation of bronchi and bronchioles, which causes excessive secretion of mucus into the airway, leading to narrowing and obstruction of the bronchial tree.

Causes tobacco smoking is the leading cause. Other less common causes include exposure to pollutants (ammonia, bromine, hydrogen sulfide), dust, and repeated bout of acute bronchitis

Si/Sx: cough and sputum occur **daily for 3 months for at least 2 consecutive years**, dyspnea, wheezing

Diagnosis:

- ABG shows **hypoxia with increased pCO2**
- Chest x-ray shows **increased pulmonary marking**
- Pulmonary function test shows **decreased** FEV1, FVC, & EFV1/FVC, and **increased** TLC and RV. Diffusion lung capacity of carbon dioxide (DLCO) is **normal**
- Diagnosis is confirmed with lung biopsy, which shows **increased Reid index** (bronchial wall thickness increases more than .04)

Treatment: as follow

Acute exacerbation treatment: Oxygen, inhaled beta-agonist (albuterol), anticholinergic (ipratropium), IV steroids and antibiotics (ceftriaxone and macrolides such as azithromycin, clarithromycin).

Chronic treatment:

- Smoking cessation
- First-line treatment is an **anticholinergic medicine** (tiotropium or ipratropium). If it is ineffective, then add **beta-agonists** (inhaled albuterol). If patient is still not responding, then **add theophylline**

Home oxygen lowers the mortality in COPD patients. It is given when:

- PO2 is < 55 mmHG or pulse oxygen saturation is <88 %
- Patient with cor pulmonale with signs of right heart failure, elevated hematocrit, PO2 < 59 mmHG or pulse oxygen saturation < 90 %

4b. EMPHYSEMA

Emphysema is characterized by loss of elasticity of terminal airway, leading to permanent abnormal enlargement of terminal bronchioles, and destruction of the alveolar wall.

Cause: Tobacco smoking is the leading cause. In rare case, alpha1-antitrypsin deficiency,

Types of emphysema
- **Centrilobular emphysema** is associated with tobacco smoking. It predominantly affects the upper half of the lungs
- **Panlobular emphysema** associated with **alpha1-antitrypsin deficiency**. It uniformly affects entire alveolus.

Diagnosis:
- ABG shows hypoxia with increased pCO_2
- Chest x-ray shows flat diaphragm and increased anterior posterior diameter of lungs
- Pulmonary function test shows **decreased** FEV1, FVC, & EFV1/FVC, and **increased** TLC and RV. Diffusion lung capacity of carbon dioxide (DLCO) is **decreased**

Note: DLCO is decreased in emphysema and normal in chronic bronchitis

Treatment: same as chronic bronchitis. However, patient with panlobular are also given alpha-1 antitrypsin infusion

RESTRICTIVE LUNG DIEASE
Restrictive lung disease is a group of disorders that restrict lung expansion, which results in decreased lung volume and inadequate oxygenation.
Diagnosis: Diagnosis depends on the specific cause. However, all restrictive lung diseases show:
- Decreased total lung capacity (TLC), functional residual capacity (FRC), residual volume (RV
- Increased or normal FEV1/FVC

1.   INTERSTITIAL LUNG DISEASE

Disease	Risk factors	Diagnosis
Asbestos	Mining, welding, shipyard, plumbing, boilers	• Chest x-ray shows pleural thickening, pleural plaques and calcification in lower lungs • Lung biopsy shows **barbell shaped asbestos fiber**
Silicosis	Pottery barns, brickyards, sandblasting	• Chest x-ray shows **eggshell calcification** in upper lungs • Lung biopsy shows **barbell shaped asbestos fiber**
Pneumoconiosis	Metal mining, dust	• Chest x-ray **shows irregular opacities**
Coal miner's lung disease	Coal mining	• Chest x-ray shows **circular densities in apical lungs**
Berylliosis	Electronics, ceramics, dental work	• Lung biopsy shows **noncaseating granuloma**

Compilation of interstitial lung disease:
- Asbestos increases the risk of adenocarcinoma
- Silicosis increases the risk of Tuberculosis (TB)

Treatment: there is no treatment for interstitial lung treatment, other than berylliosis, which is treated with steroids

2.   SARCOIDOSIS

Sarcoidosis is characterized by abnormal collection of chronic inflammatory cell (granulomas). It can affect any organ, but lungs are commonly affected.

Cause: there is no known cause of sarcoidosis

Risk factors: African-American, women, and age 20-40

Symptoms: fever, dry cough, malaise, shortness of breath, weight loss, arthritis, raised red firm skin sore (erythema nodosum) on lower legs

Diagnosis:
- Chest X-ray shows bilateral hilar adenopathy
- Biopsy of lungs or other involved shows noncaseating granuloma
- Increased Angiotensin converting enzyme (ACE)
- Hypercalcemia, which is secondary to increase in vitamin D production by granuloma
- Increased alkaline phosphatase

Treatment: Steroids

3. EXTRAPULMONARY DISEASE

Extrapulmonary diseases that can lead to restrictive disease are Myasthenia gravis, Guillain barré, kyphosis, chest wall deformities, diaphragmatic hernia, and ascites

Treatment: supportive

PLEURAL EFFUSION

Pleural effusion is an abnormal accumulation of fluid in pleural space (thin layer between lungs and chest cavity)

Types:
- **Transudate** is low in protein content, which is caused by CHF, cirrhosis
- **Exudates** is in high protein content, which is caused by lung infection, TB, lung cancer and rheumatic disease

Si/Sx: fever, chest pain, cough, shortness of breath, dullness to percussions, decreased tactile fremitus

Diagnosis:
- Chest x-ray shows blunting of the costophrenic angle
- **Thoracocentesis**: pleural fluid is removed from the chest with a needle. Fluid is then analyzed to determine the type of effusion by LDH, protein content, and cause by gram stain and cultures, acid-fast stain, cell count, pH, glucose

Transudate and exudate labs

	Exudate	Transudate
LDH effusion	> 200 IU/ml	<200 IU/ml
LDH effusion/serum ratio	> 0.6	< 0.6
Protein effusion/Serum ratio	> 0.5	< 0.5

Treatment: Drain the fluid and treat the underlying cause

ADULT RESPIRATORY DISTRESS SYNDROME (ARDS)

Adult respiratory distress syndrome is a life-threatening condition in which fluids accumulates in air sacs that prevents oxygen diffusion from lungs to blood

Cause: trauma, aspiration, septic shock, pneumonia, inhalation of toxic fumes, and near drowning

Si/Sx: dyspnea, resistance hypoxia, tachypnea, and diffuse alveolar infiltrate

Diagnosis:

- ABG shows hypoxemia with normal CO_2
- Chest x-ray shows fluid in air sacs
- Pulmonary artery catheterization shows normal capillary wedge pressure (12 -18)

Note: Capillary wedge pressure is high (> 18) in cardiogenic shock

Treatment: oxygen, Positive end-expiratory pressure (PEEP) to keep alveoli open, diuretics and dobutamine

PULMONARY EMBOLISM

Pulmonary embolism is sudden blockage in a lungs artery by fat droplet, blood clot, air bubble or tumor cells

Cause: most common cause is a blood clot in the deep veins of the proximal legs. Other less common causes may include fat droplets, amniotic fluids, air bubble

Risk factor: Virchow's triad (endothelial damage, hypercoagulable, and stasis), estrogen-containing hormonal contraception, genetic thrombophilia (factor V Leiden, protein C deficiency, protein S deficiency, antithrombin deficiency, prothrombin mutation), antiphospholipid syndrome, nephrotic syndrome, cancer

Si/Sx: chest pain, sudden dyspnea, tachypnea, tachycardia, leg pain and swelling

Diagnosis:
- ABG shows respiratory alkalosis
- Chest X-ray
- EKG may show S wave in lead 1, Q wave in lead II, and T wave in lead III
- Sinus tachycardia
- Leg ultrasound to check for deep venous thrombosis
- V/VQ scan

Treatment: as follow
- Oxygen, heparin and warfarin for a **stable patient** with **no active bleeding**
- Inferior vena cava filter for a **stable patient** with **active bleeding**
- tPAs for an **unstable** patient with **no active bleeding**
- Embolectomy for an **unstable** patient with **active bleeding**

SOLITARY PULMONARY NODULE

If solitary nodule is found incidentally on a chest X-ray, next best step in management is to get an old chest x-ray and compare it with current one. Management is as follow:

1. If old x-ray is available then compare the size:
   - **Benign** nodule doubles in **<1 month or more than 480 days**
   - **Malignant** nodule **doubles in > 1 month or < 480 days.**
2. If old x-ray is **not available**, then use the following to determine if nodule is cancerous or a benign:

Characteristic of benign and cancerous nodule

Benign nodule	Cancerous nodule
• Non-smoker • < 35 years of age, • Calcification of nodule • Nodule <2 cm • Nodule has smooth margin	• Smoker • 50 years of age, • No calcification of nodule • Nodule> 2 cm • Nodule has irregular margin

Treatment: Benign tumor is followed-up in 3-6 months. Get CT and sputum cytology for malignant tumor

Differential diagnosis of lung cancer

Cancer	Characteristic
Squamous cell carcinoma	• Centrally located tumor • Most common in smokers • Secrets PTH-like peptide that causes **hypercalcemia**
Small cell carcinoma	• Centrally located tumor • Most common in smoker • Can lead **to SIADH, Lambert-Eaton syndrome**
Large cell carcinoma	• Peripherally located tumor • Highly anaplastic, undifferentiated tumor
Adenocarcinoma	• Peripherally located tumor • Most common cause of lung cancer in non-smokers
Bronchoalveolar syndrome	• Peripherally located tumor • Subtype of adenocarcinoma

Diagnosis:
- Chest X-ray
- CT guided fine-needle aspiration
- Thoracoscopic biopsy

Treatment:
- Surgical resection and radiation for localized tumor or non-small cell carcinoma
- Chemotherapy and radiation for small cell carcinoma and metastatic cancer

SMOKING CESSATION

All patients should be screened and counseled against smoking at each visit

Treatment: Best initial step is to assess if the patient is **willing to quit** smoking, because if the patient is not willing to quit smoking, then the treatment may not be successful. However, if the patient is willing to quit, then following treatment options may be used

- Nicotine **patch and gums** are controlled release nicotine thus help reduce abrupt effects of nicotine withdrawal
- **Bupropion** is the best initial treatment for patients with depressed mood and wanting to quit smoking. However, it is **contraindicated** in patients with **seizures or epilepsy** because it lowers the seizure threshold.
- **Varenicline** can be safely used in patients with seizures and epilepsy

PULMONOLOGY INFECTIOUS DISEASES

PNEUMONIA

Pneumonia is an infection of lungs caused by bacteria, virus or fungi.

Typical and atypical pneumonia

	Typical pneumonia	Atypical pneumonia
Symptoms	• Abrupt onset of high fever (>102 F) • Chills • Progressive cough • Thoracic pain	• Progressive onset of fever (<102 F) • No chill • Dry cough • Myalgia, • Headache
Prodrome	Short duration (<2 days)	Long duration (> 2 days)
Chest x-ray shows	Lobar or segmental involvement	Multilobar or diffuse Involvement
Cause	S. Pneumoniae, H. influenza, S. aureus	Mycoplasma pneumonia, Legionella pneumonia, chlamydia

DIFFERENTIAL DIAGNOSIS OF PNEUMONIA

1. TYPICAL PNEUMONIA

Organism	Association
	Typical bacterial pneumonia
Streptococcus pneumonia	• Most common cause of typical pneumonia
Pseudomonas	• Common in cystic fibrosis
Klebsiella	• Common in alcoholics, diabetics • Associated with "current jelly" sputum
Anaerobes	• Seen in patient with altered consciousness, poor dentition, dementia

2. ATYPICAL PNEUMONIA

Organism	Characteristics
Legionella	• Common in patient exposed to contaminated water source, such as air conditioner • Si/Sx: **altered mental status, hyponatremia, diarrhea, high LDH** • **Diagnosis**: charcoal extract, urine antigen test or direct fluorescent antibodies
Mycoplasma	• Common in young adults (College students) • **Diagnosis: PCR, cold agglutinin**
Chlamydia pneumonia	• Common in elderly • Si/Sx: sore throat, hoarseness, • **Diagnosis:** serology titer
Chlamydia Psittaci	• Contracted from bird
Coxiella burnetii	• Contracted from farm animals (cattle goats), ingestion of infected milk
Actinomyces	• Common in Immunocompetent patient with dental or facial trauma • **Diagnosis**: gram stain • **Treatment**: penicillin
Nocardia	• Common in Immunocompetent patients, mimic TB • **Gram-positive acid-fast aerobe** • **Treatment**: Bactrim

Diagnosis:
- Best initial test is chest x-ray
- Most accurate test is sputum gram stain and culture

Treatment: empiric treatment is started until gram stain and culture results are available. Empiric treatment can be **outpatient or inpatient** (discussed below)

> Patient is treated in hospital (Inpatient) if patient has any of the following: Mnemonic- **CURB 65**
> * Confusion
> * Uremia
> * Respiratory rate >30/minute
> * Blood pressure: systolic <90 mmHG or diastolic <60 mmHG
> * Age >65

Inpatient empiric treatment regimen
* IV ceftriaxone and azithromycin
  Or
* IV fluoroquinolone such as levofloxacin, gatifloxacin, or moxifloxacin

Outpatient empiric treatment regimen
* Oral fluoroquinolone such as levofloxacin, or gatifloxacin, or moxifloxacin
  Or
* Oral macrolides: Azithromycin, or clarithromycin

3. **HOSPITAL ACQUIRED PNEUMONIA / HEALTHCARE ASSOCIATED PNEUMONIA**
Pneumonia that starts **within 48 hours of admission or within 90 days after hospitalization**
Risk factor: hospitalized patient that are alcoholics, have chronic lung disease, immunocompromised, or had major surgery
Treatment: combination **of 2 drugs** with IV piperacillin/tazobactam or fluoroquinolone with imipenem or meropenem

4. **VENTILATOR ASSOCIATED PNEUMONIA**
This is sub-type of hospital-acquired pneumonia develops **within 48 hours** or longer **after** receiving **mechanical ventilation**
Treatment: 3 drugs combination: Imipenem, gentamicin and vancomycin or linezolid

5.   FUNGAL PNEUMONIA

Organism	Characteristics
Pneumocystis carinii	• Common in AIDS patient with CD 4 cells count < 200 • **Diagnosis**: Increased LDH, sputum silver stain • **Treatment**: Bactrim (TMP/SMX)
Histoplasmosis	• Common in people living in wet areas such as Mississippi river valley, and Ohio • Associated with bat droppings • **Diagnosis:** Urine antigen is most sensitive test • **Treatment**: Itraconazole
Blastomycosis	• Common in people living in southeast and south-central Unites States • **Diagnosis**: sputum cytology shows **broad-based budding yeast** • **Treatment**: oral itraconazole
Coccidioides immitis	• Common in people travel to southwest desert • **Diagnosis:** sputum cytology shows **budding yeast** • **Treatment**: itraconazole
Aspergillus	• Common in neutropenic patient • **Diagnosis**: chest X-ray shows **"fungus ball"** with cavitation • **Treatment**: Amphotericin B/ itraconazole

TUBERCULOSIS (TB)

Tuberculosis is an infection caused by mycobacterium tuberculosis.
Si/Sx: depends on the type
   • **Latent tuberculosis** has no symptoms
   • **Active tuberculosis**: cough, fever, night sweat, weight loss

1.   Latent tuberculosis

Si/Sx: Patients usually are asymptomatic

Diagnosis: as follow

- First get PPD test, It is considered positive if: (see table below)

Induration	Considered positive in population
≥ 5 mm induration	HIV positive, close contact with active TB, taking immunosuppressive medicine
≥ 10 mm induration	Alcoholics, homeless, prisoners, prisoners, healthcare worker, new immigrant
≥ 15mm induration	General population

- If PPD test is positive, then **get chest X-ray.** If chest X-ray also shows active TB, then get 3 acid –fast bacilli (AFB) sputum stain

Treatment: as follow

- If **PPD test is positive**, but **chest x-ray is negative**, then treat the patient with Isoniazid (INH) plus Vitamin B 6 for 9 months
- If **PPD is positive** and **chest x-ray is positive, then** treat the patient as active TB (discussed below)

2. ACTIVE TB

Si/Sx: fever, night sweats, weight loss, hemoptysis

Diagnosis:

- **Best initial test** is chest X-ray
- Diagnosis is confirmed with **acid-fast sputum stains and culture**

Treatment: see table below on the next page

Active TB treatment

Treatment	Duration	Side effects
Rifampin	6 months	Turns **bodily fluids orange**
Isoniazid	6 months	Peripheral neuropathy *
Ethambutol	First 2 months	Optic neuritis
Pyrazinamide	First 2 months	Hyperuricemia

*Vitamin B6 is given with Isoniazid to prevent peripheral neuropathy

All TB medicines are hepatotoxic

Notes:

PULMONARY SURGERY

OPEN PNEUMOTHORAX
Open pneumothorax is characterized by a defect in the chest wall that draws the air during inspiration
Si/Sx: shortness of breath, **decreased breath on the affected side,** hypotension
Diagnosis:
- Clinical diagnosis
- Chest x-ray shows **trachea is in midline**

Treatment: Intubation, positive pressure ventilation and tape on three sides, as this will allow excessive pressure to escape
Complication: tension pneumothorax

TENSION PNEUMOTHORAX
Tension pneumothorax is a life-threatening condition in which large amount of air enter in the plural space, but cannot escape
Cause: penetrating or blunt trauma to chest
Si/Sx: shortness of breath, **decreased or absent sounds on the affected side,** hypertympanic breath sound, **JVD,** hypotension
Diagnosis:
- Clinical diagnosis
- Chest X-ray shows **trachea shifted to opposite side of the chest**

Treatment: needle thoracentesis in the 2nd intercostal space at the mid-clavicular line

HEMOTHORAX
Hemothorax is the collection of blood in the pleural cavity
Si/Sx: decreased breath sounds in the affected side, dullness on percussion, hypotension, **collapsed neck veins**
Diagnosis: clinical diagnosis
Treatment: IV fluids and chest tube

SLEEP APNEA

Sleep apnea is characterized by infrequent breathing during sleep

Types and causes:

- **Obstructive sleep apnea**, in this condition there is a partial or complete collapse of upper airway. This type of apnea is more in overweight people
- **Central sleep apnea**, there is no known cause of central sleep apnea, but it is often caused by poor ventilatory drive in conditions such as CNS disease, alcohol, hypnotic medicines

Diagnosis: Sleep study (polysomnography)

Treatment:

- **Obstructive sleep apnea:** best initial treatment is weight loss, continuous positive airway pressure (CPAP), if it ineffective, then surgical resection of palate, uvula and pharynx
- **Central sleep apnea:** avoid alcohol, hypnotic medicines before going to sleep. Other treatment options include oxygen, acetazolamide or medroxyprogesterone.

ENDOCRINOLOGY

DIABETES
Diabetes is a metabolic condition, which can be caused by too little insulin, insulin resistance or both

Type of diabetes: there are two types of diabetes: type 1 and type 2 diabetes (discussed in details below)

TYPE-1 DIABETES
Cause: autoimmune destruction of pancreatic β –cell, which leads to insulin deficiency

Si/Sx: Polyuria, polydipsia, polyphagia and weight loss

Diagnosis: Any one of the following can be used to diagnose type

- Fasting blood sugar > 125 mg/dl on two separate occasions
- One random blood sugar > 200 mg/dl, with polyuria, polydipsia, polyphagia
- Glucose > 200 mg/dl, after 2-hours postprandial test with 75 mg oral glucose tolerance test
- Hemoglobin A1c > 6.5%

Treatment: type 1 diabetes is treated with **insulin**

Insulin profile

Type of insulin	Onset	Peak effect	Duration
Rapid-Acting insulin (Aspart, lispro, & gluisine)	10- 30 minutes	0.5 – 3 hours	3-5 hours
Short- Acting insulin (Regular insulin)	30- 60 minutes	2-5 hours	5- 8 hours
Intermediate-Acting insulin (NPH insulin)	2-4 hours	6-7 hours	Up to 12 hours
Long-Acting insulin (Detemir, glargine)	1-2 hours	1-2 hour	Up to 24 hours

Note: Oral hypoglycemics such as metformin or sulfonylurea, do not work in type 1 diabetes because they work by stimulating insulin release from the pancreatic beta-cells, which are destroyed in type 1 diabetes

NPH insulin and regular insulin's dose adjustment

- **Regular insulin:** It is **usually given before a meal** to **prevent postprandial hyperglycemia** (2-4 hours after a meal). If a patient develops postprandial hypoglycemia, it means high dose of regular insulin was prescribed. It is managed by **lowering the dose of regular insulin before** a meal, and vice versa.
- **NPH insulin:** It is given **to control the blood sugar between meals, overnight, and while fasting.** If a patient develops hypoglycemia around 7AM or 5 PM, it means high dose of NPH insulin was prescribed. It is managed by **lowering the dose of NPH insulin** in the evenings or mornings, and vice versa.

Dawn phenomenon and Somogyi effect

- **Dawn phenomenon** is characterized by early morning (≅ 3AM) **euglycemia.** It is caused by normal secretion of growth hormone and **decreased insulin effectiveness.** Patient is hyperglycemic around 7AM. It is **managed by increasing NPH insulin dose at dinnertime.**
- **Somogyi effect** is characterized by early morning (≅ 3AM) **hypoglycemia.** It is caused by **high dose of NPH insulin at the dinnertime.** Body responds to this by releasing epinephrine, which causes hyperglycemia around 7AM. Somogyi effect is **managed by lowering the dose of NPH insulin at dinnertime.**

Bottom line is if a patient have hyperglycemia around 7AM, and then have the patient check his glucose level at 3AM

DIABETIC KETOACIDOSIS
Diabetic ketoacidosis is an **acute life-threating** complication of diabetes mellitus. It mostly occurs in type 1 diabetes
Cause: infection (UTI, influenza, gastroenteritis, pneumonia), missed treatment, stress, trauma, illegal drugs, alcohol
Si/Sx: Kussmaul hyperpnea, abdominal pain, dehydration, vomiting, fruity odor, increased anion gap metabolic acidosis, hyperkalemia. In severe condition patients may altered mental status
Treatment: Normal saline, insulin, potassium replacement (only if potassium is < 4), and treat the underlying cause.

Serum bicarbonate **is measured to** determine the **severity of diabetic ketoacidosis**

TYPE 2 DIABETES

Type 2 diabetes is **caused by insulin resistance**
Si/Sx: polyuria, polydipsia, polyphagia, weight loss, fatigue
Diagnosis: same as Type 1 diabetes
Treatment: is as follow

- Best initial treatment is **lifestyle modification** (diet, weight loss and exercise) and **metformin**, if it is ineffective, then add GLP-1 agonist or DDP-4 inhibitor, and if dual is ineffective, then add sulfonylurea or Thiazolidinedione's. If even triple therapy is ineffective, then add long-acting insulin.
- If a patient with Type-2 DM has kidney failure, then start the patient on insulin

ORAL HYPOGLYCEMICS PROFILE

Medicine	Mechanism	Side effects
Metformin	Blocks hepatic gluconeogenesis	Lactic acidosis, renal insufficiency
Sulfonylurea (Glipizide, glyburide, glimepiride)	Increases the insulin release from the pancreas	Hypoglycemia, SIADH, weight gain
Thiazolidinedione's (Rosiglitazone, Pioglitazone)	Improves peripheral insulin sensitivity	CHF exacerbation
Alpha-glucosidase inhibitor (Acarbose, miglitol)	Inhibits alpha-glucosidase enzyme in the small intestine	Bloating, abdominal cramps
GLP-1 agonist (Exenatide)	Increases insulin and decreases glucagon	Pancreatitis
DDP-4 inhibitors (Sitagliptin, saxagliptin)	Inhibits the enzyme that metabolizes GLP-1 agonists	Sitagliptin-pancreatitis, allergic reaction Saxagliptin-allergic reaction,

HYPEROSMOLAR DIABETIC COMA

Hyperosmolar diabetic coma is an acute complication of diabetes mellitus. It mostly occurs in **type 2 diabetes**

Cause: illness, stress, dehydration, infection, and non-compliance with medicine

Si/Sx: high blood sugar level >1,000 mg/dl **without acidosis**, excessive thirst, change in mental status, vision loss

Treatment: aggressive IV fluids and insulin

CHRONIC COMPLICATIONS OF DIABETES (TYPE 1 AND TYPE 2)

1. **Cardiovascular:** Patients with diabetes are at increased risk of MI. Patients should be instructed to be compliant with diabetic medication. In addition, blood pressure should be kept **< 130/80 mmHg**, and **LDL < 100** in a patient with DM alone or LDL **< 70** in a patient with **DM plus CAD**. Treat **high BP with ACE inhibitors, and high LDL with statins**. Patients **>30 years of age** should be started on **low-dose aspirin**.

2. **Eye exam:** Patients with **DM 2** should have an **annual eye exam** after they are diagnosed with DM2. However, patients with **DM1** should have their **first eye exam 5 years after they are diagnosed with DM1**, **then annually thereafter.** If proliferative retinopathy is seen during eye exam, then treat it with **photocoagulation**.

3. **Nephropathy:** Patients are at risk of developing diabetic nephropathy. Patients should be annually screened for microalbuminuria (normal urine albumin are 30- 300mg in 24 hours). If microalbuminuria is present, then start patient on **ACE inhibitors or ARBs to prevent further renal damage.**

4. **Gastroparesis:** this develops years after DM, in which stomach takes a long time to empty its content. Food may turn into a hard mass, which may cause early satiety, nausea, vomiting, abdominal pain and constipation. Treatment: **diet modification**- high protein, low fiber and low fats. If **diet modification is ineffective**, then metoclopramide **or erythromycin.**

5. **Neuropathy:** High blood sugar can injure nerve fibers throughout the body, but nerves in legs and feet are most commonly affected first. Late complications of neuropathy include impotence, orthostatic hypotension and mononeuropathy (mononeuropathy involves damage to specific nerve, it can lead to wrist drop, foot drop, isolated cranial nerve palsies – CN III or CN IV).
Treatment for neuropathy: All patients with DM should be instructed to do **regular self-feet exam**. Gabapentin is given to the patient, who has the burning sensation in hands or feet.

HYPOGLYCEMIA

Hypoglycemia is a medical emergency; it is characterized by low blood sugar
Cause: Insulinoma, exogenous insulin abuse, sulfonylurea, alcohol abuse
Si/Sx: dizziness, change in mental status, loss of consciousness, palpitations, shakiness, anxiety, sweating
Diagnosis:
- Fingerstick usually shows blood glucose < 70mg/dl
- Blood test to check the level of insulin, c-peptide, proinsulin (see table below)
- UA to check for urine sulfa (see table below)
- Abdomen CT, in cases Insulinoma is suspected

Differential diagnosis of hypoglycemia

	Insulinoma	Exogenous insulin abuse	Sulfonylurea medicine
Insulin	**High**	**High**	**High**
C-Peptide	**Increased**	Low or nml	**Increased**
Proinsulin	**Increased**	Low or nml	nml
Urine sulfa	Absent	Absent	**Present**

Treatment: raise the blood sugar. Fruit juice, glucose tablet or candy usually treats mild symptoms. Patients with severe symptoms may need injection of glucagon or IV glucose.

THYROID DISORDER

Thyroid gland secretes hormones that are essential to regulate the rate of metabolism, growth and development. Over production of the thyroid hormones leads to hyperthyroidism, and underproduction of thyroid hormones leads to hypothyroidism.

Si/Sx: Usually all forms of hypo/hyperthyroidism have similar symptoms. (Discussed below)

Hyperthyroidism	Hypothyroidism
Heat intolerance	Cold intolerance
Weight loss	Weight gain
Warm skin	Cold and pale skin
Nervousness	Weakness
Irritability	Lethargy, fatigue
Emotional liability	Memory impairment, dementia
Tachycardia, atrial fibrillation	Bradycardia

Cause and types: There are lots of conditions that can lead to over or underproduction of thyroid hormones. Level of thyroid hormones (T3, free T4 (fT4), TSH), and Radioiodine uptake scan (RAIU) help determine the cause or type hyperthyroidism. (Discussed below)

Hyperthyroidism differential diagnosis

Condition	T3	Free T4	TSH	RAIU
Grave's disease	High	High	Low	Increased **diffuse** uptake
Pituitary tumor	High	High	**High**	Increased **diffuse** uptake
Subacute thyroiditis	High	High	Low	**Decreased uptake**
Silent thyroiditis	High	High	Low	**Decreased uptake**
Exogenous thyroid hormone abuse	High	High	Low	**Decreased uptake**
Plummer's disease (Toxic multinodular goiter)	High	High	Low	**Increased uptake in hot nodules with cold background**

Other specific characteristic of causes of hyperthyroidism

1. **Subacute thyroiditis** is caused by **viral infection** such as influenza, mumps. Most obvious symptoms of subacute thyroiditis are **neck pain, and jaw pain**. Physical examination may show tender thyroid gland. Labs may show **increased ESR**.
2. **Exogenous thyroid hormone abuse** is commonly seen in health care workers or someone with access to exogenous thyroid hormones. Physical exam may show **atrophy of thyroid gland**.
3. **Graves's disease** is the most common cause of hyperthyroidism. Physical exam shows **ophthalmology, onycholysis**, and **dermopathy**. Labs show **antimicrosomal** and **antithyroglobulin** antibodies.
4. **Plummer's disease (Toxic multinodular goiter)** is common in elderly; it is caused by multiple foci of thyroid tissues that stop responding to T4 feedback inhibition.
5. **Pituitary adenoma** can cause hyperthyroidism by excessive production of TSH. It is the only hyperthyroidism in which TSH is increased. Diagnosis **confirmed by MRI** of head

Diagnosis: T3, T4, TSH and RAIU scan are mentioned on the previous page, and other labs are mentioned with specific characteristics

Treatment:
It is necessary to **control adrenergic symptoms** (tachycardia, palpitations, tremors, and anxiety) before initiating the treatment for a specific cause of hyperthyroidism. **Propranolol**, non-selective beta-blocker, is the best initial treatment to decrease these symptoms; it also blocks the peripheral conversion of T4 to T3.
Treatment for specific cause of hyperthyroidism is as follow:
- Pituitary adenoma: **Surgery**
- Subacute thyroiditis: **NSAIDs**
- Silent thyroiditis: **Propranolol**
- Graves's disease**: Propylthiouracil (PTU) or methimazole**, both of these decreases the peripheral conversion of T4 to T3. However, methimazole should not be given to pregnant women because it causes congenital aplasia cutis. Definitive treatment for Graves's disease is **subtotal thyroidectomy** or **radioactive iodine ablation**.

6. THYROID STORM

Thyroid storm is a life-threatening condition of hyperthyroidism, which is caused by sudden **release of large amount of thyroid hormones**

Cause: severe infection or illness, severe stress, recent treatment with radioiodine, over-dose of thyroid hormones

Si/Sx: fever, tachycardia, decreased mental status, nausea, vomiting, dehydration

Treatment is given in the following order; IV fluids, steroids, beta-blockers, PTU and iodine

HYPOTHYROIDISM

Hypothyroidism is caused by decreased production of thyroid hormones

Si/Sx: Discussed on 86

Causes: Hashimoto's disease, pituitary adenoma, post-ablative surgery or radioiodine, iodine deficiency, drugs such as lithium, amiodarone, interferons, sulfonamide

1. HASHIMOTO'S DISEASE

Hashimoto's disease is an autoimmune disease; it is the most common cause of hypothyroidism. Women are affected more than men, with female to male ratio (8:1).

Diagnosis:
- Labs show low T3, low T4 and high TSH
- Diagnose is confirmed by antithyroid peroxidase antibodies (TPO), and anti- microsomal antibodies.

Treatment: Levothyroxine

2. MYXEDEMA COMA

Myxedema coma is a life-threatening form of hypothyroidism

Cause: severe infection or illness, severe stress, untreated hypothyroidism, trauma

Si/Sx: altered mental status, respiratory depression, hypothermia,

Treatment: IV hydrocortisone and IV levothyroxine

THYROID NODULES

Majority of the thyroid nodules are discovered incidentally during physical exam.

Management of thyroid nodule is as follow:

Initial step is to **check TSH Level** and further management is as follow:

1. If TSH is **low,** then get a **radionuclide uptake scan (RAUI)**
   1a. If a radionuclide scan shows **hot nodule** (increased uptake), then treat the patient with **PTU**
   1b. If a radionuclide scan shows **cold nodule** (decreased uptake), then do **ultrasound-guided fine-needle aspiration (FNA)** (discussed below)

2. If TSH is **normal or high**, then management is as follow:
   2a. **Nodule ≤ 1cm** and patient has **no risk factors for thyroid cancer,** then do **regular follow-up.** However, if patient **has risk factors for thyroid cancer,** then do **FNA** (discussed below)
   2b. **Nodule > 1cm,** then do **FNA** (discussed below)

FNA results and treatment options:

- If FNA shows **malignancy,** then do **surgery or radioiodine ablation**
- If FNA shows **benign cytology,** then treat the patient with **levothyroxine** and follow-up. If tumor is regressing, then **continue the treatment.** However, it tumor is still the same, then **repeat the FNA or surgical excision**
- IF FNA shows **non-functioning or cold nodule,** then repeat **RAUI,** if scan shows increased uptake, then treat the patient with **PTU.** However, if scan shows decreased uptake, then **do surgery or radioiodine ablation**

THYROID CANCERS

1. PAPILLARY CARCINOMA

Papillary carcinoma is the **most common thyroid cancer.** It is a slow growing tumor, and **spreads via lymph node**

Cause: It is associated with radiation exposure to head and neck area

Diagnosis: Histopathology of biopsy shows **ground-glass orphan Annie nucleus & psammoma bodies**

Treatment: Surgery and patients should be placed on levothyroxine after surgery

2. FOLLICULAR CARCINOMA

Follicular carcinoma is the **second most common** thyroid cancer. It **metastasizes to lungs and bone via blood**
Treatment: same as papillary cancer

3. ANAPLASTIC CARCINOMA

Anaplastic carcinoma is a highly malignant carcinoma. It **spreads by direct extension.**
Anaplastic carcinoma has worst prognosis, almost all patients die within 5 year after developing

4. MEDULLARY CARCINOMA

Medullary carcinoma arises from parafollicular cells of the thyroid. It produces calcitonin.
It is a component of MEN type IIa, and MEN type IIb

MULTIPLE ENDOCRINE NEOPLASIA (MEN) SYNDROMES

Multiple endocrine neoplasia syndromes is group of disorders that affects the multiple endocrine glands
Types: discussed below

Types	Associated disorders
MEN Type 1 (Wermer's syndrome)	• Pituitary • Pancreases • Parathyroid tumor
MEN Type IIa (Sipple syndrome)	• Pheochromocytoma • Medullary thyroid cancer • Parathyroid hyperplasia
MEN Type IIb	• Pheochromocytoma • Medullary thyroid cancer • Neuroma

HYPERPARATHYROIDISM

Hyperparathyroidism is characterized by overactivity of the parathyroid gland, which leads to increased production of parathyroid hormone (PTH). PTH is the main hormone that regulates the calcium and phosphate level.

Types and causes: hyperthyroidism is of two types:

- **Primary hyperparathyroidism** is caused by dysfunction in the parathyroid **gland itself.** Most common cause is the **solitary adenoma** (80%), 2nd common cause is **four-gland hyperplasia** (19%), and the least common cause is **parathyroid cancer** (1%).
- **Secondary hyperparathyroidism** is caused by chronic kidney failure, severe vitamin D deficiency and severe calcium deficiency

Si/Sx: there are no specific symptoms of hyperparathyroidism. Most of the cases are asymptomatic, but some patient may have symptoms similar to symptoms hypercalcemia such as bone pain, kidney stone, constipation, and psychiatry problems

Diagnosis:

- In **primary hyperparathyroidism,** both PTH and **ionized serum calcium** levels are **elevated,** but **phosphate levels are very decreased** (<2.5 mg/dL).
- In **secondary hyperparathyroidism,** PTH is elevated and **ionized calcium level is low-to-normal.** Phosphate level may vary; phosphate level is **low in vitamin D deficiency,** but **high in renal failure.**

Treatment:

- Primary hyperparathyroidism - **Parathyroidectomy** is standard care. Calcimimetic or bisphosphonates are given when surgery is not possible.
- Secondary hyperparathyroidism - **Treat the underlying cause**

HYPOADRENALISM

Hypoadrenalism also referred as adrenal insufficiency, is a condition in which adrenal glands **do not produce sufficient steroid hormones** (mainly cortisol) and aldosterone. Aldosterone is the main hormone that regulates sodium, potassium and water retention.

Cause:

- Primary adrenal insufficiency is caused by destruction of all three layers of the adrenal gland, due to conditions such as Addison's disease (is the most common cause), Tuberculosis, fungal infection, AIDS, and metastatic cancer.
- Secondary adrenal insufficiency is caused by pituitary and hypothalamic failure.

Si/Sx: weakness, fatigue, anorexia, weight loss, nausea, vomiting, hypotension, and sparse body hair. Patients with primary adrenal insufficiency also have increased skin pigmentation, which is due to high POMC, a precursor of ACTH

Diagnosis:

- **Lab shows** Hyponatremia, hyperkalemia, metabolic acidosis, hypoglycemia, and ACTH; ACTH is **high in primary** adrenal insufficiency but **low in secondary** adrenal insufficiency.
- **Cosyntropin stimulation test:** Cortisol levels are measured before and after the administration of cosyntropin. **Cortisol will remain low in primary adrenal** insufficiency, but would be **increased** in **secondary** adrenal insufficiency

Treatment:

- **Primary adrenal insufficiency** is treated with glucocorticoids and mineralocorticoid
- **Secondary adrenal insufficiency** is treated with glucocorticoids alone

Acute adrenal crisis is seen in people who are **suddenly removed from long-term steroid therapy**. Patient present with altered mental status, profound hypotension and fever. It is managed by giving **100mg hydrocortisone**

HYERALDOSTERON

Hyperaldosteronism is characterized by **overproduction** of aldosterone

Cause:

- Primary hyperaldosteronism is caused by Conn syndrome (unilateral adrenal adenoma), adrenocortical carcinoma, and bilateral carcinoma
- Secondary hyperaldosteronism is caused by renal artery stenosis, adrenal tumor

Si/Sx: Muscle weakness, hypertension, polyuria, polydipsia

Diagnosis:
- Both primary and secondary hyperaldosteronism show low potassium and metabolic acidosis
- Aldosterone and plasma renin level help differentiate primary and secondary hyperaldosteronism. (See table below)

TYPE	Aldosterone	Plasma renin level
Primary hyperaldosteronism	High	Low
Secondary hyperaldosteronism	High	High

- CT scan of adrenals to check for adrenal tumor

Treatment:
- Unilateral adrenal tumors are removed surgically
- Bilateral hyperplasia or unresectable tumors are treated with oral potassium sparing medicines such as spironolactone or eplerenone

PHEOCHROMOCYTOMA

Pheochromocytoma is a neuroendocrine tumor of adrenal medulla; it secretes high levels of catecholamines, norepinephrine and epinephrine

Si/Sx: Episodic hypertension, palpitation, headaches, sweating, tremors, flushing, nausea, vomiting, diarrhea

Diagnosis:
- Best initial test is 24-hour urinary metanephrines (VMA and HVA).
- Diagnosis is confirmed with CT/MRI.
- 10 % of pheochromocytoma is extra-adrenal. If CT or MRI does not detect a tumor, **then do MIBG scan**. MIBG scan is a nuclear isotope scan, which detects the extra adrenal pheochromocytoma.

Treatment: Treat the patient in the following order:
- First control the hypertension with alpha-blocker such as phenoxybenzamine or phentolamine, then give beta-blockers (propranolol) or calcium channel blockers to control the hypertension and prevent reflex tachycardia
- Once the patient is stabilized, then pheochromocytoma is surgically removed

CUSHING'S SYNDROME

Cushing's syndrome is a condition in which high levels of cortisol is secreted.
Cause: pituitary tumor (also referred as Cushing disease), small cell cancer of lungs, and adrenal tumor/hyperplasia
Si/Sx: discussed in table below

Physical findings	Moon faces, buffalo hump, truncal obesity, osteoporosis, purple striae
Psychological	Depression, psychosis
Metabolic changes	Hyperglycemia, hyperlipidemia
Lab. Abnormalities	Low potassium, high aldosterone, metabolic alkalosis
Reproductive organs abnormalities	Menstrual abnormality in women Impotence in men

Diagnosis: diagnosis is as follow:

1. Best initial test is **24 hours urine cortisol or 1mg overnight** dexamethasone suppression test
   1a. Elevated **24-hour cortisol** level **confirms** the Cushing syndrome.
   1b. **1 mg overnight dexamethasone** is usually done, when 24-hours urine cortisol is not an option. **Normal person** should have suppressed **cortisol levels suppressed** after 1mg overnight dexamethasone test. Cortisol suppression excludes the Cushing syndrome.

Important: Dexamethasone is metabolized faster with drugs (phenytoin, rifampin) or physical stress (depression, anorexia, or depression). So it is necessary to check if patient's 1mg overnight dexamethasone test was **false negative** due to any of theses.

---

2. If 1 mg overnight dexamethasone suppression test does not suppress **cortisol levels, then 8 mg dexamethasone** is given and **cortisol levels are measured again,**

    2a. If cortisol levels are suppressed after the test– Dx. **Pituitary tumor** (Cushing's disease)

    2b. If cortisol levels are not suppressed after the test, then measure ACTH levels:

- If ACTH level is > 20 –Dx. **Small cell cancer**
- If ACTH level is < 8 –Dx. **Adrenal tumor or hyperplasia**

3. **Confirm** the diagnosis as following:

- Pituitary tumor is confirmed with **MRI of the head.** If MRI does not detect any tumor, **then do inferior petrosal venous sinus sampling**
- Small cell cancer of lungs is confirmed with **CT chest**
- Adrenal tumor or hyperplasia is confirmed with **CT abdomen**

Treatment:

- Pituitary tumor, small cell cancer of lungs and adrenal tumor or hyperplasia are **surgically resected**
- If tumor is unresectable, then give oral **ketoconazole or metyrapone**

PROLACTINOMA

Prolactinoma is characterized by **increased prolactin level**

Cause: Pituitary tumor, drugs (methyldopa, metoclopramide, Tricyclic antidepressants), pregnancy, lactation, hypothyroidism (high TRH levels stimulates prolactin secretion), seizures, nipple stimulation, and chronic renal failure

Si/Sx: Headaches, diplopia, CN III palsy, other gender specific symptoms are as follow:

Men	Impotence, gynecomastia, decreased libido
Women	Amenorrhea, galactorrhea, infertility

Diagnosis:
- Prolactin level (usually > 200 mg/ml in prolactinoma)
- **After measuring the prolactin level** and **before doing MRI or CT of the head,** rule out other causes such as pregnancy medicine, hypothyroidism
- MRI or CT head to confirm the pituitary tumor

Treatment: Treatment of prolactinoma **depends on the cause**
- If a prolactinoma is caused by pituitary tumor, then treat it with **dopamine agonist** (cabergoline or bromocriptine), but if dopamine agonist is ineffective, then do **transsphenoidal surgery.**
- Radiation is for a nonresectable pituitary tumor
- If a prolactinoma is caused by other causes such as dopamine antagonist, or hypothyroidism, in that case treat the underlying cause.

ACROMEGALY

Acromegaly is characterized by **excess secretion of growth hormone**
Cause: Acromegaly is almost always caused by **pituitary adenoma**
Si/Sx: are discussed below

Symptoms of acromegaly

Physical	Deep voice, coarse facial feature, thick skinfold, increase in shoes size, hat size, gloves size, ring size
Cardiovascular	CHF, Cardiomegaly, HTN
Metabolic	Glucose intolerance or diabetes
Reproductive organs	Amenorrhea in women, and impotence in men
Others	Carpel tunnel syndrome, colonic polyps

Diagnosis:

- Best initial diagnostic test is insulin-like growth factor-1 (IGF-1)
- Diagnosis is **confirmed with glucose intolerance test**: 100 mg glucose is given to a patient, normal person shows suppressed growth hormone, but a patient with acromegaly shows growth hormone levels > 5ng/ml
- MRI of head to locate the tumor

Treatment:

- Best initial treatment is **transsphenoidal surgery**
- Medicine is used in patients with refractory tumors. Medicines such as **dopamine agonists** (cabergoline) inhibit the growth hormone (GH) release, Somatostatin **analogues** (octreotide, lanreotide) inhibit the GH release, or **Pegvisomant** is a GH receptor antagonist.

SIADH

Inappropriate secretion of antidiuretic hormone **(SIADH)** is characterized by excess release of antidiuretic hormone. It causes euvolemic hyponatremia

Cause: SSRI, sulfonylureas, small cell cancer, **CNS** abnormality

Diagnosis:

- Urine osmolality > 20 mEq/L
- Plasma osmolality <100 mOsm/kg
- Low serum osmolality <290 mEq/L
- Urine Na> 20

Treatment:

- Water restriction
- Vasopressin receptors antagonist (Tolvaptan or conivaptan) are used in emergency situation, to raise the sodium in euvolemic hyponatremia
- Demeclocycline is used in chronic SIADH, it works by inhibiting the ADHs action on the collecting ducts of the kidneys
- Treat the underlying cause

DIABETES INSIPIDUS

Diabetes insipidus is characterized by excessive thirst and excretion of diluted urine

Types and cause: two types of diabetes insipidus are:

1. **Central diabetes** insipidus, it is caused by lack of ADH secretion from the pituitary gland. Risk factors include brain tumor, head injury, infection, ischemia and autoimmune disease
2. **Nephrogenic diabetes** insipidus is caused by kidney's resistance to circulating ADH. Risk factors include kidney disease, hypercalcemia, hypokalemia, and drugs such as lithium, amphotericin B, and demeclocycline

Si/Sx: polyuria, polydipsia, excessive thirst, lethargy, irritability, muscle pain

Diagnosis:

- Water deprivation test: patient excretes dilute urine after restricted water intake
- **Vasopressin test: patient urine osmolality is checked after the dose of ADH**. Patient with central **diabetes insipidus** shows increased urine osmolality after the test. Whereas, patient with **nephrogenic diabetes insipidus** shows no change in urine osmolality after the test.

Treatment:

- Treat the underlying cause
- Central diabetes insipidus is treated with vasopressin (IM, IV, or spray, other than oral)
- Nephrogenic diabetes is treated with salt restriction; increase water intake and correct hypercalcemia, hypokalemia. Diuretics (hydrochlorothiazide or amiloride) or NSAIDs may be used for refractory cases.

ELECTROLYTES

SODIUM
Normal range of sodium (Na+) is 135 - 145 mEq/L

HYPERNATREMIA
Hypernatremia refers to the condition in which body's sodium is >145mEq/L

Si/Sx: weakness, lethargy, and neurologic abnormalities such as seizure, irritability, confusion, or coma

Causes
- Central diabetes insipidus
- Nephrogenic diabetes insipidus
- Diuretic, DKA
- Infection

Diagnosis: sodium levels, urine osmolality

Treatment of hypernatremia: depends on patient's condition
- If the patient has **acute hypernatremia** or **low blood pressure, then** give **IV normal saline** to expand the volume and correct the blood pressure
- If the patient is **unstable** or has **neurologic abnormalities**, then give IV D5W or ½ normal saline, with maximum correction rate of 1 mEq/hour, otherwise, patient may develop cerebral edema
- If patient is stable and has normal blood pressure, **then give oral water and treat underlying cause**

HYPONATREMIA
Hyponatremia refers to the condition in which body's sodium is <135mEq/L

Si/Sx: confusion, convulsion, fatigue, irritability, coma, headache, vomiting

Cause:
- **Pseudohyponatremia:** Every 100mg/dl glucose above the normal limit, decrease sodium by 1.6 mEq/L
- **Hypervolemia:** CHF, cirrhosis, nephrotic syndrome
- **Hypovolemia:** diarrhea, vomiting, sweating, renal insufficiency, low aldosterone

- **Euvolemic**: hypothyroidism, psychogenic, polydipsia, SIADH, oxytocin

Treatment:
- If the patient is **stable**, then **restrict the water intake to 1 L/day**
- If the patient is **confused** or has **mild symptoms**, then give **normal saline and loop diuretics**
- If the patient has **severe symptoms** (seizure, coma), then give **3 % hypertonic saline, but** don't exceed >0.5mEq/hour or 12mEq in a day otherwise patient may develop central pontine myelinolysis
- A stable patient with pseudohyponatremia is treated by **correcting the glucose level**

POTASSIUM
Normal range of potassium (K+) is 3.5 - 5.5 mEq/L

HYPERKALEMIA
Hyperkalemia refers to the condition in which body potassium is >5.5 mEq/L

Si/Sx: weakness, muscle weakness and palpitation. High potassium may cause cardiac arrhythmias or sudden cardiac death

Causes of hyperkalemia include:
- Acidosis, aldosterone deficiency, ACE inhibitors, ARBS
- Beta-blockers
- Crush injury
- Digitalis, insulin deficiency
- Renal, RTA type IV

Diagnosis:
- Blood potassium level
- EKG usually shows **peaked T wave, absent P wave and prolong PR interval**

Treatment: depends of EKG
- If EKG shows arrhythmias **or cardiac abnormality, then** give **calcium gluconate** (it stabilizes the cardiac cell membrane) followed by **IV Insulin** (drives K+ into the cell) + **glucose** (given to prevent hypoglycemia), IV **sodium bicarbonate** (shifts K+ into the cell) and **kayexalate** (removes potassium from the body)

- If **EKG** is normal, then give **IV Insulin, glucose, sodium bicarbonate and kayexalate**
- If patient has a renal failure or medicines are ineffective, then do **dialysis**

Note: beta-blockers also drive potassium into the cell, and may be given when other choices are not available

Pseudohyperkalemia refers to a condition in which potassium is >5.5 mEq/L, but patient has no symptoms of hyperkalemia. It is commonly caused by hemolysis during venipuncture. No treatment is required; just repeat the blood potassium level.

HYPOKALEMIA (K+< 3.5)
Hypokalemia refers to the condition in which body potassium is < 3.5mEq/L
Si/Sx: muscle weakness, spasm, constipation, fatigue, palpitations
Causes of hypokalemia includes:
- Amphotericin, Hyperaldosterone
- Batters syndrome
- Diuretics, Distal RTA
- Proximal RTA

Diagnosis:
> Blood potassium level
> EKG usually show U wave

Treatment:
- If the patient is **unstable, has arrhythmia or ileus, then** give **IV K+**. However, don't exceed IV K >0 .5 mEq /hour and make sure patient is attached to the EKG, to monitor the EKG changes
- If the patient is **stable,** then give **oral potassium replacement**. There is no max or minimum limit for oral K replacement

Complication: Rhabdomyolysis

Note: Avoid giving dextrose-containing fluids to a patient with hypokalemia because dextrose drive K+ into the cell and may worsens the hypokalemia

CALCIUM
Normal calcium range is 8.5- 10.5 mEq/L

HYPERCALCEMIA
Hypercalcemia is the condition in which body's calcium is > 10.5 mEq/L
Cause:
- **Primary hyperparathyroidism** (most common cause)
- Familial **hypocalciuric** hypercalcemia
- Malignancy: **squamous cell carcinoma (PTH-like protein)**
- Granulomatous disease (Sarcoidosis)
- **TB, berylliosis, histoplasmosis**
- Thiazide, **vitamin D intoxication**

Si/Sx: symptoms includes:
- Neurologic: **decreased mental activity**
- GI: **constipation, anorexia**
- Renal: nephrogenic **diabetes** insipidus, **kidney stone**
- Cardiac: **decreased QT interval**

Diagnosis: check serum calcium, serum PTH, serum vitamin D level, and urine calcium
Treatment: depends on the followings:
- **If the patient is unstable, symptomatic or calcium >14 mg/dl,** then give **IV hydration,** followed by **furosemide.** If this is ineffective, or there is a need to lower the calcium fast, then give **calcitonin**
- **If the patient is stable patient or asymptomatic, then** give **oral bisphosphonates** (pamidronate)
- **If a stable** patient has a **granulomatous disease,** then give **steroids and fluids**

HYPOCALCEMIA
Hypocalcemia refers to the condition in which calcium is <8.5mEq/L
Cause
- Parathyroidectomy
- Hypomagnesemia
- Hyperphosphatemia
- Pseudohypoparathyroidism (kidney resistance to parathyroid - patients have short 4th figure, mental retardation)
- Renal failure
- Vitamin D deficiency

Symptoms: symptoms includes:
- Seizure, depression
- Cramping, Tetany (Chvostek sign, Trousseau sign)
- Cardiac: increased **QT interval**

Diagnosis: calcium level, calcium bound to albumin, EKG

Management:
- **Oral** calcium replacement
- If hypocalcemia is due to **vitamin D deficiency, then treat the patient with** vitamin D and **calcium** replacement
- If hypocalcemia is due to **hyperphosphatemia, then** treat the patient with **phosphate binder and calcium replacement**

Note: In renal failure, ca2+ is low and phosphate is high, whereas ca2+ and phosphate are both low in vitamin D deficiency

MAGNESIUM
Normal magnesium range is 1.5 -2.5 mEq/L

HYPOMAGNESEMIA
Hypomagnesemia is the condition in which body's magnesium is < 1.5 mEq/L

Symptoms: abnormal eye movement, fatigue, convulsion, muscle spasm, muscle weakness, numbness

Cause: causes includes:
- Alcohol withdrawal
- Drugs: loop diuretics, gentamicin, cisplatin

Treatment: magnesium replacement

Complications: hypocalcemia, torsades de pointes

HYPERMAGNESEMIA
Hypermagnesemia is the condition in which magnesium is >2.5 mEq/L

Symptoms: muscle weakness; loss of deep tendon reflexes (DTR), hypotension, hypocalcemia, arrhythmia, bradycardia

Cause:
- Magnesium containing laxative
- **MgSo4 (**seizure prophylaxis given during labor and delivery)
- **Real failure**
- DKA, adrenal insufficiency

Management:
- ABCs and intubated patient, if needed
- IV saline
- Last resort is dialysis

HEAT DISORDERS

1. HEAT CRAMPS
Heat cramps is a mild heat disorder that occurs due to loss of large amount of water and salt during exercise
Si/Sx: painful, involuntary muscle contraction, muscle tenderness. **Normal body temperature**, patient is able to **sweat and has no neurological** abnormalities
Treatment: rest, oral hydration and electrolyte replacement

2. HEAT EXHAUSTION
Heat exhaustion is a severe heat disorder
Si/Sx: muscle and abdominal cramps, weakness, fatigue and dizziness. Body temperature may be **slightly elevated**; patient is able to sweat and may have **mild neurological abnormalities** such as headaches, anxiety
Treatment: rest, oral hydration and electrolyte replacement. Patients with severe weakness may require IV fluids

3. HEAT STROKE
Heat stroke is a life-threatening condition
Si/Sx: body temperature is **elevated (>104 F); lost the ability to sweat, severe neurological abnormalities** such as confusion, disorientation, and blurry vision
Diagnosis: clinical diagnosis, but labs shows increased BUN/Cr, increased WBCs, hemoconcentration
Treatment: IV fluids, rapid cooling, place the patient in a cool environment, spray water and fanned to evaporate the fluids. Chlorpromazine or diazepam may be used to control shivering.

Note: Do not immerse the patient in ice water because that can result in overcooling and hypothermia

HYPOTHERMIA

Hypothermia is a medical emergency in which body's core temperature falls below the required temperature (95.0 F) for normal metabolism and body function

Cause: alcohol, water immersion

Si/Sx: mild hypothermia can cause shivering, HTN, tachycardia, and tachypnea. **Moderate hypothermia** causes violent shivering, muscle incoordination and mild confusion. **Severe hyperthermia** causes altered consciousness and arrhythmia, which can lead to death.

Diagnosis:

- Core body temperature
- EKG usually shows arrhythmia, most characteristic feature of hypothermia is an elevation of J point, also knows as Osborn J wave, which can be mistaken for ST elevation MI

Treatment: Rewarming measures such as a warm bed, warm bath or covering patient in a warm blanket. Warm IV fluids can be used in severe hypothermia. CPR should be continued during rewarming.

SHOCK

Shock is a life-threating condition in which there is an inadequate blood flow and perfusion.

Causes and symptoms

1. **Cardiogenic shock** is caused by heart problems such as MI, CHF. Patient usually presents with **JVD, pale and cold skin**
2. **Hypovolemic shock** is caused by fluid loss, in conditions such vomiting, diarrhea, use of diuretics. Patients usually present with **cold and pale skin**
3. **Septic shock** is caused by infections such as E.coli, S. aureus. Patients usually have **fever, and warm skin**
4. **Neurogenic shock** is caused by damage to the nervous system. Patients usually have **warm skin.**

Differential diagnosis of shock

Type of shock	HR	CO	PCWP	SVR
Septic shock	Increased	**Increased**	Decreased	Decreased
Cardiogenic shock	Increased	Decreased	**Increased**	**Increased**
Hypovolemia shock	Increased	Decreased	Decreased	**Increased**
Neurogenic shock	Increased	Decreased	Decreased	Decreased

HR = heart rate, CO= cardiac output, PCWP= pulmonary capillary wedge pressure, SVR= Systemic vascular resistance

Treatment: maintaining ABCs (airway, breathing and circulation) is the primary goal. Give bolus of fluids and reassess the patient. If fluids do not increase the blood pressure, then vasopressor may be required. Mechanism of vasopressors is as follow:

- Norepinephrine increases the peripheral vascular resistance and maintains the organ perfusion
- Dopamine at low dose keep the kidneys perfused, at high dose it increases the heart contractility, and at the highest dose it causes vasoconstriction
- Dobutamine increases the heart contractility

ANAPHYLAXIS
Anaphylaxis is a life-threatening allergic reaction that occur within seconds or minutes after exposure of allergen, such as bee stings, medicines or peanuts
Si/Sx: **wheezing, difficulty breathing, hypotension, weak rapid pulses**
Treatment: Immediately secure the airway, subcutaneous epinephrine, corticosteroids and H1 antihistamine

ACID-BASE DISORDERS

How is acid based disorder recognized?
A pH value helps determine, if the patient has an alkalosis or acidosis. To determine if the patient has a metabolic or respiratory acid-base disorder, look at CO2 and bicarbonates values

CO2
Normal CO2 value is 40 mmHg
- **High CO2** means either the person has **respiratory acidosis** (pH<7.4) or compensating for **metabolic alkalosis** (pH>7.4)
- **Low CO2** means either the person has **respiratory alkalosis** (pH>7.4) or compensating for **metabolic acidosis** (pH<7.4)

Expected CO2 level increase in compensation can be calculated by this formula = 1.5(HCO3-) +8

Bicarbonate
Normal bicarbonate value is 24 mEq/L
- **High bicarbonate** means either the person has **metabolic acidosis** (pH<7.4) or compensating for **respiratory alkalosis** (pH>7.4)
- **Low bicarbonate** means either the person has **metabolic alkalosis** (pH>7.4) or compensating for **respiratory acidosis** (pH<7.4)

Practice examples:
1) pH 7.36, PCO2 46, PO2 81, HCO3 29= _____
2) pH 7.10, PCO2 41, PO2 81, HCO3 8=_____
3) pH 7.35, PCO2 62, PO2 71, HOC3 29=_____

Answers:
1) Metabolic alkalosis with respiratory acidosis
2) Metabolic acidosis with no respiratory compensation
3) Respiratory acidosis with metabolic alkalosis

MIXED ACID-BASE DISORDERS

In a primary acid-base disorder with compensation, **CO2 and bicarbonate** values go in the **same direction**. Means, high CO2 causes respiratory acidosis, and to compensate that, the kidneys start to retain more negatively charged bicarbonate. However, in a **mixed disorder,** CO2 and **bicarbonat**e values go in the **opposite directions** and causes mixed disorders (respiratory and metabolic acidosis or alkalosis). Mean, when high CO2 causes respiratory acidosis, then the kidneys start to loss negatively charged bicarbonate.

NEPHROLOGY

ACUTE RENAL FAILURE

Acute Renal failure is characterized by sudden decline in kidney's function, which leads to abnormal clearance of waste products, fluids and electrolytes.

Cause: three main causes of acute renal failure are:

- Prerenal failure
- Intrarenal failure
- Postrenal failure

Differential diagnosis of acute renal failure

Test	Prerenal failure	Intrarenal failure	Postrenal failure
BUN/Cr ratio	> 20	< 15	> 15
Urine Na	< 20	> 20	> 40
Urine fractional Na excretion	< 1%	> 2%	> 4%
Urine osmolality	> 500	< 350	< 350
Urine analysis	Hyaline cast	Muddy brown cast, RBC cast, or eosinophils	White cell casts

PRERENAL FAILURE

Prerenal failure is an abrupt loss of renal function that is caused by decreased blood flow to the kidneys

Cause: causes of prerenal failure are:

- Dehydration is the most common cause
- Heart failure
- Liver failure (Cirrhosis)
- Toxic shock
- Renal artery stenosis
- Hepatorenal syndrome
- Drugs: ACE inhibitor, Diuretics
- Burns
- Pancreatitis

Diagnosis: labs, as discussed on the previous page
>   Treatment:

- Fluid and electrolytes replacement, diuretic to prevent volume overload
- Treat the underlying cause
- Dialysis, if needed

POSTRENAL FALIURE

Postrenal failure occurs when an obstruction in the urinary tract below the kidneys interrupts the urine flow and wastes build up in the kidneys.

Cause: causes of postrenal failure are:

- Obstruction of ureters by stones, stricture, or blood clots
- Benign prostatic hyperplasia
- Cervical cancer
- Retroperitoneal fibrosis
- Neurogenic bladder (multiple sclerosis, spinal cord injury)

Diagnosis: labs, as discussed on the previous page

Treatment:

- **Best initial step is to relieve the obstruction with a foley catheter**
- Fluids and electrolytes replacement
- Treat the underlying cause
- Dialysis, if needed

INTRARENAL FAILURE

Intrarenal failure is caused by direct damage to the kidneys due to accumulation of the toxic metabolites

Cause: causes of intrarenal failure are

- Acute tubular necrosis (the most common cause)
- Allergic interstitial nephritis
- Atheroemboli disease
- Glomerulonephritis

Diagnosis: labs, as discussed on the previous page

- Urinary **muddy brown casts** suggests **acute tubular necrosis**
- Urinary **RBC casts** suggests **glomerulonephritis**
- Urinary **eosinophils** suggests **acute allergic interstitial nephritis or atheroembolic disease**

Treatment:
- If the patient has allergic interstitial nephritis, then discontinue the offending medicine
- Fluid and electrolyte abnormalities
- Treat the underlying cause
- Dialysis, if needed

Indications for urgent dialysis are: Mnemonic: **AEIOU**
- **A**cid-base disorder
- **E**lectrolyte abnormality
- **I**ntoxication
- **V**olume overload
- **U**remia (uremic encephalopathy, uremic pericarditis)

ACUTE TUBULAR NECROSIS (ATN)

ATN is a condition in which renal tubular epithelial cells are damaged or destroyed. ATN is the most common cause of intrarenal failure

Cause: there is no exact known to cause ATN, but risk factors may include trauma, rhabdomyolysis, sepsis, hemorrhage, radiocontrast dye, and drugs such as aminoglycosides, amphotericin

Diagnosis
- Labs: Same as intrarenal failure labs (see page 109)
- Urinalysis shows **muddy brown casts**

Treatment: IV fluids, monitor electrolyte, treat the underlying cause

How can ATN be prevented?

There is no known exact cause of ATN, but there are lots of risk factors. Only way to prevent ATN is to control the risk factors or carefully monitor the kidney functions after starting medicines known to cause ATN. However, two frequently asked preventable causes on USMLE are:

1. Radiocontrast dye induced ATN is prevented by:
   - Hydrate the patient with normal saline, 1mL/Kg/hour, before the procedure
   - If a patient is taking metformin, advise the patient to stop taking it at least 48 hours prior to the contract procedure and give IV hydration before the procedure

2. Tumor lysis syndrome induced ATN is prevented by:
    *   IV hydration plus allopurinol before initiating
        chemotherapy

ACUTE INTERSTITIAL NEPHRITIS (AIN)

Acute interstitial nephropathy is characterized by inflammatory infiltrate
and edema in the renal interstitium.

Cause: infections, or reaction to the medicine, but reaction to medicine
accounts for 71-92% cases. Medicines that cause this reaction are:

*   Penicillin
*   Sulfonamide
*   Diuretics
*   NSAIDs
*   Phenytoin
*   Rifampin
*   Allopurinol
*   H2 blockers

Si/Sx: Fever, **maculopapular rash**, flank pain, swelling of the body, change
in mental status

Diagnosis:

*   Labs: same as intrarenal failure (see page 109)
*   Urinalysis shows pyuria (WBCs without bacteria), hematuria
*   Urinalysis with **Hansel or Wright stain** shows eosinophiluria

Treatment: In most of the AIN spontaneously resolve after removing the
offending drug or treating the underlying infection. However, if the
patient continues to have renal failure, then give steroids.

Main differences in nephrotic and nephritic syndrome

	Nephrotic syndrome	Nephritic syndrome
Si/Sx	Hematuria, hypertension, oliguria, azotemia	Protein urea, hypoalbuminemia, hyperlipidemia, generalized edema
UA	Fatty casts in urine	RBC and granular casts in urine

NEPHRITIS SYNDROME

Nephritis syndrome is a group of conditions, which causes inflammation of the internal structures of the kidney.

1. **POSTSTREPTOCOCCAL (POSTINFECTIOUS) GLOMERULONEPHRITIS (PSGN/PIGN)**

   PSGN/PIGN is a nephritis syndrome that can occur after any infection, but commonly occurs after infection with **streptococcus bacteria: 1-2 weeks after pharyngitis or 3-6 weeks after impetigo**.

   Si/Sx: Periorbital edema, **smoky-brown urine**, oliguria, hypertension

   Diagnosis:
   - Urinalysis shows RBCs casts, azotemia
   - Blood test shows low serum C3 complement level, anti-DNase antibodies, and increased antistreptolysin O (ASO)
   - **Most accurate** is **renal biopsy**, which shows lumpy-bumpy granular deposits of IgG and C3 in the basement membrane

   Note: Biopsy is rarely required to diagnose PSGN; blood tests are sufficient to make diagnosis

   Treatment: there is no specific treatment for PSGN/PIGN. Treatment is directed towards symptoms, which as follow:
   - Antibiotics such as penicillin, is given for streptococcal bacteria
   - Anti-hypertensive medicines such as calcium channel blockers or ACE inhibitors, may be needed for hypertension
   - Diuretics to prevent fluid overload

2. GOODPASTURE SYNDROME

Goodpasture syndrome is an **autoimmune disorder** that affects the **kidneys and lungs**

Si/Sx: hematuria, hemoptysis, shortness of breath

Diagnosis

- CBC shows iron deficiency anemia
- Best initial test is blood test, which shows anti-basement membrane antibodies
- **Most accurate test is a biopsy of lungs or kidney.** Biopsy of lungs shows hemosiderin-laden macrophage, and biopsy of kidney shows smooth linear deposits of IgG

Treatment: Plasmapheresis

3. IgA NEPHROPATHY

IgA nephropathy is also known, as Berger disease is the most common cause of glomerulonephritis in the world.

Si/Sx: Episodic hematuria that occurs after infection such as upper respiratory infection, urinary tract infection

Diagnosis:

- Blood test shows normal C3
- **Best initial test is urine immunoelectrophoresis** to measure IgA, but IgA levels are increased only in half of the patients
- **Most accurate test** is a kidney biopsy, which shows proliferation of the mesangium with IgA deposit on immunofluorescence or electron microscope.

Treatment: There is no specific treatment to cure IgA nephropathy. Approximately 50% of the patient will progress to end-stage renal failure. Treatment is given to slow the progression to chronic renal failure, which is as follow:

- Angiotensin-converting enzyme (ACE) inhibitors are given to patients with severe proteinuria
- Steroids are given to patient with acute flares, these works by suppressing the immune system

4.   WEGNER'S GRANULOMATOSIS

Wegner's granulomatosis is a systemic vasculitis (causes inflammation of the blood vessels) of small and medium sized vessels in many organs. It mainly affects the kidney, upper and lower respiratory tract, but it can also affect other organs such as skin, eyes, GI, joints and CNS.

Cause: unknown etiology

Si/Sx: fever, cough, **sinusitis, hemoptysis, hematuria**, joint ache

Diagnosis:

- Chest X-ray shows cavities in lung
- Best initial test is blood test to detect anti-neutrophil cytoplasmic autoantibodies (ANCA)
- Most accurate test is a **biopsy of the affected organ** such as kidney, lungs or skin. Biopsy of the kidney shows segmental necrotizing glomerulonephritis.

Treatment: prednisone plus immunosuppressive (azathioprine, methotrexate, or cyclophosphamide)

5.   POLYARTERITIS NODOSA

Polyarteritis nodosa is a systemic vasculitis (causes inflammation of the blood vessels) of small-and medium sized vessels in many organs. It mainly affects the kidney; it can also affect any other organ such as skin, eyes, GI, joints and CNS, but it spares lungs

Cause: unknown etiology, but it can be associated with hepatitis B or C

Si/Sx: Fever, hematuria, abdominal pain, abdominal pain, decreased appetite

Note: Unlike Wegner's granulomatosis, patient with polyarteritis nodosa don't have hemoptysis or sinusitis

Diagnosis:

- Blood test shows increased WBCs, ESR, and C-reactive   protein
- Angiography shows aneurysm or narrowing of affected blood vessels
- Most accurate test is biopsy of the **kidney or sural nerve**
- All patient should also be **tested for Hepatitis B and C**

Treatment: prednisone plus immunosuppressive (Azathioprine, methotrexate, or cyclophosphamide)

6. ALPORT SYNDROME

Alport syndrome is a genetic defect of type IV collagen; it causes glomerulonephritis, hearing and visual disturbance

Si/Sx: hematuria, hearing loss, decreased vision or vision loss

Diagnosis: renal biopsy: electron microscope shows glomerular **basement membrane splitting**

Treatment: There no specific treatment for Alport syndrome, treatment is directed towards symptoms

NEPHROTIC SYNDROME

1. MINIMAL CHANGE DISEASE

Minimal change disease is the most common cause of nephrotic syndrome in children

Cause: unknown etiology, but risk factors include NSAIDs, tumors, vaccinations, and viral infections

Diagnosis: kidney biopsy: electron microscope shows **fusion of foot process**

Treatment: Prednisone

2. FOCAL SEGMENTAL GLOMERULOSCLEROSIS

Focal segmental glomerulosclerosis is kidney disease in which some parts ("segmental") of the glomerulus are sclerosed

Cause: idiopathic, heroin, HIV, diabetes, sickle cell disease, diabetes

Diagnosis: kidney biopsy shows **sclerosis in capillary tufts**

Treatment: Prednisone and cyclophosphamide

Prognosis: More than half of the patients advances to end stage renal disease

3. MEMBRANOUS GLOMERULONEPHRITIS

Membranous glomerulonephritis is the most common cause of nephrotic syndrome in adults. It is characterized by basement membrane thickening

Cause: causes include:
- Cancers, specially lung and colon cancer
- Infection: HBV, HCV, syphilis, malaria
- Medicines: gold salts, penicillamine
- Autoimmune disease: SLE, rheumatoid arthritis, Graves' disease

Diagnosis: diagnosis is confirmed with kidney biopsy; electron microscopy shows **"spike and dome"** appearance, which is due to IgG and C3 immune, complex in a basement membrane
Treatment: Prednisone and cyclophosphamide
Prognosis: 50% of the patients progress to end-stage kidney failure

4. MEMBRANOPROLIFERATIVE GLOMERULONEPHRITIS (MPGN)

MPGN is characterized by deposits in the glomerular mesangium and glomerular basement membrane thickening. It can present with **nephritis or nephrotic features**
Cause: HBV, HCV, CLL, SLE
Type: two types of MPGN are:

- Type 1 MPGN is characterized by subendothelial and mesangial immune deposits
- Type 2. MPGN is less common than type 1. It is associated with autoantibodies against C3 nephritic factor (C3 convertase)

Diagnosis: diagnosis is confirmed with **kidney biopsy**

- Type 1 MPGN shows **immune complex deposits** and abnormal mesangial cell proliferation between glomeruli basement membrane and endothelial cells, which gives " **tram-track** " appearance of the capillary wall
- Type 2 MPGN shows **dense deposits** along glomeruli basement membrane

Treatment: There is no cure for MPGN. Treatment is given to control the symptoms and slow the disease progression, which is as follow:

- Steroids plus cyclophosphamide
- Anti-hypertensive medicine and diuretic

Screening: Screen all patients for HBV and HCV infection
Prognosis: MPGN has a poor prognosis. It often slowly progresses to chronic kidney failure

5. DIABETIC NEPHROPATHY

Diabetic nephropathy also known as Kimmelstiel-Wilson syndrome is the most common cause of ERSD in United States. It is generally caused by long-standing **poorly controlled diabetes**

Diagnosis:
- UA shows microalbuminuria
- Kidney biopsy with light microscopy shows mesangial expansion but sometimes is may show nodules, mesangial hypercellularity, and glomerular basement membrane thickening.

Treatment: Strict glucose control, ACE inhibitor to slow the renal progression to ESRD

6. RENAL AMYLOIDOSIS

Amyloidosis is a group of conditions in which abnormal proteins are deposited in the extracellular space of organs. Renal amyloidosis is result of **amyloidosis deposits in the renal**.

Association: it is associated with immune cell disorder such as multiple myeloma, inflammatory diseases

Diagnosis: biopsy of affected organ or fat pad; stain biopsied tissue with Congo red; stain shows **apple -green birefringence**

Treatment: Prednisone and Melphalan. Renal transplant is reserved for refractory disease

7. LUPUS NEPHRITIS

Systemic lupus erythematosus (SLE) is an autoimmune disease that can affect any organ. Lupus nephritis is a **complication of SLE**

Diagnosis:
- Blood test detects the presence of **antinuclear antibody and anti-double stranded DNA**
- Most accurate test is renal Biopsy. World health organization has classified lupus nephritis in 5 types based on the biopsy findings. (Discussed on the next page)

Treatment: treatment depends on type of lupus nephritis, discussed on the next page

Lupus nephritis stages and treatment

Type	Biopsy finding	Treatment
Type I	Normal appearing kidney	None
Type II	Mesangial proliferation	Symptomatic treatment only
Type III	Focal segmental proliferation	Prednisone and mycophenolate
Type IV	Diffuse proliferative • May present with combination of nephrotic and nephritic disease • Light microscope shows wire-loop abnormality	Prednisone and mycophenolate
Type V	Membranous disease	There is no clear beneficial treatment. Prednisone may help

END-STAGE RENAL DISEASE (ESRD)

End-stage renal failure defined as a complete kidney failure; that they no longer able to work at the level required to for day-to-day life. People often need dialysis or kidney transplant

Cause: Two most common causes are diabetes and high blood pressure; other causes may include glomerulonephritis, polycystic kidney disease, pyelonephritis, renal artery stenosis, long-term NSAIDs use

Si/Sx: Headaches, anorexia, fatigue, convulsion, pericarditis, bruising

Treatment for ESRD: salt and water restriction, protein restriction, dialysis to correct the acid-base or electrolytes abnormalities, and treat the other complications

Complications: discussed on next page

Indications for urgent dialysis are:	Mnemonic: **AEIOU**
• Acid-base disorder • Electrolyte abnormality • Intoxication • Volume overload • Uremia (uremic encephalopathy, uremic pericarditis)	

Complication of ESRD

Complication	Cause/ characteristic	Treatment
Anemia	Normochromic normocytic anemia, due to **decreased** production of **erythropoietin**	Erythropoietin
Coagulopathy	Platelet count is normal, but bleeding is prolonged because of **defect in platelet degranulation**	DDAVP
Osteomalacia	Decreased conversion of **25hydroxycholecalciferaol** to **1,25-dihydroxy** leads to hypokalemia and hyperphosphatemia	Vitamin D replacement and calcium carbonate
Hyperphosphatemia/ hypocalcemia	Due to decreased active vitamin D and renal failure	Oral phosphate binder such as calcium carbonate or calcium acetate
Hypermagnesemia	Due to decreased clearance from the kidney	Restrict food high in magnesium, laxatives
High circulating insulin	Insulin is high because insulin **clearance is decreased**	Decrease the dose of oral hypoglycemics in diabetics
Decreased libido and impotence in men	Decreased testosterone	Testosterone replacement

NEPHROLITHIASIS

Nephrolithiasis also known as Kidney stones or renal calculi is a solid mass that is made up of tiny crystals.

Types: Calcium oxalate stones are the most common kidney stones, but other less stones include calcium phosphate, struvite, uric acid and cystine stones

Si/Sx: sudden colicky flank pain that may radiate to ipsilateral tests or labia, nausea, vomiting

Diagnosis:

- UA shows gross or microscopic hematuria. However, absence of microhematuria does not exclude kidney stone because 10-15% of the patients do not have hematuria
- Urinary pH (normal urine pH is 5.85)
- Abdominal x-ray to look for stone (renal **ultrasound for pregnant women**)
- Renal ultrasound to check for any obstruction

Differential diagnosis of kidney stones

Type	Association	Treatment
Calcium oxalate or calcium phosphate stones	• Calcium oxalate is the **common cause of kidney stones** (80- 85%) • Most common cause is idiopathic hypercalciuria. Other causes include increased absorption, decreased clearance • Abdominal X-ray shows **radiopaque stones**	Hydration, thiazide diuretics
Struvite stones	• 2nd most common cause of kidney stones (9%) • **Large staghorn or struvite calculus** • Associated with **urease-producing organisms** such as Proteus, pseudomonas, Klebsiella, or staphylococcus • Urine pH > 7.2 • Abdominal X-ray shows **radiopaque stones**	Hydration, treat the underlying infection
Uric acid stones	• 3rd most common causes of kidney stones (7%) • Associated with gout, hyperuricemia, myeloproliferative disease, • Urine pH is < 5.5 (acidic) • Abdominal X-ray shows **radiolucent stone**	Hydration, alkalinization of urine, treat the underlying cause
Cystine stones	• Least common type of kidney stones (1%) • Associated with abnormal renal excretion of cystine, ornithine, lysine and arginine • **Hexagonal** shaped kidney stones • Abdominal X-ray shows **radiopaque stone**	Hydration, alkalinization of urine

Treatment: hydration, pain relievers, and a particular treatment depend
on the stones (as mentioned in the table on the previous page). However,
bigger stones such as 5-10mm are removed with extra-corporeal shock
wave lithotripsy, and stones >10mm are removed with laser lithotripsy or
basket extraction.

RENAL ARTERY STENOSIS
Renal artery stenosis is narrowing of an artery that carries blood to the
kidney
Cause: fibromuscular dysplasia is the most common in young patients
(<30 years), and atherosclerosis is the most common cause in old patient
(>50 years)
Si/Sx: refractory hypertension, deterioration of kidney function when
treatment with ACE inhibitors is initiated
Physical exam may show audible abdominal bruit on the affected side
Diagnosis:
- Labs: same as pre-renal failure plus low potassium
- Best initial test is Doppler ultrasound or Magnetic resonance
  angiogram (MRA)
- Most accurate test is angiography
Treatment: Angioplasty

POLYCYSTIC KIDNEY DISEASE (PKD)
Polycystic kidney disease is an inherited disease. It is characterized by
presence of fluid-filled cysts in the kidney.
Type: two types of PKD are:
- Autosomal dominant PKD (ADPKD): This is the most common
  type PKD. Symptoms usually develop after 30 years of age.
- Autosomal recessive PKD (ARPKD): This is less common, but
  severe form of PKD. Most of the patients are infants or young
  children.
Associations: PKD is associated with the following conditions:
- Aortic aneurysm
- Cysts in liver, pancreas, spleen (Liver cysts are most common
  cysts site outside the kidney)
- Diverticula
- Mitral valve prolapse

Si/Sx: Pain, hematuria, kidney stones, UTI, hypertension
Diagnosis: Abdominal CT or ultrasound
Treatment: there is no specific treatment for PKD. Treatment is directed towards symptoms such as, treat HTN, UTI and kidney stones.
Prognosis: it slowly progresses to ESRD, and renal failure is the most common cause of death

BENIGN PROSTATE HYPERTROPHY (BPH)
Benign prostate hypertrophy is a hyperplasia of prostate cells. It is a normal condition in males over 50 years of age.
Si/Sx: weak urine stream, incomplete emptying of bladder, dribbling at the end of urinating,
Diagnosis:
- Urinalysis and urine culture, to rule out infection
- Creatinine level, to check kidney function
- Digital rectal exam
- Prostate–specific antigen (PSA) level to screen for prostate cancer

Treatment:
- **Mild symptoms** are treated with **reassurance and lifestyle modifications** such as avoiding fluids within 2 hours of bedtime, pelvic muscle strengthening exercises, avoid decongestants or antihistamines because these drugs increase the BPH symptoms.
- **Mild to moderate symptoms** are treated with **alpha 1-blockers** (terazosin, prazosin) or **5-alpha reductase** (Finasteride)
- **Moderate to severe symptoms** can be treated with **surgical procedures** such as Transurethral resection of the prostate (TURP), or simple prostatectomy

ERECTILE DYSFUNCTION
Erectile dysfunction is a sexual dysfunction that is characterized by an inability to keep or maintain erection that is firm enough to have intercourse.
Cause: Psychological, marital problems, medications (beta-blockers, digoxin, antidepressant), disease (diabetes, HTN, thyroid disorder, multiple sclerosis, Parkinson's disease), nerve damage, low testosterone

Diagnosis:
- Clinical diagnosis
- Check testosterone and gonadotropin levels
- Rule out endocrine abnormalities such as prolactin level

Treatment:
- **Best initial management** is to **rule out psychological or marital problems**
- Treat the underlying condition, if applicable
- Phosphodiesterase -5 (PDE5) inhibitors such as Sildenafil (Viagra), Vardenafil (Levitra) or tadalafil (Cialis) – these medications increase the blood flow to corpora cavernous.
- If PDE5 inhibitors are ineffective, then any of the following may be used; Penis pumps, penile implants or intercavernous Injection
- Testosterone replacement may be used in patients with low testosterone levels

ANION GAP

Anion gap is the difference in the measure cations and anion in serum, plasma or urine. It is measured to **determine the cause of metabolic acidosis.**

It is calculated with the equation = $[Na^+] - ([Cl^-] + [HCO_3^-])$

It is classified as either normal anion gap (4-12 mEq/L), high (> 12 mEq/L), or in are cases, low.

- Normal anion gap metabolic acidosis is seen in conditions such RTA or diarrhea.
- High Anion gap metabolic acidosis in conditions such as uremia, ethanol toxicity (discussed on the next page)

1. RENAL TUBULAR ACIDOSIS (RTA)

Renal tubular acidosis is a medical condition, which is caused by kidney's insufficiency to reabsorb bicarbonate or excrete H+ that results in non-anion metabolic acidosis

Type: Three main types of RTA are type I, II and IV.

Differential diagnosis of RTA

Type	Type I (Distal)	Type II (Proximal)	Type IV
Defect	Distal tubule defect	Proximal tubule defect	Decreased aldosterone or decreased aldosterone effect on the kidney
Cause	• Autoimmune disease • Sickle cell anemia • Amphotericin • Analgesics • Lithium	• Multiple myeloma • Amyloidosis • Fanconi syndrome • Carbonic anhydrase inhibitors	• Diabetes • Hypertension • HIV • Hyporeninemic hypoaldosteronism
Blood K+	Low	Low	High
Urine pH	> 5.4	> 5.4 in early; <5.5 as acidosis worsens	< 5.4
Test	Ammonium chloride	Sodium bicarbonate	Urine sodium (which will be high)
Treatment	Oral bicarbonate plus oral potassium citrate	Bicarbonate plus thiazide	Oral fludrocortisone
Complications	Kidney stones	Rickets, Osteomalacia	Hyperkalemia

2. HIGH ANION GAP METABOLIC ACIDOSIS

High anion gap metabolic acidosis (> 12 mEq/L) occurs due to increased production of anions such as lactate or acetate, and secondary loss of bicarbonate. Classic mnemonic to remember the causes is **MUD PILES**

High anion gap causes and treatment

Condition	Treatment
Methanol glycol poisoning	Fomepizole, dialysis
Uremia	Dialysis
Diabetic ketoacidosis (DKA)	IV fluids and insulin
Pyrazinamide	Stop the drug
Isoniazid	Stop the drug
Ethanol glycol poisoning	Fomepizole, dialysis
Salicylic acid	Alkalinization of urine, dialysis

Notes:

INFECTIOUS DISEASES

URINARY TRACT INFECTION (UTI)

Urinary tract infection is the infection of urinary tract (kidney, ureters, bladder or urethra). Infection of the bladder is called **cystitis,** infection of the kidney is called **pyelonephritis,** and infection of urethra is called **urethritis.**

Cause: E. coli is the most common cause of UTI, but other causes may include Enterobacter, Serratia, Klebsiella pneumonia, S. saprophytes, Pseudomonas, and proteus mirabilis.

Risk factor: female gender (women tend to get more UTIs than men because they have shorter urethra), diabetes, having a urinary catheter, surgery or instrumentation of urinary tract, kidney stones, enlarged prostate, pregnancy

Si/Sx, diagnosis, and treatment: discussed under cystitis, pyelonephritis and urethritis.

CYSTITIS

Cystitis is inflammation of the bladder

Cause: discussed in UTI section

Si/Sx: urgency, frequency, burning, suprapubic tenderness, hematuria

Diagnosis:

- **Urine analysis** shows increased urinary nitrites, increased leukocyte esterase, pyuria, bacteriuria
- **Urine culture:** positive for offending bacteria with colony count exceeding 10 x 5/ml

Treatment:

- Women with uncomplicated UTI are treated with TMP/SMX for 1-3 days
- Complicated UTIs are treated with TMP/SMX for 7 days. Complicated UTIs means; male with UTIs, diabetics, urinary obstruction, renal transplant, immunosuppressed, pregnancy

Note: A patient with a **complication UTIs, secondary to obstruction** should be abdominal CT or ultrasound, before starting medication

Prophylactic antibiotic: single dose TMP/SMX, taken daily or after every intercourse, **is** given to women, who get 3 or more UTI per year.

PYELONEPHRITIS
Pyelonephritis is inflammation of the kidney
Causes: discussed in UTI section
Si/Sx: urgency, frequency, dysuria, fever, chills, flank pain, costovertebral angle (CVA) tenderness
Diagnosis:

- Urine analysis: same as cystitis **plus** presence of **white cell casts**
- Urine culture: same as cystitis
- Renal ultrasound or CT, it is done to check for stones or other source of obstruction

Treatment:

- Outpatient treatment with oral ciprofloxacin
- Inpatient treatment with IV ampicillin and gentamicin. Inpatient treatment is given to pregnant women, unstable or those who cannot take oral medicine due to nausea vomiting

URETHRITIS
Urethritis is swelling and inflammation of the urethra.
Symptoms: purulent discharge, urgency, frequency, burning while urinating,
Cause: two most common causes are Neisseria gonorrhea and Chlamydia trachomatis
Diagnosis:

- Best initial test: **urethral swab** for gram stain, culture. Also culture all possible sites of sexual contact such as oral, anal, vagina
- Most effective test: **Nucleic acid amplification test**

Treatment:

- Neisseria gonorrhea urethritis is treated with **single** shot **IM ceftriaxone** or **single dose oral cefixime**
- Chlamydia trachomatis urethritis is treated with **single** dose of **oral azithromycin** or **7 days doxycycline**

ASYMTOMATIC BACTERIURIA

Asymptomatic bacteriuria is characterized by presence of significant number **of bacteria (> 10,000 mL) in the urine,** but **no UTIs symptoms** are present

Treatment: no treatment required. However, amoxicillin is given to pregnant women, kidney transplant recipient or if a patient is going for a urinary tract surgery.

BACTERIAL PROSTATITIS

Bacterial prostatitis is the inflammation of the prostate, which can be caused by any urinary tract infection. In **acute bacterial prostatitis** symptoms starts quickly. However, if symptoms or infection lasts for **3 or months,** then it is called **chronic bacterial prostatitis.**

Si/Sx: fever, chills, dysuria, low back pain, perineal pain

Treatment: TMP/SMX or ciprofloxacin **(4-6 weeks for acute prostatitis,** and **6-8 weeks for chronic prostatitis)**

EPIDIDYMITIS

Epididymitis is characterized by inflammation of epididymis. It is common in young men between 19-35 years of age

Causes: gonorrhea and chlamydia are the most common cause, but other causes may include regular use of a urethral catheter, recent surgery of urinary tract

Si/Sx: testicular pain with fever, pyuria, painful scrotal swelling

Diagnosis:

- Physical exam shows tests at normal position, tenderness around epididymis
- Urinalysis and urine culture

Treatment: bed rest and antibiotics

Sexually Transmitted Disease Differential Diagnosis

Disease	Characteristic	Diagnosis	Treatment
Chancroid	Painful soft ulcer with sharply defined borders	Urethral swab to culture	IM ceftriaxone or oral azithromycin
HSV	Painful multiple vesicles on genital or mucous membrane	Best initial test is Tzanck smear, most accurate test is viral culture	Acyclovir
Granuloma inguinale	Raised beefy-red ulcer	Clinical exam, biopsy	Doxycycline
Lymphogranuloma venereum	Enlarged lymph nodes may develop draining sinuses tracts	Serology	Azithromycin or doxycycline
Gonococcal urethritis	Purulent discharge, urgency, frequency, migratory arthritis	Urethral swab for gram stain and culture	IM ceftriaxone or cefixime
Non-Gonococcal urethritis	Purulent discharge, urgency, frequency, arthritis	Urethral swab for gram stain and culture	Azithromycin or doxycycline
Syphilis Primary syphilis	Painless chancre that appears within 2-3 weeks after the exposure of infection and disappears within 10-90 days	Initial test is VDRL or PRP Accurate test is darkfield exam	Oral Penicillin*
Secondary syphilis	Pinkish or pale rash in palms or sole in a white person, or copper colored rash in palm or sole in a black person, alopecia, condylomata lata	Initial test is VDRL or RPR, and confirmatory test is FTA	Oral Penicillin*
Tertiary syphilis	Tabes dorsalis, gammas, Argyill-Roberston pupils	Initial test is VDRL or RPR and confirmatory test is FTA	IV Penicillin*

* Note: If the patient with a primary or secondary syphilis is **allergic to penicillin,** then treat the patient with **doxycycline**. However, if a **pregnant women** or patient with **tertiary syphilis** is allergic to penicillin, **then desensitize them** with penicillin, and treat them with penicillin

RENAL SURGERY

RENAL CELL CARCINOMA
Renal cell carcinoma is a kidney cancer that starts in the tubules of the kidney.
Risk factors: smoking, polycystic kidney disease, family history, Von Hippel-Lindau disease
Si/Sx: hematuria, flank pain, flanks mass, fever, secondary polycythemia
Diagnosis: Ultrasound or abdominal CT shows heterogenic solid mass
Treatment: Surgery

BLADDER CANCER
Bladder cancer is the second most common urologic cancer; usually transitional cell carcinoma
Risk factor: male gender, cigarette smoking, aniline dye, cyclophosphamide, schistosomiasis
Si/Sx: Painless gross hematuria is the most common finding, but most of the patients are asymptotic in the early stages,
Diagnosis:
- UA often shows hematuria
- CT or ultrasound is performed to detect local invasion and distance metastases
- Most accurate test is cystoscopy with biopsy

Treatment: Surgery

PROSTATE CANCER
Prostate cancer is the most common cause of cancer in men, and the second most common of cancer-related death in men
Si/Sx: prostate cancer is usually asymptomatic; most of the tumors are discovered incidentally on prostate digital rectal exam. Some patient may present with urinary hesitancy, weak stream, urinary retention
Diagnosis:
- Palpable hard nodule on digital rectal exam
- Increased PSA
- CT scan is performed to detect any malignancy
- Most accurate is the biopsy of the prostate gland

Treatment:
- Surgery and radiation for localized cancer
- Flutamide plus leuprolide for metastatic cancer

TESTICULAR CANCER
Testicular cancer is the cancer of testes that may affect one or both testes.
Risk factor: cryptosporidium, abnormal testicle development, Klinefelter syndrome, history of testicular cancer
Type: Two most common types of testicular cancers are seminoma and non-seminoma
- Seminoma cancer is slow growing cancer
- Non-seminoma cancer is fast growing cancer. It is made up of one or more types of cells and identified based on cell type: choriocarcinoma, teratoma, embryonal carcinoma, yolk sac tumor

Si/Sx: painless lump, pain or discomfort in testes, feeling of heaviness in the scrotum,
Diagnosis:
- Testicular ultrasound
- Tumor markers: AFP, LDH, beta-HCG
- Most accurate test is biopsy
- Imaging such as X-ray or CT of abdomen and pelvis is performed to check for metastasis

Treatment:
- **Seminoma** cancer is treated with **orchiectomy and radiation**
- **Non-seminoma** cancer is treated with **orchiectomy and chemotherapy**

GASTROENTEROLOGY

ESOPHAGUS DISORDERS

ACHALASIA

Achalasia is a failure of the lower esophageal smooth muscles fibers to relax that causes lower esophageal sphincter to remain closed during swallowing

Causes: loss of the nerve plexus, but there is no known cause for loss of nerve plexus. A small percentage of cases occur secondary to other conditions such as Scleroderma, Chagas' disease

Si/Sx: chest pain, weight loss, **non-progressive dysphagia to solids and liquids simultaneously**, regurgitation of undigested food

Diagnosis:

- Chest X-ray may show dilated esophagus and no air in the stomach. However, Chest X-ray is not sensitive or specific to diagnose achalasia and further tests are required.
- **Barium swallow** is the **best initial test**. It shows dilated esophagus with a tapered narrowing of the lower end, referred as " **bird beak**".
- **Esophageal manometry** is the **most accurate test**. It shows high pressure in the lower esophageal sphincter (LES) at rest, and failure of LES to relax with swallowing.
- Endoscopy is another helpful diagnostic test. It allows direct visualization of the inside of the esophagus. Endoscopy is a useful to exclude the malignancy

Treatment: There is no cure for achalasia. Treatment is given to reduce the pressure in the LES and allow the passage of food into the stomach

- **Pneumatic dilatation** is the **best initial treatment**. In this procedure, endoscopy tube with a balloon in the end is placed across the lower esophageal sphincter and the balloon is inflated. This is effective in 80 to 85% of the patients. Complications of pneumatic dilations are chest pain, GERD, esophageal perforation.
- **Myotomy** is performed **when pneumatic dilation fails**. In this procedure, LES muscle fibers are cut and weakened. Complication of myotomy is GERD

- **Botulin toxin injection** is given if the patient does not want to have pneumatic dilation and myotomy. It relieves the obstruction by **temporarily paralyzing the nerve** that contracts the LES. Botulin toxin is **not a primary treatment** because the effect of the injection is short-lived (3 months to 1 year), and re-injections are required.

ESOPHAGEAL SCLERODERMA

In esophageal scleroderma, normal esophageal tissue is replaced with fibrous tissue. LES it becomes immobile, and valves does not close

Si/Sx: non-progressive dysphagia to solids and liquids, some patients may have GERD symptoms

Diagnosis:

- **Barium swallow** is the **best initial test**
- **Esophageal manometer** is the **most accurate diagnostic test**. It shows **immobile esophagus** and **decreased LES resting pressure**

Treatment: There is no cure for scleroderma. Proton pump inhibitors (PPIs) are given for life to relieve GERD

ZENKER DIVERTICULUM

Zenker diverticulum is the out-pouching of posterior pharyngeal constrictor, at the junction of the pharynx and esophagus

Si/Sx: non-progressive dysphagia, bad breath, **regurgitation of previously eaten food**

Diagnosis: Barium swallow shows diverticulum in proximal esophagus

Treatment: Surgical resection of diverticulum

Note: Endoscopy and nasogastric tube should be avoided in patients with Zenker diverticulum because of fear of pharynx perforation

ESOPHAGEAL RING AND WEBS

Esophageal rings and webs are thin folds of tissue that leads to partial or complete obstruction of the esophagus.

Types: Plummer-Vinson syndrome, Peptic stricture, and Schatzki's ring.

Differential diagnosis of esophageal ring and webs

Disease	Symptoms	Diagnosis	Treatment
Plummer-Vinson syndrome	Dysphagia, chest pain, acid reflux, **iron deficiency anemia**	Barium swallow shows **proximal esophageal** stricture	**Iron replacement**
Peptic stricture	Dysphagia, chest pain, acid reflux **(GERD)**	Barium swallow **distal esophageal** stricture	Pneumatic dilation
Schatzki ring	Dysphagia, chest pain, acid reflux, **intermittent dysphagia to solids**	Barium swallow ring in the **mid-esophagus**	Pneumatic dilation

DIFFUSE ESOPHAGEAL SPASM

Diffuse esophageal spasm is **uncoordinated contractions** of esophageal muscles. These contractions prevent forward movement of food from esophagus to stomach

Si/Sx: dysphagia, chest pain felt right **after meals or after drinking a cold beverage. Chest pain that may mimic myocardial infarction,** but has no effect with exertion

Diagnosis:

- Barium study may show " corkscrew" pattern during the time of spasm
- Esophageal manometry will show high-intensity uncoordinated contractions

Treatment: Calcium-channel blockers or nitrates are given to relax the esophageal muscles

ESOPHAGITIS

Esophagitis is irritation or inflammation of esophagus

Cause: Infection (virus, yeast, fungi), medicine, GERD, surgery or chest radiation

Si/Sx: Painful swallowing, difficulty swallowing, sore throat, hoarseness, heartburn

Management: as follow:

For step 2, most important thing is to figure out the cause of esophagitis and management

1) Most common **drugs responsible** for esophagitis are iron sulfate, vitamin C, NSAIDs, doxycycline, bisphosphonates (alendronate, risedronate)

   Treatment for drug induced esophagitis: advise the patient **to sit upright** then take medicine with **lots of water** and **stay upright for 30 minutes after taking the medicine**

2) Most common **viruses responsible** for esophagitis are HIV, Herpes simplex virus (HSV), and Cytomegalovirus (CMV)

   Treatment for viral induced esophagitis is as follow:

   • **Candida** is the most common cause of esophagitis in an immunocompromised patient. **HIV-positive patient with CD 4** count < 100 are usually started on **fluconazole**. If the patient is getting better, then **continue treating the patient with fluconazole**. However, if the patient is not getting better, then **endoscopy** should be done (endoscopy findings and treatment options discussed below)

   • If the patient is **HIV-negative**, then do **endoscopy biopsy** (endoscopy findings and treatment options discussed below)

Endoscopy findings	Most likely diagnosis	Treatment
Multiple punched-out ulcer	Herpes simplex virus (HSV)	Acyclovir
Single large ulcer or intracytoplasmic inclusion	Cytomegalovirus (CMV)	Ganciclovir plus acyclovir

MALLORY-WEISS SYNDROME

Mallory-Weiss syndrome is a tear in the mucus membrane at the gastroesophageal junction

Cause: retching, vomiting, binge drinking

Si/Sx: Painless bloody vomiting

Treatment: IV fluid is the **best initial treatment**, and in most cases bleeding will stop spontaneously. However, if bleeding does not stop cauterization or epinephrine injection near the bleeding site may be given to close the bleeding blood vessels.

BOERHAAVE SYNDROME

Boerhaave syndrome is spontaneous esophageal perforation

Cause: iatrogenic, binge drinking, during medical instrumentation such as an endoscopy or paraesophageal surgery

Si/Sx: Severe retching and bloody vomiting followed by retrosternal chest pain and upper abdominal pain

Diagnosis:

- Chest X-ray shows mediastinal or free peritoneal air
- Water-soluble contrast esophagram (Gastrografin) can be used to confirm the diagnosis

Treatment: IV fluids, IV antibiotics and surgery

Note: Barium swallow is not used to diagnose Boerhaave syndrome because the spillage of barium into the mediastinal and pleural cavity can induce inflammation and may cause fibrosis. However, if Gastrografin study is negative, then barium study can be performed.

ESOPHAGEAL VARICES

Esophageal varices are abnormally dilated sub-mucosal veins in lower third of the esophagus. They are often caused by portal hypertension and cirrhosis (liver disease). These veins can leak or even rupture and cause life-threating bleeding.

Si/Sx: Painless bloody vomiting and signs of liver disease such as gynecomastia, splenomegaly, spider angiomata and palmar erythema.

Diagnosis: Endoscopy

Treatment:

- **IV fluids, blood** transfusion (if hematocrit is < 30 % in an older individual and < 25% in a young individual), **fresh frozen plasma** to correct PT or INR, and platelet transfusion if the platelet count is < 50,000.
- **Octreotide** is given to lower the portal hypertension and **antibiotics** (quinolone or ciprofloxacin) are given to prevent infection from gram-negative bacteria that can cause spontaneous bacterial peritonitis.
- After above measures, **endoscopy is done**. Endoscopy is **diagnostic and therapeutic**. Endoscopy with band ligation obliterates the bleeding vessels. However, if the **patient continues to bleed,** then do **transjugular intrahepatic portosystemic shunt (TIPS)**. In TIPS, a small tube is placed between the portal vein and hepatic vein that carries blood from the liver to the heart, which reduces the portal pressure.

Complication: rebleeding (propranolol is recommended to help prevent rebleeding).

GASTROESOPHAGEAL REFLUX DISEASE (GERD)

GERD is a condition in which stomach content (food, acid) refluxes back into the esophagus

Cause: Alcohol, smoking, abnormal lower esophageal sphincter relaxation, hiatal hernia, scleroderma, pregnancy and medicines

Si/Sx: Metallic taste in mouth, nocturnal cough, sore throat, burning chest pain, wheezing, hoarseness

Diagnosis:

- GERD is diagnosed **based on signs and symptoms**. However, if the diagnosis is not clear, then 24-hour pH monitoring is performed.

Treatment:

- **Lifestyle modification** is the best initial treatment for all the patients with GERD:
  - Weight loss
  - Elevate head of bed 6-8 inches
  - Avoid alcohol, nicotine, caffeine
  - Avoid chocolate, spicy food, fatty food and peppermint
  - Avoid eating within 3 hours of bedtime
- If lifestyle modification is ineffective, then **PPIs are used**. If PPIs are ineffective as well, then **Nissen fundoplication or endocinch** procedure may be performed to tighten the lower esophageal sphincter.

Complication: Patient with long-standing GERD is at risk of developing Barrett's esophagus. Therefore, patient should have serial monitoring with endoscopy starting 5 years after they were first diagnosed with GERD.

BARRETT'S ESOPHAGUS

Barrett's esophagus is caused by **long-standing GERD (> 5 years)**. In this condition **lower esophageal epithelium** (squamous cell epithelium) is replaced by **columnar epithelium**. Barrett's esophagus is a premalignant condition. It can lead to adenocarcinoma of the lower esophagus.

Diagnosis: Endoscopy biopsy

Treatment: depends on endoscopy biopsy. (Discussed below)

Endoscopy biopsy findings	Treatment
Barrett's esophagus or columnar metaplasia	PPIs and repeat endoscopy every 2-3 years
Low-grade dysplasia	PPI and repeat endoscopy every 3-6 months
High-grade dysplasia	Distal esophagectomy

ESOPHAGEAL CANCER

Esophageal cancer is a malignancy of esophagus. Two most common esophageal cancers are squamous cell cancer and adenocarcinoma. Squamous cell cancer arises from the cells of the upper part of the esophagus. Adenocarcinoma arises from the cells of the lower part of the esophagus.

Risk factors:
- Risk factors for the **squamous cell carcinoma** are **smoking, ethanol** and **Plummer venison syndrome.**
- Risk factor for the **adenocarcinoma** is **Barrett's esophagus**

Si/Sx: Progressive dysphagia initially to solids, and later to liquids, weight loss, heartburn, coughing, hoarseness

Diagnosis:
- Barium swallow to rule out obstruction
- Endoscopy biopsy is performed to **confirm the diagnosis**
- X-ray or CT of the chest is performed to check for **metastases**

Treatment: depends on location of the tumor
- **Localized tumors** are treated with **surgical resection** and chemotherapy.
- **Metastatic tumors** are treated with **radiation and chemotherapy**.
- **Metal stent** is placed to keep esophagus open for palliation and improve dysphagia

STOMACH DISEASE

GASTRITIS

Gastritis is a condition in which the inner lining of the stomach becomes inflamed

Cause: NSAIDs, alcohol, Helicobacter pylori, pernicious anemia

Si/Sx: Black stool, vomiting blood, nausea, vomiting, pain in the upper part of the abdomen, loss of appetite

Treatment: Treat the underlying cause

PEPTIC ULCER DISEASE (PUD)

Peptic ulcer is a condition in which lining of the stomach or duodenum is affected. A peptic ulcer in the stomach is called a gastric ulcer, and peptic ulcer in the duodenum is called a duodenal ulcer.

Cause: Helicobacter pylori (H. pylori) is the **most common cause** of peptic ulcer, but causes may include NSAIDs, alcohol, smoking, burns, head trauma and Zollinger-Ellison syndrome.

Si/Sx: Gastric ulcer and duodenal ulcer both cause epigastric pain, bloating, nausea, hematemesis and melena. In **gastric ulcer pain increases soon after eating and gets better 2-3 hours after eating.** In **duodenal ulcer pain occurs 2-3 hours after eating and relieves soon after eating.**

Diagnosis:
- **Endoscopy** helps determine the location of the ulcer
- **Urease breath test and stool antigen detection test** are the **best initial tests**. These tests are non-invasive tests, but make sure that the patient is not taking PPIs for at least two weeks prior to performing these tests otherwise tests may come out false positive.
- **IgG serology** is the **most sensitive test**. If IgG serology test is negative, then one can safely exclude the possibility of H. pylori infection. However, if the serology test is positive for H. pylori, then this test has no value because once serology is positive, it stays positive for life. Therefore, the positive test will not differentiate old infection from new infection
- **Endoscopy biopsy** is the **most accurate test**

Treatment for H.pylori
- **Best initial treatment** is the combination of **three medicines -** PPIs, Amoxicillin and clarithromycin. If a patient is **allergic to penicillin,** then replace amoxicillin with tetracycline drugs.
- H.pylori is capable of **developing resistance to antibiotics**. If a patient is not responding to initial treatment, then perform urease breath test or stool antigen test to see if H.pylori is present. If any of the test is positive for H.pylori, then treat the patient with a **combination of 4 antibiotics – PPIs, metronidazole, tetracycline and bismuth.** However, if urease breath test or stool antigen test is negative for H.pylori, then check gastrin level to check for **Zollinger-Ellison syndrome**

Complication of PUD: Perforation, gastric outlet obstruction, and hemorrhage

ZOLLINGER-ELLISON SYNDROME (ZES)

Zollinger-Ellison syndrome is a small tumor of pancreas or duodenum in which a large amount of gastrin is secreted. High level of gastrin increases the production stomach acid.

Si/Sx: patient often present with recurrent signs and symptoms of peptic ulcer disease

Diagnosis:

- **Gastrin level** is best **initial test**
- If **gastrin levels** are **inconclusive**, then do **secretin stimulation test**. In this test, a small amount of secretin is injected, and gastrin hormone and gastric acid output are rechecked. In a normal person, these are suppressed. However, in a patient with ZES, gastrin hormone and gastric acid output remains high.
- Once the diagnosis is confirmed, it is important to localize the tumor. **Abdominal CT, MRI, or ultrasound** is performed first to **localize the tumor**. If these fail to locate the tumor, then **endoscopic ultrasound** is performed **detect metastatic ZES**. **Nuclear somatostatin scan** (nuclear octreotide scan) is useful to find metastatic ZES.

Treatment: depends on location of the tumor

- **Localize** tumor is **surgically removed**.
- **Metastatic** ZES is treated with **lifelong PPIs**

GASTROPARESIS

Gastroparesis is a condition in which forward movement of food from the stomach to the small intestine is slowed or stopped.

Cause: nerve damage or loss of nerve sensitivity, in conditions such as diabetes, gastrectomy, systemic sclerosis, or anticholinergic medicines

Si/Sx: abdominal distension, early satiety, postprandial nausea, and unintentional weight loss

Diagnosis: Gastroparesis is a clinical diagnosis. It can be confirmed with gastric emptying scan, but often not necessary

Treatment: Initial treatment for gastroparesis is **diet modification**- high protein, low fiber and low fats. If **diet modification is ineffective,** then drugs such as **erythromycin or metoclopramide** may be given, these increase the GI motility.

DUMPING SYNDROME

Dumping syndrome is a condition in which ingested food bypass the stomach and enters small intestine undigested.

Cause: It is seen in patients who had surgery to remove all or some part of stomach, or patients with stomach bypass surgery to help lose weight

Si/Sx: Symptoms of dumping syndrome are seen during the meal or within 15-30 after the meal. Symptoms include nausea, vomiting, **sweating, flushing, lightheadedness, heart palpitations, confusion, and fainting**

Diagnosis: Dumping syndrome is a clinical diagnosis. Gastric emptying scan can be used to confirm the diagnosis

Treatment: Initial treatment for gastroparesis is **diet modification-** eat multiple small meals that are high in protein, high fats and low carbohydrates. If diet modification is ineffective, then **somatostatin (Octreotide)** may be given to slow down the emptying of food into the intestine.

INFLAMMATORY BOWEL DISEASE (IBD)

Inflammatory bowel disease is an inflammatory condition of all or part of the digestive tract. Two types IBD are Crohn's disease (CD), and ulcerative colitis (UC)

Si/Sx of CD and UC

	Ulcerative colitis	Crohn's disease
History	**Bloody diarrhea** Tenesmus Lower abdominal pain	**Watery diarrhea** Weight loss Abdominal pain
Extraintestinal manifestation	Toxic megacolon Erythema nodosum Pyoderma nodosum Arthralgia Uveitis	Same as ulcerative colitis **plus** the followings: Kidney stone Gallstones Vitamin B12 deficiency

Diagnosis: Barium study is the **best initial test**, and **endoscopy biopsy** is the **most accurate test**. If the diagnosis is still not clear, then serology test is performed. Results discussed below

Diagnostic findings of UC and CD

	Ulcerative colitis (UC)	Crohn's disease (CD)
Barium study	Diffuse and continuous involvement, Lead-pipe colon, edema, pseudopolyps	Skip lesion, creeping fat, cobblestoning, stricture
Endoscopy biopsy	Transmural granuloma	Crypt abscess
Serology	Antineutrophil cytoplasmic antibody (ANCA)	Antisaccharomyces cerevisiae antibody (ASCA)

Treatment:

- Best **initial treatment** for UC is **sulfasalazine or 5-ASA (mesalamine)**
- Best **initial treatment** for CD is **sulfasalazine**
- High dose steroids are useful in acute exacerbation of both UC and CD.
- Azathioprine and 6-mercaptopurine are given if the patient develops acute flare-up of IBD while weaning the patient off of steroids.
- Tumor necrosis factors (TNF) such as infliximab is given if a patient with CD develops fistula

COLON CANCER SCREENING

Condition	Screening
No family history of colon cancer or general population	Start colonoscopy at age 50, then every 10 years
IBD (Crohn's disease, Ulcerative colitis)	Start colonoscopy **8 years after the diagnosis of IBD**, then every year thereafter
One family member with colon cancer	Start colonoscopy at **40 or 10 years prior** to the age at which the youngest family member was diagnosed with colon cancer (**Which ever come first**), then every 10 years
Colon cancer in three family members, in two generations, one death before the age of < 50	Start **colonoscopy** at age **25 or 10 years prior** to at which the youngest family member was diagnosed with colon cancer, then every **1-2 years thereafter**
Turcot's syndrome, Gardner syndrome, Familial adenomatous polyposis	Start **sigmoidoscopy 10-12 years** of age then **every year** thereafter

- Turcot's syndrome is characterized by the presence of multiple adenomatous colon polyposis with increased risk of colorectal cancer and increased risk of **medulloblastoma**
- Gardner's syndrome characterized by the presence of multiple adenomatous colon polyposis, **desmoid tumors**, and **osteomas of the skull or mandible**

DIARRHEA

INFECTIOUS DIARRHEA

Infectious diarrhea is characterized **fever, bloody diarrhea and WBC** in stool.

Differential diagnosis of infectious diarrhea

Organism	Association	Diagnosis	Treatment
Campylobacter	Person to person spread, contaminated food	**Best initial test** is **fecal leukocytes** Most **accurate test** is **stool culture and sensitivity**	Hydration for mild diarrhea. Ciprofloxacin for severe diarrhea
Yersinia	Pets, contaminated food	Same as above	Same as above
Shigella	Person to person spread, contaminated food	Same as above	Same as above
Salmonella	Contaminated eggs milk, poultry	Same as above	Same as above
Entero-hemorrhagic E.coli (0517:H7)	Under cooked beef	Same as above	Hydration **No antibiotics**
Giardia	Fresh water streams	ELISA stool antigen	Metronidazole
Cryptosporidium	Fresh water stream	Stool oocysts	Supportive
Entamoeba histolytica	Contaminated food or water	Stool oocysts	Metronidazole
Clostridium difficile	Is associated with antibiotics	C. difficile toxin test	Metronidazole, or oral vancomycin if metronidazole is ineffective

OSMOTIC DIARRHEA
Osmotic diarrhea caused by **ingestion of nonabsorbable solutes**, which remains in the bowel and draws water from the body.
Cause: Lactose intolerance, mannitol, oral magnesium
Diagnosis:
- Stool osmotic gap > 50 mOsm/kg
- Stop ingesting offending agent or **fasting will stop diarrhea**

Treatment: Stop ingesting offending agent

> Stool osmotic gap is calculated by: 290 - 2 Na+ K

SECRETORY DIARRHEA
Secretory diarrhea is characterized as loose stool; electrolytes and water are actively secreted or are not absorbed from luminal content
Cause: Cholera toxin, enteric virus
Diagnosis:
- Stool osmotic gap is <50 mOsm/kg
- **Fasting will not stop diarrhea**

Treatment: Supportive

EXUDATIVE DIARRHEA
Exudative diarrhea is characterized by the presence of **blood and pus** in the stool
Cause: Crohn's disease, Ulcerative colitis
Diagnosis and treatment: see Crohn's disease and Ulcerative colitis

CARCINOID SYNDROME
Carcinoid syndrome is a group of symptoms associated with carcinoid tumor, which secretes high amount of serotonin.
Si/Sx: Diarrhea, heart palpitation, **wheezing, flushing**
Diagnosis: Best initial test is 5-HIAA levels
Treatment: Octreotide

MALABSORPTION DIARRHEA

Malabsorption diarrhea is characterized inability to absorb nutrient form gastrointestinal tract

Si/Sx: Bulky stools, fatty stools, bloating, failure to thrive, weight loss, muscle wasting

Cause: discussed below

Differential diagnosis for malabsorption diarrhea

Type	Specific symptoms	Diagnosis	Treatment
Celiac disease	Malabsorption symptoms, iron deficiency anemia, **vesicular rash on extensor surface of skin**	Best **initial test**: anti-endomysial, anti-gliadin, and anti-transglutaminase antibody. **Most accurate** test is **small bowel biopsy**	Gluten free diet, iron replacement, Vitamin B12 replacement
Tropical spruce	Same as above + **recent travel to tropical**	Small bowel biopsy will show microorganism	Oral tetracycline
Whipple disease	Malabsorption symptoms plus **arthralgia, neurological abnormality, ocular abnormality**	Small **bowel biopsy** will PAS positive microorganism Or **PCR of stool** for Tropheryma whippelii	Tetracycline
Chronic pancreatitis	Malabsorption symptoms **plus history of chronic pancreatitis**	**Initial test** is amylase **and lipase. Most accurate test is Secretin stimulation test**	Oral pancreatic enzyme replacement

Q. **What is the purpose of D-xylose test?**

A. D–xylose is a simple sugar that does not require enzymes for digestion prior to absorption. D-xylose test is used to **determine if malabsorption diarrhea is caused by the small intestine disease** (Celiac spruce, Tropical spruce, Whipple disease) or **chronic pancreatitis.** Oral D-xylose is given to the patient and then checked in blood or urine sample. **D-xylose is not absorbed** if the patient has any of the **small intestine disease** that affects its ability to absorb nutrients. In contrast, **D-xylose absorption** is **normal** in **chronic pancreatitis.**

Q. **What is the purpose secretin stimulation test?**

A. Secretin stimulation test measures the ability of the pancreas to release pancreatic enzyme in response to secretin in the small intestine (duodenum). In this test nasogastric tube is inserted through the nose into the duodenum. Secretin is given intravenously. Duodenum content is collected in NG tube over next 1-2 hours. **Normal person** shows **increased pancreatic enzyme in NG tube.** In contrast, person with **chronic pancreatitis** shows **no or low pancreatic enzyme** in NG tube.

IRRITABLE BOWEL SYNDROME (IBS)
Irritable bowel syndrome is a functional GI disorder characterized by abdominal pain and altered bowel habits without any organic cause. It is more common in young females than males
Si/Sx: abdominal pain is relieved by defecation; pain is less at night, alternating bowel habits of constipation and diarrhea
Diagnosis: IBS is a diagnosis of exclusion
Treatment: Reassurance, high fiber diet or antispasmodics may help

GI BLEEDING

Differential diagnosis for GI bleeding

	Upper GI bleeding	Lower GI bleeding
Location	Proximal to ligament of treitz	Distal to the ligament of treitz and superior to the anus.
Cause	Esophageal varices, esophagitis, Mallory-Weiss tear, Gastric ulcer, Gastritis, duodenal ulcer,	Anal fissure, IBD, hemorrhoids, diverticulosis, colonic polyps, colon cancer
Stool	Black, **"tarry "** feces (melena)	**Bright red blood** in stool (Hematochezia)

Management of GI Bleeding
- Check if the patient needs **fluid resuscitation**
- **Most common cause** of GI bleeding is **upper GI bleeding**
- Start workup with **NG tube** followed by **endoscopy**
- Then, do **anoscopy** to exclude hemorrhoids
- Further diagnostic testing depends on the quantity of the bleeding:
  - Do **colonoscopy** If bleeding is **< .05 ml/min**
  - Do **angiography** if bleeding is **> 2ml/min**
  - Do **tagged red cell scan**, if bleeding is **between .05 - 2 ml/min**

HEMORRHOIDS
Hemorrhoids are swollen and inflamed veins in the lower rectum and anus that can cause pain and or bleeding
Cause: Straining during bowel movement, increased pressure in vein
Si/Sx: Internal hemorrhoids are usually painless, but these tend to bleed easily. External hemorrhoids are painful.
Treatment: conservative treatment includes high fiber diet, sitz bath, stool softener. **Definitive treatment** for **internal** hemorrhoids is **rubber band ligation**, and for **external** hemorrhoids is **surgical hemorrhoidectomy**.

LIVER DISEASES

CIRRHOSIS
Cirrhosis is advanced liver disease, in which fibrosis and nodules replace the normal liver tissue

Cause: Most common causes of cirrhosis are **alcohol, hepatitis B and hepatitis C,** other less common causes include primary biliary cirrhosis, primary sclerosis cholangitis, hemochromatosis, Wilson disease, autoimmune hepatitis, and nonalcoholic steatohepatitis.

Si/Sx: all forms of cirrhosis have following characteristics:
- Low albumin levels
- Portal hypertension
- Gynecomastia
- Spider angiomata
- Thrombocytopenia (increased PT time)
- Jaundice
- **Ascites**
- Palmar erythema
- Asterixis
- Hepatic encephalopathy
- Esophageal varices

Ascites is the accumulation of fluid in the peritoneal cavity. It results from high pressure in the portal system and low albumin. Most common causes of ascites are cirrhosis and severe live disease, but other causes may include CHF, cancer, pancreatitis, and portal vein thrombosis.

Diagnosis:
- Ultrasound
- Paracentesis (needle aspiration of peritoneal fluid)– it is performed if the patient develops new ascites, abdominal pain and tenderness or fever. Fluid is checked for its **gross appearance, protein level, albumin, and cell count.**
- SAAG (Serum ascites albumin gradient) is the difference between serum albumin and ascites albumin (discussed on the next page)

Differential diagnosis for ascites

SAAG = Serum albumin – ascites albumin	
<1.1 g/dL	>1.1g/dL
• Infection (TB, bacterial fungal, parasitic) • Malignancy (Pancreatic cancer, ovarian cancer) • Hypoalbuminemia (Nephrotic syndrome, protein losing enteropathy, malnutrition)	• Budd-Chiari syndrome • Portal hypertension • CHF • Constrictive pericarditis

Treatment:

There is no specific treatment for cirrhosis. Treatment is directed towards managing the complications and treating the underlying cause. (discussed below)

Cirrhosis complications	Treatment
Ascites and edema	Spironolactone and other diuretic
Hepatic encephalopathy	Neomycin, lactulose
Portal hypertension	Propranolol

SPONTANEOUS BACTERIAL PERITONITIS

Spontaneous bacterial peritonitis is a life-threating complication of ascites
Cause: E coli
Si/Sx: Fever, abdominal pain and bloating, abdominal tenderness
Diagnosis:
- Abdominal ultrasound or CT
- Best initial test is WBCs count, from the sample of peritoneal fluid
- Most accurate test is peritoneal fluid culture

Note: WBCs > 500 or neutrophil >250 confirm the infections and antibiotics should be started immediately without waiting for culture results to avoid complications
Treatment: IV cefotaxime or ceftriaxone. Additionally, IV albumin is added to the treatment to maintain renal perfusion pressure

SPECIFIC CAUSES AND MANAGEMENT OF CIRRHOSIS

1. PRIMARY BILIARY CIRRHOSIS
Primary biliary cirrhosis is an autoimmune disease of the bile duct of the liver. Bile builds up in the liver and leads to slow progressive liver damage, and ultimately causing scarring, fibrosis and cirrhosis. It is much more in females than male; 9:1(females to male)
Si/Sx: Fatigue, pruritus, jaundice, xanthoma (cholesterol deposit in the skin), and xanthelasma (cholesterol deposits around eyes)
Diagnosis:
- Blood shows normal bilirubin, increased alkaline phosphatase and increased IgM-antibodies
- Most **accurate test** is the blood test **Anti-mitochondrial antibody and liver biopsy**

Treatment: Ursodeoxycholic acid

2. PRIMARY SCLEROSIS CHOLANGITIS
Primary sclerosis cholangitis is a chronic bile duct disease that causes inflammation and obstruction of bile duct, inside and outside the liver. Bile builds up in the liver and leads to slow progressive liver damage, and ultimately leads to scarring, fibrosis and cirrhosis
Cause: Autoimmune diseases, but it is more common in patients with Ulcerative colitis (UC)
Si/Sx: Fatigue, pruritus, jaundice
Diagnosis:
- Blood test shows increased bilirubin, increased alkaline phosphate and increased Gamma-glutamyl transferase or gamma-glutamyl transpeptidase (GGTP).
- Most **accurate test** is endoscopic retrograde cholangiopancreatography **(ERCP)**, showing " **beads on a string**" appearance, which is narrowing and dilation of biliary tract

Treatment: Ursodeoxycholic acid or cholestyramine

3. HEMOCHROMATOSIS
Hemochromatosis is an abnormal accumulation of iron in the body
Cause:
- Primary hemochromatosis is autosomal recessive disease that is caused by mutation in HFE gene.
- Secondary hemochromatosis is found in patients with thalassemia, excess iron intake, receiving multiple blood transfusions

Si/Sx: Excessive iron deposited in the body leads to **darkening of skin, diabetes, pseudogout, restrictive cardiomyopathy**, and **infertility**
Diagnosis:
- **Iron studies** show **increased** iron, increased ferritin level, increased transferrin and low total iron binding capacity (TIBG)
- **Most accurate test is liver biopsy**

Treatment: Phlebotomy. Deferoxamine is useful in patients who are refusing phlebotomy or cannot undergo phlebotomy.

4. WILSON DISEASE
Wilson disease is an autosomal recessive disorder in which copper accumulates in the body tissues. It affects liver, kidney, nervous system and blood cells
Si/Sx: Tremors, psychosis, seizure, cirrhosis, **hemolytic anemia**, renal tubular acidosis
Diagnosis:
- **Best initial tests** are **slit-lamp examination of eyes** for Kayser-Fleischer ring (dark circle around the eye that may be visible to the naked eye) and **low ceruloplasmin level**.
- **Most accurate test** is liver biopsy

Treatment: best initial treatment is penicillamine; it binds to the copper and increases its urinary excretion. Other treatment options include zinc acetate that blocks the copper absorption in the intestine; Trientine that binds to copper and increased urinary excretion of copper

5. AUTOIMMUNE HEPATITIS
Autoimmune hepatitis is an inflammation of the liver that occurs when body's own immune system attacks liver
Type: two main types of autoimmune hepatitis are:

- **Type I autoimmune hepatitis**: this is the most common. It can occur at any age. Most of the patients have other autoimmune disorders. Diagnosis: **ANA and anti-smooth muscle antibodies**
- **Type II autoimmune hepatitis**: this is most common in young girls. Diagnosis: **anti-liver-kidney-muscle antibody**

Treatment: prednisone and or azathioprine for both types

6. ALCOHOL HEPATITIS

This is the most common cause of liver disease in US

Diagnosis:

- Clinical diagnosis
- AST: ALT = 2:1 is highly suggestive of alcohol liver disease

Treatment: Abstain from alcohol can reverse the disease

7. NONALCOHOLIC STEATOHEPATITIS (NASH)

Nonalcoholic steatohepatitis (NASH) is liver inflammation caused by accumulation of fat in the liver. It **resembles alcoholic liver disease, but it affects** people who drinks **little alcohol or do not drink** at all. It is seen in **obese, diabetics or patient with hyperlipidemia**

Diagnosis: liver biopsy is the **most accurate test**, which shows microscope fat deposits.

Treatment: Treat the underlying cause; lose weight, treat diabetes or hyperlipidemia.

HEPATITIS

Hepatitis is swelling and inflammation of the liver

Cause: Virus, drugs, alcohol, autoimmune

AST and ALT in hepatitis

- **Viral** hepatitis - **ALT > AST**
- **Drug** hepatitis - **AST > ALT**
- **Alcohol** hepatitis – **AST>ALT= 2:1**

HEPATITIS A

Hepatitis A is the most **common cause of hepatitis**. It is usually transmitted by fecal oral route

Diagnosis -IgM anti-hepatitis A virus

Treatment: Self-limited

HEPATITIS B

Hepatitis B is transmitted by exposure of blood or body fluids contaminated with hepatitis B infection such as blood transfusion, sexual contact or re-use of contaminated needle

Diagnosis: hepatitis B is diagnosed based on serology (discussed below)

Stage	Surface antigen (HBsAg)	e-antigen (HBeAg)	Core-antibody (HBcAb)	Surface antibody (HBsAb)
Acute disease	**Present**	**Present**	**Present**	Absent
Window phase	Absent	Absent	**Present**	Absent
Recovered	Absent	Absent	**Present**	**Present**
Vaccinated	Absent	Absent	Absent	**Present**
Chronic disease	**Present**	**Present**	**Present**	Absent

Note: Acute and chronic hepatitis B has same serology. Only way to differentiate them is to look at the duration of HBsAg. If **HBsAg** is present for < 6 months, then it is diagnosed as acute hepatitis. If HBsAg is present for > 6 months, then it is diagnosed as chronic hepatitis

Treatment:
- **Acute hepatitis** B is self-limited
- **Chronic hepatitis B** is treated with lamivudine. If lamivudine is ineffective, then entecavir, telbivudine, adefovir or interferon may be used

HEPATITIS C

Hepatitis C is transmitted by blood transfusion, or re-use of contaminated needle

Diagnosis
- Best initial test is **hepatitis C antibody,** but it may negative for 4-10 weeks after the infection
- Most accurate test is hepatitis C **PCR-RNA,** and it can be found within 1-2 weeks after the infection
- **Liver biopsy** is usually done to check the extent of the liver damage

Treatment: Interferon plus ribavirin

PANCREATITIS

Acute and chronic pancreatitis

	Acute pancreatitis	Chronic pancreatitis
Definition	Sudden inflammation of pancreas	Longstanding damage to the pancreas
Cause	Gallstone, alcohol, trauma, surgery, mumps, medicine, Hyperlipidemia, ERCP	Hereditary pancreatitis, hyperparathyroidism, Cystic fibrosis
Si/Sx	**Epigastric pain radiation to the back**, nausea, vomiting, fever, shock, Physical exam may show; **Grey turner sign, Cullen sign**	Nausea, vomiting, constant epigastric pain, **malabsorption**
Diagnosis	Increased amylase and lipase, Sentinel loop on X-ray. **Most accurate test is CT abdomen**	Increased amylase and lipase, abdominal CT **Most accurate test is secretin stimulation test**
Treatment	Supportive management, IV fluids, pain medicine, NG suction, If CT abdomen **shows > 30% necrosis of pancreas** then add IV antibiotics (Imipenem, meropenem or meperidine)	Oral pancreatic enzyme replacement
Complication	Pancreatic abscess, pancreatic pseudocyst	Malnutrition, pancreatic cancer

Pancreatic abscess and pancreatic pseudocyst

	Pancreatic abscess	Pancreatic pseudocyst
Time line	Within 10 days of the episode of acute pancreatitis	5 weeks after the episode of pancreatitis
Si/Sx	Fever and shock	Fever and shock
Diagnosis	CT abdomen	CT abdomen
Treatment	CT-guided percutaneous drainage plus antibiotics	If a cyst is present from < 6 weeks and is < 6cm in size, then just observe. If a cyst is present for > 6weeks or is > 6cm in size, then do percutaneous drainage

PANCREATIC CANCER

Adenocarcinoma of the head of pancreas is the most common type of pancreatic cancer

Risk factors: cigarette smoking, chronic pancreatitis, first-degree relative with pancreatic cancer, high fat diet and diabetes mellitus.

Si/Sx: painless progressive jaundice, loss of appetite, weight loss, diarrhea, Trousseau's sign, and Courvoisier's sign

Diagnosis: Increased bilirubin increased liver function test, **CT scan.**
Future diagnostic tests depend on CT findings:

- If a **CT scan shows a mass** on pancreas, then perform **percutaneous biopsy**
- If a CT scan shows **no mass** on pancreas, then perform Endoscopic retrograde cholangiopancreatography **(ERCP)**

Treatment: Pancreaticoduodenectomy (Whipple procedure)

GASTROENTEROLOGY SURGERY

RIGHT UPPER QUADRANT (RUQ) PAIN

1. BILIARY COLIC

Biliary colic is a transient pain that is felt when something blocks the outflow of bile from the gallbladder

Cause: Gallstones is the most common cause, other less common causes are strictures and tumor

Si/Sx: Sharp colicky RUQ pain felt within 30-60 minutes after meals, particularly **after eating food high in fats**. Pain usually lasts for 1-6 hours.

Diagnosis: Abdominal ultrasound

Treatment: Cholecystectomy

2. CHOLECYSTITIS

Cholecystitis is inflammation of the gallbladder

Cause: Obstruction of the cystic duct with gallstones leads to bile buildup in the gallbladder, which causes inflammation

Si/Sx: sharp RUQ pain **radiating to the right shoulder or back**, positive **Murphy sign** (RUQ palpitation during inspiration causes sharp pain and respiratory arrest)

Diagnosis: Abdominal Ultrasound will show gallstones, pericholecystic fluid and thickened gallbladder wall. If ultrasound is inconclusive, then get **HIDA scan**

Treatment: NPO, NG suction, IV fluids and IV antibiotics. Emergency cholecystectomy is performed if the patient's condition is worsening or if the patient is not responding to the treatment

3. ASCENDING CHOLANGITIS

Ascending cholangitis is a bacterial infection of the biliary tract

Si/Sx: RUQ pain, high fever (104°-105°), jaundice, change in mental status and shock

Diagnosis: high alkaline phosphatase, abdominal ultrasound shows dilation of common bile duct

Treatment: NPO, NG suction, IV fluids and IV antibiotics. Endoscopic retrograde cholangiopancreatography (ERCP) or Percutaneous transhepatic cholangiography (PTC) is done to decompress the biliary tree and remove obstructing stone

4.   CHOLEDOCHOLITHIASIS
Choledocholithiasis is the presence of gallstone in the common bile duct
Si/Sx: RUQ pain, jaundice, increased conjugated bilirubin, increased alkaline phosphate
Diagnosis: Ultrasound
Treatment: Laparoscopy cholecystectomy

5.   HEPATIC ADENOMA
Hepatic adenoma is a benign liver tumor
Risk factors: OCPs with high estrogen or anabolic steroids
Si/Sx: most of the hepatic adenomas are asymptomatic, but some patients may have RUQ pain
Diagnosis: MRI
Treatment: Stop OCPs or anabolic steroids. Symptomatic tumor is surgical resected

6.   PYOGENIC LIVER ABSCESS
Pyogenic liver abscess is the pus-filled area in the liver
Cause: Bacteria, abdominal infection, trauma
Si/Sx: RUQ pain, fever, enlarged liver
Diagnosis: CT or Ultrasound
Treatment: Percutaneous drainage

7.   AMOEBIC LIVER ABSCESS
Amoebic liver abscess is liver abscess caused by amebiasis
Si/Sx: RUQ pain, fever, weight loss, liver tenderness
Diagnosis: CT or ultrasound
Treatment: Metronidazole. If metronidazole is ineffective, then do percutaneous drainage

LEFT UPPER QUADRANT (LUQ) PAIN

1. ACUTE MESENTERIC ISCHEMIA

Acute mesenteric ischemia is a condition in which reduced blood flow in mesenteric blood vessels lead to ischemia and eventually necrosis of the bowel wall

Cause: Strangulation, arterial thrombosis, arterial embolism, surgery

Si/Sx: Weight loss, postprandial pain, abdominal pain

Diagnosis:
- Labs show metabolic acidosis and increased amylase
- Most accurate test is angiography

Treatment: Surgical resection of affected bowel

2. SPLENIC RUPTURE

Cause: Blunt abdominal trauma, enlarged spleen

Si/Sx: LUQ pain, LUQ tenderness, confusion, Kehr's sign (LUQ pain referred to the left shoulder pain)

Diagnosis: Physical exam, abdominal CT

Treatment: Splenectomy

RIGHT LOWER QUADRANT (RLQ) PAIN

1. APPENDICITIS

Appendicitis is inflammation of appendix

Cause: occurs when appendix is obstructed by feces, foreign object or in the rare case tumor

Si/Sx: fever, nausea, vomiting, periumbilical pain, rebound tenderness, Rovsing's sign

Diagnosis:
- Appendicitis is a clinical diagnosis; fever and leukocytosis (10,000-15, 000 WBC predominantly neutrophils)
- Most accurate test is abdominal CT

Treatment: NPO, IV fluids, IV antibiotics, and then Laparoscopy surgery

LEFT LOWER QUADRANT (LLQ) PAIN

1. DIVERTICULOSIS AND DIVETRICULITIS

Condition	DIVERTICULOSIS	DIVERTICULITIS
Cause	Is a condition in which **pouches form** in the wall of the colon	Is a condition in which pouches form in the wall of the **colon become inflamed** or infected
Si/SX	LLQ abdominal pain, **lower GI bleeding** (bright red blood per rectum)	Nausea, vomiting, fever LLQ abdominal tenderness
Diagnosis	**Colonoscopy**	**Abdominal CT**
Treatment	High- fiber diet	Ciprofloxacin and metronidazole

Note: Colonoscopy is not done in diverticulitis because of fear of colon rupture

2. SIGMOID VOLVULUS

Sigmoid volvulus is twisting of sigmoid colon around its mesenteric attachment. It is the most common form of volvulus of the GI tract.
Si/Sx: Crampy LLQ pain, abdominal distention, constipation
Diagnosis: Abdominal X-ray shows " **parrot beak**" appearance
Treatment: Rigid proctosigmoidoscopy

ABDOMINAL TRAUMA AND MANAGEMENT

1. Patient with **gunshot wounds** should be taken directly for **exploratory laparotomy**
2. Management of a patient with **blunt abdominal trauma** depends on the patient's condition:
   - If a patient is **hemodynamic unstable,** then proceed directly for **laparotomy**
   - If a patient is **hemodynamically stable,** then do Diagnostic Peritoneal Lavage (DPL) or Focused Assessment with Sonography for Trauma (FAST).

Small bowel and large bowel obstruction

	Small bowel obstruction	Large bowel obstruction
Si/ Sx	**Intermittent crampy abdominal pain**, vomiting, abdominal distension, constipation, focal tenderness, **hyperactive bowel sounds**	Constipation, abdominal distension, cramping, **feculent vomiting**
Cause	Adhesion from prior surgery, hernia, IBD, volvulus, stricture	Diverticulitis, colon cancer, volvulus
Diagnosis	Abdominal x-ray show **multiple air-fluid** level	Abdominal X-ray show **dilated bowel with gas**, haustra, may have a cut-off point
Treatment	NPO, IV fluids & electrolyte replacement, nasogastric decompression and surgical resection	NPO, nasogastric decompression and treat the underlying cause. Surgery is reserved for refractory cases

GROIN HERNIA

Differential diagnosis for groin hernias

Types	Description	Treatment
Direct inguinal hernia	The indirect hernia protrudes **medial** to the inferior epigastric vessels. It is more common in males than females	Surgical repair for symptomatic patient
Indirect inguinal hernia	The indirect hernia passes **lateral to inferior epigastric artery into the spermatic cord**. It is the most common type of hernia	Surgical repair for symptomatic patient
Femoral hernia	Femoral hernia protrudes **below the inguinal ligament**. It is more common in females than males	Surgical repair for symptomatic patient

Notes:

RHEUMATOLOGY

OSTEOARTHRITIS

Osteoarthritis (OA) is the most common form of arthritis around the world. It is a slowly progressive non-inflammatory, asymmetric arthritis **caused by destruction of cartilage due to wear-and-tear of joints.** Incidence of osteoarthritis increases with age. Most commonly affected joints are weight bearing joint such as hip and knee.

Si/Sx: Joint pain, crepitations with joint motion, stiffness lasting less than 20 minutes, which increases with exercise and relieves with rest.

Diagnosis:

- Physical exam may show **Heberden's nodes** (swelling on DIP joints of hands), **Bouchard's nodes** (swelling on PIP joints of hands)
- X-ray of affected joints shows osteophytes (bony spurs) and unequal joint space loss.
- Aspiration of synovial fluid shows straw colored fluid, WBC < 2000 cell/μL, PMNs < 25%.

Treatment:

- Best initial treatment is weight loss and muscle strengthening exercises
- Acetaminophen is the first-line treatment. NSAIDs are 2nd line. NSAIDs are not used as primary treatment because of their toxicity
- Interarticular steroids are used if a patient presents with severe pain or if the treatment is ineffective
- Joint replacement is reserved for refractory disease

RHEUMATOID ARTHRITIS

Rheumatoid arthritis (RA) is a chronic inflammatory arthritis that mainly affects the synovium of joints. It involves symmetric joints. **Inflammatory reaction** can lead to **synovial hypertrophy and a pannus formation** that can cause cartilage destruction, bone erosion and joint deformity. It is more common in women than men.

Si/ Sx: Joint pain and stiffness lasting for at least 30 minutes and present for > 6 weeks, it effects metacarpophalangeal joint (MCP) and proximal interphalangeal joints (PIP), ulnar deviation of fingers, rheumatoid nodules (presents in < 50% of the patients)

Labs:

- Rheumatoid factor (RF) is IgM antibodies against Fc portion of IgG. However, **RF is not specific** for RA because it is present in 70-80% of the patients with RA
- **Anti-cyclic Citrullinated peptide** (anti-CCP) is more **sensitive** and **specific** for RA
- ESR is elevated
- Aspiration of synovial fluid shows cloudy fluid, WBC between 200- 50,000 ml, PMNs > 50%
- Joint X-ray shows joint erosion

Treatment:

- NSAIDs are used to control pain
- Prednisone is used in acute RA flare-ups
- Disease modifying antirheumatic drugs (DMARDs) should be started early to **slow the disease progression** or if X-ray **shows joint erosion**

Disease modifying antirheumatic drugs (DMARDs)

Medicine	Indications	Side effects
Methotrexate	First-line treatment for RA	Elevated LFTs, bone marrow suppression
TNF inhibitor (Infliximab, adalimumab, etanercept)	First-line treatment for RA If patient is not responding to methotrexate	Reactivation of TB
Hydroxychloroquine	Used as a monotherapy for mild RA or combined with other DMARDs	Macular damage
Rituximab	Combined with DMARDs when they fail to control symptoms	Immune reaction, infection

Note: TNF inhibitors can reactivate TB granuloma. All patients should have PPD test prior to starting TNF inhibitors. Patients on hydroxychloroquine should have yearly eye exam.

Other important facts of RA:
- Coronary artery disease (CAD) is the most common cause of death in patients with RA
- RA patient has a subluxation of C1 and C2 of the spine. It is imperative to get patient's lateral cervical spine X-ray before intubating otherwise patient may develop quadriplegia.

Key features of Felty syndrome and Caplan syndrome

Felty syndrome	Caplan syndrome
• Rheumatoid arthritis • Splenomegaly • Neutropenia	• Rheumatoid arthritis • Pneumoconiosis

SERONEGATIVE ARTHROPATHIES
Seronegative arthropathies are group disorders that **affect joints**, but do **not have rheumatoid factor**. Seronegative arthropathies disorders include:
- Psoriatic arthritis
- Reactive arthritis
- Ankylosing spondylitis

Common characteristics of seronegative arthropathies disorders are:
- Involve sacroiliac joint and lower back
- Negative rheumatoid factor (RF)
- Negative anti-nucleic acid (ANA)
- Associate with HLA- B27

1. ANKLOSING SPONDYLITIS
Ankylosing spondylitis is an inflammatory disease that causes some of the vertebrae in the spine to fuse together, which makes the spine less flexible. It is more common in men, in mid 20s.

Si/Sx: Low back **pain and stiffness after waking up**, which usually lasts more than an hour and **relieves with activity**

Diagnosis:
- **Schober's test**: this test is used to measure the flexibility of the spine. A mark is made approximately at L5, and then one mark is 5 cm below this mark and another 10 cm above this mark. The patient is asked to touch his toes without bending knees. In a normal person the distance between these dots should increase more than 5cm
- **Best initial test** is X-ray of spine and hip that shows " **bamboo stick spine**" which is fusion of intervertebral discs and sacroiliitis
- **MRI** is the **most accurate test**; it detects the disease even before X-ray

Treatment: Encourage physical activity and NSAIDs. If patient is not responding to NSAIDs, then give TNF inhibitors
Complications: Uveitis, restrictive lung disease and aortitis

2. PSORIATIC ARTHRITS

Psoriatic arthritis is a form of arthritis that affects some people who have psoriasis
Si/Sx: Nail pitting, sausage shaped digits, arthritis of distal interphalangeal (DIP) joints
Diagnosis:
- Elevated ESR
- Best initial test is plain X-ray of joints, which shows "**pencil-in-cup deformity**" at the DIP joints

Treatment:
- **Best initial** treatment is **NSAIDs**
- DMARDs such as methotrexate are used in **severe disease or when patient is not responding to NSAIDs.** DMARDs slow or stop the joint damage and progression of psoriatic arthritis.
- Anti-TNF (etanercept, adalimumab, infliximab) is used, when **DMARDs fail** to control symptoms. These stop the inflammation by suppressing TNF.

Key to differentiate RA, OA and Psoriatic arthritis
- **Rheumatoid arthritis** affects **MCP joints** and **PIP** joints
- **Osteoarthritis** affects **DIP** joints and **PIP** joints
- **Psoriatic arthritis** affects **DIP** joints

---

3. REACTIVE ARTHRITIS

Reactive arthritis develops **in reaction to an infection in another part** of the body such as GI or genitourinary tract infection. Most common bacteria are **Chlamydia, Salmonella, Shigella, Yersinia, and Campylobacter**

Si/Sx: Joint pain, **uveitis, conjunctivitis, urethritis**, mouth ulcers, skin rash

Treatment: There is no specific treatment for reactive arthritis; treatment is directed towards **symptoms**

- **NSAIDs** are given to control inflammation and joint pain.
- Interarticular corticosteroids help reducing the inflammation in severe pain or acute flare-ups
- **Doxycycline** is added to NSAIDs if patient is suspected to have reactive arthritis from **chlamydia infection**

SYSTEMIC LUPUS ERYTHEMATOUS (SLE)

SLE is an autoimmune disease in which body's immune system mistakenly attacks own healthy tissues. It can affect any organ. It is much more common in females than males (9:1). African-American females are often affected more than other races.

Si/Sx: Non-specific symptoms fatigue, fever, anorexia weight loss, joint pain

Diagnosis: Need 4 of the following to diagnose SLE:

Mnemonic: **DOPAMINE RASH**

1.   Discoid rash: raised rim with central necrosis and atrophy
2.   Oral ulcers
3.   Photosensitivity
4.   Arthritis
5.   Malar rash: butterfly pattern on cheeks
6.   Immunologic criteria (discussed below)
7.   Neurologic disorder (Psychosis, seizures, or personality changes)
8.   Elevated ESR
9.   Renal disease (nephrotic or nephritic syndrome)
10. ANA positive
11. Serositis (pericarditis, pleurisy)
12. Hematologic disease (hemolytic anemia, thrombocytopenia, leukopenia)

Diagnostic tests: immunologic are as follow:
- ANA is found in > 98 % of cases, it is **sensitive but not specific**
- **Anti-ds DNA and Anti-smith antibodies** are **specific** for SLE
- Complement levels (C 3 & C 4) are decreased during SLE flare-up

Treatment:
- NSAIDs are given to patients with mild joint pain
- Steroids and hydroxychloroquine are given to patients with acute SLE flare-ups

If the patient with **SLE has glomerulonephritis**, first get the renal biopsy and then **treat the patient based on biopsy findings**. Treatment is as follow:
- No treatment is needed if biopsy shows sclerosis
- Prednisone is given if the biopsy shows early and non-proliferative disease
- Prednisone and mycophenolate is given if biopsy shows advance and proliferative disease

DRUG-INDUCED LUPUS
Lupus can also be triggered such as **hydralazine, procainamide, isoniazid, and quinidine**
Diagnosis: Anti-histone antibody
Treatment: Stop the offending drug and symptoms usually resolve in one to two weeks

SCLERODERMA
Scleroderma is a group of disorders in which normal tissue is replaced with thick fibrous tissue
Type: two types of scleroderma are:
- Diffuse scleroderma, which involves almost all organs.
- Limited scleroderma is known as CREST syndrome, it affects some organs (discussed on the next page)

1. Diffuse scleroderma
Diffuse scleroderma primarily affects skin, but may also involves lungs, renal, cardiovascular system, genitourinary system (GU), and, gastrointestinal system (GI)

Si/Sx: symptoms are as follow:

- Raynaud's phenomenon is spam in small blood vessels of fingers and toes in response to cold and emotional stress; they become numb then turn white, then blue and then red.
- Skin: hardening of skin in hands, arms, face, trunk and legs
- Gastrointestinal: esophageal dysmotility, GERD
- Renal: Malignant hypertension and renal failure
- Lungs: pulmonary fibrosis and pulmonary hypertension

Diagnosis:

- ANA
- Anti-topoisomerase antibodies (anti-scl-70)

Treatment: There is no specific treatment for scleroderma. Treatment is directed towards symptoms

- Raynaud's phenomenon: Tx. Nifedipine
- Skin thickening: Tx. D- Penicillamine
- GERD and esophageal dysmotility: Tx. Proton pump inhibitors (PPIs) for life
- Hypertension: TX. ACE-inhibitors
- Pulmonary hypertension: Tx. Bosentan (endothelin inhibitor), epoprostenol, treprostinil (prostacyclin analogues), or sildenafil

2. CREST syndrome

CREST represents Calcinosis of fingers, Raynaud's phenomenon, Esophageal dysmotility, Sclerodactyly, and Telangiectasia
Diagnosis: Anticentromere antibodies
Treatment: D-penicillamine

Note: CREST syndrome does not involve joints, kidney and lungs. Involvement of any of these organs excludes CREST syndrome.

POLYMYOSITIS AND DERMATOMYOSITIS
Polymyositis and dermatomyositis are chronic inflammatory disease of proximal muscles. In addition to muscles dermatomyositis also affects the skin.

Si/Sx: symptoms of polymyositis and dermatomyositis

Polymyositis	Dermatomyositis
• Progressive muscle weakness • Difficult swallowing (dysphagia) • Difficulty speaking • Mild joint or muscle tenderness • Fatigue • Shortness of breath	Same as dermatomyositis **plus** following skin finding: • Purple discoloration of face • Scaly lesions over knuckles • Erythematous neck and shoulder area

Diagnosis:
- ANA
- **CPK and aldolase** are the **best initial tests**
- **Muscle biopsy** is the **most accurate test**

Treatment: Prednisone

Complications: patients are at increased risk of developing cancer especially of the cervix, lungs, pancreas, breasts, ovaries and gastrointestinal tract

POLYMYALGIA RHEUMATICA
Polymyalgia rheumatica is an inflammatory disease that causes **pain and stiffness in shoulder, neck, upper arm and hips**

Si/Sx: **pain and stiffness in proximal muscle** with difficulty getting up from seated position. Other general symptoms include fever, fatigue, unintentional weight loss, and depression

Diagnosis:
- Increased ESR (>100)
- Other labs such as CPK, aldolase and muscle biopsy **are normal**

Treatment: Low dose prednisone

Complication: Polymyalgia rheumatica is often associated with temporal arteritis, also as known as giant cell arteritis. It is possible to have both of these conditions together. Symptoms of temporal arteritis are headache, temporal tenderness, jaw claudication and visual disturbance.

FIBROMYALGIA

Fibromyalgia is a disorder of unknown etiology

Si/Sx: Patient usually presents with **widespread body pain and tenderness** with **trigger points** in joints, muscles, tendons and other soft tissues. Other symptoms includes fatigue, **non-refreshing sleep**, headache, depression

Diagnosis:

- There is **no specific test** to diagnosis fibromyalgia. It is diagnosed based on physical exam. Patient must have **pain and tenderness** at **least 11 of the 18 trigger points**; neck, shoulders, chest, rib cage, elbows, lower back, buttocks, thighs, knees
- Other labs such as ESR, CPK, aldolase are all normal

Treatment:

- Initial treatment involves **physical therapy, exercise and relaxation** techniques. If these fail to control symptoms then antidepressant (amitriptyline, pregabalin or milnacipran) or muscle relaxant are given.

CRYSTAL INDUCED ARTHROPATHY

1. GOUT

Gout is an inflammatory arthritis, it occurs when uric acid builds up in joints.

Etiology: Levels of uric acid can be increased by some genetic defects or acquired causes such as excessive alcohol ingestion, steroid withdrawal, drugs (diuretics, pyrazinamide, ethambutol) hemolysis, neoplasia

Si/Sx: sudden onset of intense joint pain, which is most commonly seen in first metatarsophalangeal joint (MTP).

Diagnosis: Joint fluid aspiration shows **needle shaped negative birefringent crystals**

Treatment:

Acute treatment to treat the acute attack and prevent further attacks

- NSAIDs is first line of treatment for an acute attack
- Colchicine is given to **elderly** or those who cannot tolerate NSAIDs
- Steroids are given to patients with renal failure or if the patient is not responding to NSAIDs

Chronic or maintenance treatment is given to prevent future attacks. It is combination of lifestyle modification and medications

- **Lifestyle modifications** such as weight loss, limit alcohol and low purine diet.
- **Medications: Allopurinol** is used in patients who overproduce or under-secret uric acids. It can also be used in patients with kidney failure and kidney stones. **Probenecid** is used in patients who under-secret uric acids

2. PSEUDOGOUT

Pseudogout is an inflammatory arthritis caused by accumulation of **calcium pyrophosphate** crystals in joints

Si/Sx: Severely painful, warm and swollen joint. Large joints such as knees and wrist are frequently affected

Etiology: older age, trauma, metabolic disease such as hyperparathyroidism, hemochromatosis, hypophosphatemia, and hypomagnesemia

Diagnosis:

- Joint fluid aspiration shows **positive birefringent rhomboid-shaped crystal.**
- X-ray of affected joint shows joint damage and crystal deposit in the joint cartilage

Treatment: NSAIDs are first line therapy. Steroids are given if patient is not responding to NSAIDs

Important differences in gout and pseudogout

	GOUT	PSEUDOGOUT
Joints affected	Small joints	Large joints
Type of crystals in joints	Monosodium urate crystal	Calcium pyrophosphate crystals
Shape of crystal	Needle shaped	Rhomboid shaped
Crystal birefringence	Negatively birefringent	Positively birefringent

PAGET DISEASE OF BONES (OSTEITIS DEFORMANS)

Paget disease of bones is caused by increased activity of both osteoblast (bone formation cells) and osteoclasts (reabsorbs bone) cells that results in abnormal bone formation

Si/Sx: Bone pain, diffuse bone fractures, hearing loss, bowing of legs, enlarged head and skull deformity, **high cardiac output failure**

Diagnosis:

- Best initial test is alkaline phosphate
- X-ray is the most accurate test; x-ray shows sclerotic lesions
- Bone scan is the most sensitive test

Treatment: bisphosphonates, calcitonin is second line treatment

FOOT PAIN DIFFERENTIAL DIAGNOSIS

Condition	Presentation	Treatment
Plantar fasciitis	Sharp heel pain ever time foot strikes the ground. Pain is worse in the morning	Stretching
Morton neuroma	Pain and numbness between 3rd and 4th toe	Wear appropriate shoes and pain relievers. Surgery is reserved for refractory cases

BONE TUMOR

Tumor	Age	Characteristics	Treatment
Ewing sarcoma	5 to 15	• 2nd most common tumor • Occurs at the diaphysis of long bone • X-ray shows " onion skinning"	Chemotherapy
Osteogenic sarcoma (osteosarcoma)	10-25	• The most common tumor • Occurs around the knee (distal femur and proximal tibia) • X-ray shows " sun-burst sign	Excision and local irradiation
Osteochondroma	< 25	• Benign tumor • Occurs around the knee (distal femur and proximal tibia)	Excision
Giant cell	20-40	• Benign tumor • Occurs in the epiphysis of the long bone • X-ray shows " hot-spot" at the location of the tumor	Excision and local irradiation

RHEUMATOLOGY INFECTIOUS DISEASES

SEPTIC ARTHRITS

Septic arthritis also known as infectious arthritis is caused by direct invasion of joint space by bacteria.

Cause: Septic arthritis is classified as either gonococcal or non-gonococcal.

- **Gonococcal arthritis** is caused by **Neisseria gonorrhea**; it is the most common cause in **sexually active young adults**.

- **Non-gonococcal arthritis** is caused by **staphylococcus aureus (40%), streptococcus (30%), and aerobic gram-negative rods (20%)**. It is most common in adults and children older than 2 years of age. Incidence of non-gonococcal arthritis increases with the degree of joint damage joints and prosthetic joints. Rheumatoid arthritis is the greatest risk factor.

Si/Sx: affected joint is immobile, swollen, red, warm and tender. The patient may have fever due to bacteremia

Diagnosis: Arthrocentesis (joint fluid aspiration) to get cell count, gram stain and culture. Results are as follow:

	Non-gonococcal arthritis	**Gonococcal arthritis**
WBC	>50,000 predominantly PMNs	30,000 – 50,000 cell
Gram stain	Positive in 40-70 %	Positive in 25 %
Culture	Positive in 90-95 %	Positive in 50 %

Note: Patients with gonococcal arthritis should also have a swab of all the sites of sexual contacts (urethra, anus, cervix, and oropharynx) to determine the sensitivity of bacteria

Treatment: Empiric treatment is given to the patient until the definitive cause and sensitivity are known. Empiric treatment is as follow:

- Empiric treatment for non-gonococcal arthritis is vancomycin and ceftriaxone
- Empiric treatment for gonococcal arthritis is IV or IM ceftriaxone

Q. How would you differentiate non-gonococcal arthritis from
    gonococcal arthritis based on physical findings?
A. Non-gonococcal arthritis is monoarticular (effects single joint) arthritis.
    Gonococcal arthritis is polyarticular migratory arthritis. Patient with
    gonococcal arthritis may also have rash (petechia, purpura) and
    tenosynovitis.

OSTEOMYELITIS

Osteomyelitis is the infection of the bone that is caused by microbial agent.
Bacteria can enter the bone via hematogenous spread, nearby infections or
direct contamination.

Cause: S. aureus is the most common cause; other causes may include
group B. streptococcus, and Streptococcus pneumonia

Si/Sx: Fever, chills, pain, swelling, warmth, redness over infected area

Diagnosis:

- **X-ray** is the **best initial test**. If x-ray is negative, then get MRI
- **Bone biopsy and culture** is the **most accurate test**

Treatment: Empiric treatment with IV vancomycin and 3rd generation
cephalosporin's, until culture and sensitivity results become available

Note: Patients with Sickle cell anemia are at increased risk of osteomyelitis
from salmonella, and IV drugs abusers from pseudomonas. However, S.
aureus is still the most common cause of osteomyelitis

RHEUMATOLOGY SURGERY

SHOULDER INJURIES

Injury	Characteristics	Diagnosis	Treatment
Anterior shoulder dislocation	Arm is held close to body and **externally rotated,** as if the patient is going to shake hands	X-ray of shoulder with anterior and lateral view	Close reduction
Posterior shoulder dislocation	Arm is held close to the body and **internally rotated**	X-ray of shoulder with axillary or scapular view	Close reduction
Rotator cuff injury	Patient experiences **shoulder pain** when arm is **raised from 60° to 120°**	MRI of shoulder	NSAIDs and physical therapy
Clavicular fracture	Pain over fracture site and **inability to lift arm** because of pain	X-ray	Arm sling or figure-of-eight wrap

ELBOW PAIN

Injury	Cause	Diagnosis	Treatment
Tennis elbow (**Lateral epicondylitis**)	Painful **lateral elbow** that is caused by overuse of elbow. It is most common in people playing tennis or racquet sports	**Wrist extension** and **supination** against the resistance **elicits pain**	Ice, rest, NSAIDs, bracing
Golfer Elbow (**Medial epicondylitis**)	Painful **medial elbow** that is caused by overuse of elbow. It is most common in golfers	**Pronation** of forearm and **flexion of wrist** against the resistance **elicits pain**	Ice, rest, NSAIDs, bracing

FOREARM AND WRIST INJURIES

CARPEL TUNNEL SYNDROME

Carpel tunnel syndrome is a painful hand and arm conditions caused by median nerve entrapment in the wrist.

Si/Sx: Pain and numbness in median nerve distribution (thumb, index finger, middle finger and radial half of the ring finger), which is worst at night

Diagnosis: Clinical diagnosis

- Phalen's test: wrist flexion at 60 ° for 1 minute reproduces the pain.
- Tinel's sign: tapping median nerve over along its course reproduces the pain

Treatment: Wrist splint and NSAIDs. Surgery is reserved for refractory cases

FOREARM AND WRIST INJURY CONTINUED

Injury	Characteristics	Diagnosis	Treatment
Colles fracture	**Distal radius fracture** results from the fall **onto an outstretched hand**. It is most common in **elderly** (osteoporosis makes bone very fragile	X-ray	Closed reduction and long arm case
Scaphoid fracture	Scaphoid bone is **located at the base of the thumb**. Scaphoid fracture results from fall on a outstretched hand with weight on the palm	X-ray, but may be negative for first 3 weeks	If x-ray is negative - **spica cast** If x-ray shows displaced and angulated fracture - **open reduction and internal fixation**
Monteggia fracture	**Direct hit on ulna** results in fracture of the proximal third of the ulna with dislocation of the head of the radius	X-ray	Fractured joint - open reduction and internal fixation Dislocated joint - closed reduction
Galeazzi fracture	**Direct hit on radius** results in fracture of the radius with dislocation of the distal radioulnar joint	X-ray	Same are Monteggia fracture
Nightstick fracture	**Isolated fracture of ulna** associated with direct trauma to the forearm	X-ray	Splint for minor fracture Open reduction and internal fixation for significantly displaced fractures

FINGER INJURIES

Injury	Cause	Physical exam	Treatment
Trigger finger	One of the finger or thumb gets **locked in a bent position**	Clinical diagnosis: patient have flexed fingers, which are hard to extend without using other hand	Steroid injection
De Quervain tenosynovitis	Painful condition occurs when the tendons around the **base of the thumb are affected**	Clinical diagnosis; have the patient **hold the thumb in closed fist then force the wrist towards ulnar side reproduces** the **pain on the radial side** of the wrist and thumb	Steroid injection
Dupuytren contracture	**Thickening of the fibrous** tissue layer underneath the skin of the palms and fingers	Physical exam shows **fingers are flexed towards the palms and tender nodules in the palms**	Surgery
Jersey finger	Injury to **flexor tendon of distal interphalangeal** joint. It is often seen in athletes when one player grabs another player's jersey with the tip of the finger(s) while that player is running away.	Inability to actively flex the distal knuckle of the injured finger	Splint
Mallet finger	Injury to the **extensor tendon of distal interphalangeal joint**. It occurs when ball or other objects strikes the tip of the finger.	Inability to extend distal knuckle of the injured finger	Splint

HIP AND LEG INJURIES

Injury	Cause	Leg appearance	Treatment
Hip dislocation	**Motor vehicle accident** is the most common cause of hip dislocation	Leg is shortened and **internally rotated**	Closed reduction
Hip fracture	Most common from **fall** or **direct trauma.** Some medical conditions such as osteoporosis weakens the bone and make person susceptible to break bones easily	Leg is shortened and **externally rotated**	Open reduction and pinning
Femoral shaft fracture	Direct trauma to the femur	Injured leg is shorter than the other leg	Intramedullary rod fixation
Tibial fracture	Direct trauma to the tibia		Casting **Intramedullary nailing** for open fractures, multiple bone fragments and large degree of displacement

KNEE INJURY

1. ANTERIOR CRUCIATE LIGAMENT (ACL)

ACL injury is usually caused **hyperflexion** of knee, stopping suddenly while running, or direct trauma to the knee

Si/Sx: Pain, swelling, difficulty walking

Diagnosis:
- Positive **anterior drawer** sign
- MRI

Treatment: Arthroscopic repair

2. POSTERIOR CRUCIATE LIGAMENT (PCL)
PCL injury due to **hyperextension** of the knee or direct trauma to the knee
Si/Sx: Pain, swelling, difficulty walking
Diagnosis:
- Positive **posterior drawer** sign
- MRI

Treatment: Arthroscopic repair

3. MENISCAL TEAR
Meniscal tear is caused by traumatic injury to the knee
Si/Sx: Pian swelling, patient complain of catching or locking of the knee
Diagnosis:
- McMurray's test
- MRI

Treatment: Arthroscopic repair

Unhappy triad involves 3 structures of the knee: anterior cruciate ligament (ACL), medial collateral ligament (MCL), and medial meniscus or lateral meniscus

ACHILLES RUPTURE
Achilles tendon is the strongest tendon in the body. It connects calf muscles to the heel. Sudden force on the foot or ankle can rupture it.
Si/Sx: pain, inability to stand on toe on injured side, popping or pistol-shot like noise when injury occurred
Diagnosis: Thompson test: absent plantar flexion of the injured foot when examiner squeezes calf muscles
Treatment: Surgery

BACK PAIN

1. DISK HERNIATION

Disk herniation is defined as localized displacement of disk material beyond the intervertebral disk space. Most common locations are **L4-L5** and **L5-S1** part of the spine.

Si/Sx: low back pain, pain shooting down buttocks, thighs and knees which **exacerbates with coughing and sneezing**

Diagnosis:
- **Straight leg raise test**: with patient lying on his back on the examination table, the examiner lifts the patient's leg while knee is straight. This test is considered positive if the patient experience **pain when legs is raised between 30 - 70 degrees**
- MRI- may **confirm** the diagnosis

Treatment: **Bed rest and NSAIDs** are the best initial therapy. Most of the patients get better within 4 weeks. If these are ineffective, then do **nerve block**. Surgery is reserved for refractory cases.

2. CAUDA EQUINA SYNDROME

It is an emergency medical condition in which damage to the cauda equina results in an acute loss of function of the lumbar plexus, and nerve roots of the spinal cord.

Si/Sx: Severe back pain, **sudden loss of sensation** over genitals, anus and inner thighs, sexual dysfunction, bowel and bladder incontinence

Diagnosis: MRI

Treatment: immediate corticosteroids and surgery

3. METASTATIC MALIGNANCY OF SPINE

Occurs when cancer cells from primary tumor site metastasize to the bone

Si/SX: Constitutional symptoms (fever, chills, weight loss), back pain that **worst at night and is not relieved with rest**

Diagnosis: X-ray is the **best initial test**. Spine MRI is the gold standard and it is also best initial **diagnostic test**. Bone scan is most sensitive test.

Treatment: Steroids and radiations

4. SPINAL STENOSIS

Abnormal narrowing of the spinal canal that may occur at any part of the spine

Si/Sx: Pseudoclaudication = pain and discomfort in the buttocks, thighs, legs and feet with walking or prolonged standing; **pain is relieved by sitting or leaning forward.** Other symptoms include weakness, numbness, and sexual dysfunction

Diagnosis: MRI

Treatment: Mild to moderate symptoms is treated with **exercise and pain relievers. Laminectomy** is reserved for patient with disabling symptoms or refractory cases

COMPARTMENT SYNDROME

Compartment syndrome is a serious condition that occurs when the pressure in the muscle compartment increases and compromise the blood supply to the muscle and nerve cells. It is commonly seen in lower extremities after trauma to them.

Si/Sx: pain out of proportion, paresthesia, numbness, paralysis and pallor. Pulses may be present, but absence of pulses considered ominous

Diagnosis:
- Clinical diagnosis, but it can be confirmed by measuring the compartment pressure, which is usually > 30 mm Hg in compartment syndrome

Treatment: immediate fasciectomy to lower the pressure and restore tissue perfusion. Delay in fasciectomy can lead to permanent damage

NEUROLOGY

STROKE

Stroke is a condition in which blood supply to a part of the brain is reduced or blocked. This interrupted blood supply deprives brain cell of oxygen, and brain cells begin to die.

Type: Two types strokes are **hemorrhagic stroke** and **ischemic stroke**. Hemorrhagic stroke occurs when blood vessels in the brain leaks or ruptures. Ischemic stroke occurs when blood vessels in the brain are blocked or narrowed by thrombus or emboli. 85% of strokes are ischemic strokes.

Symptoms: headaches, difficulty walking, difficulty speaking and understanding, paralysis or numbness body parts, and trouble with seeing. Other symptoms depends on the site of artery occlusion (see table below)

Artery occlusion and symptoms

Artery occlusion	Symptoms
Anterior cerebral artery (ACA)	• Contralateral lower extremity weakness • Urinary incontinence
Middle cerebral artery (MCA)	• Contralateral hemiparesis • Contralateral sensory loss • Wernicke's aphasia • Broca's aphasia • Apraxia
Posterior cerebral artery (PCA)	• Agnosia • Hallucination • Contralateral homonymous • Hemianopia
Posterior inferior cerebral artery (PICA)	• Vertigo • Ataxia • Dysarthria • Ipsilateral face numbness • Contralateral body numbness
Basilar artery	• Locked- in syndrome • Only vertical eye movement is spared

How is a transient ischemic attack (TIA) different from a stroke?
Transient ischemic attack is caused by temporary decrease in blood supply
to the part of a brain. The patient may have symptoms similar to a stroke,
but symptoms resolves within 24 hours. Conversely, stroke is permanent
neurological damage

Diagnosis:
- **Best initial test is CT head without contrast**. CT scan is done to
  see if patient had a hemorrhagic stroke or ischemic stroke
- Most **accurate test is MRI** of head

Treatment: depends, if stroke is hemorrhagic or non-hemorrhagic
(discussed below)

**Treatment for hemorrhagic stroke: lower intracranial pressure to prevent
further damage:** elevate head, hyperventilation to keep pCO_2 between 25-
30 mmHG and mannitol. Surgical evacuation of hematoma is necessary if
signs of mass effect are present.

Treatment for non–hemorrhagic stroke: as follow:
- If a patient presents **<4 hours** of stroke, then give tissue
  plasminogen activators (**tPAs**). However, make sure that the
  patient has no contraindications for tpAs.
- If a patient has any **contraindications for tPAs** or patient presents
  >4 hours after onset of stroke, then give **aspirin**. However, if the
  patient is already on aspirin, then **add dipyridamole or stop the
  aspirin, and then give clopidogrel**.

Contraindication for tPAs

Absolute contraindication	Relative contraindication
<ul><li>Previous intracranial bleeding at anytime</li><li>Closed head trauma within last 3 months</li><li>Ischemic stroke within last 3 months</li><li>Brain tumor</li><li>Active bleeding disorder</li><li>Blood pressure > 180 systolic, >100 diastolic</li></ul>	<ul><li>Prolonged CPR (> 10 minutes)</li><li>Pregnancy</li><li>Active peptic ulcer</li><li>Invasive procedure in last 2 weeks</li></ul>

Further management: Once the patient has been stabilized, it is necessary to **evaluate the patient to determine the cause**. Most common causes are atrial fibrillation, thrombi emboli, and carotid stenosis.

1. EKG to check for atrial fibrillation. If EKG is normal, then get 24-48 hours Holter monitor.
2. Echocardiogram to check for valve vegetation and valve defects
3. **Carotid angiography or carotid Doppler**: do carotid angiography or Doppler to determine the extent of stenosis. Perform carotid endarterectomy if stenosis is > 70 %, but < 100%.

Prevention: Reduce the risk of recurrent stroke by followings:
- Stop smoking
- Keep blood pressure < 130/70
- Keep LDL < 100
- Control diabetes (keep HbA1C < 7 %)

MOVEMENT DISORDERS

1. PARKINSON'S DISEASE
Parkinson's disease is a neurological disorder that affects movement
Cause: depletion of dopamine. A lack of dopamine results in abnormal nerve function, that results in loss of ability to control body movements. In older patients (>50), it is usually caused **loss of dopamine** in substantia nigra. Other things that can affect the dopamine levels are **antipsychotic medicines, MTPT, stroke, encephalitis**
Si/Sx:
- **Resting tremor**
- Muscle rigidity
- Slow movements (bradykinesia)
- Posture imbalance
- Speech change
- Writing change (writing become small)

Diagnosis: Parkinson's disease is a clinical diagnosis

Treatment: Treatment for Parkinson's is based on symptoms

Mild symptoms are treated as follow:

- Anticholinergic medication (benztropine, trihexyphenidyl) is used in **patients < 60 years of age**. Side effects of anticholinergic medicines are dry mouth, blurred vision, dry cough, worsening prostate hypertrophy and constipation. Anticholinergic medicines **are not used in patients above 60 years** of age due to side effects.
- **Amantadine** is given to patients **> 60 years of age**

Severe symptoms are treated as follow:

- **Levodopa and carbidopa**: levodopa crosses the blood brain barrier and converts to dopamine. **Carbidopa prevents the peripheral breakdown of levodopa**. Side effects of levodopa and carbidopa include dyskinesia, akathisia and on-off phenomena. Side effects of levodopa and carbidopa can be controlled by **adjunct therapy** with COMT inhibitors (Entacapone, tolcapone) or MAOI inhibitors (selegiline, rasagiline).
- If adding COMT inhibitors or MAOI inhibitor is ineffective, then add **antidepressant** such as SSRIs because there is a high incidence of depression in patients with Parkinson's disease.
- **Thalamotomy or deep brain stimulation** is reserved for refractory cases

2. BENIGN ESSENTIAL TREMORS

Benign essential tremor is a movement disorder that is characterized by tremor of body parts, but hands are most commonly involved

Cause: there is no known clear cause

Si/Sx: **action tremors**, tremor gets worse with physical or mental stress, but **goes away with alcohol intake**

Diagnosis: clinical diagnosis

Treatment: Propranolol

3. CEREBELLAR TREMORS

Cerebellar tremors are also known as intention tremors, which appear at the **end of purposeful movements**

Cause: damage to cerebellum such as tumor, stroke, multiple sclerosis

Si/Sx: tremors at the end of purposeful movements

Treatment: Treat the underlying cause

4.   RESTLESS LEG SYNDROME (RLS)

Restless leg syndrome is a disorder of nervous system in which patient gets **irresistible urge to move their legs** and moving relieves the discomfort

Causes: there is no specific known cause, but risk factors include kidney failure, diabetes, iron deficiency, and pregnancy

Si/Sx: unpleasant sensation in legs that are often expressed **as crawling, creeping, and gnawing**

Diagnosis: clinical diagnosis

Treatment: treat the underlying cause. Dopamine agonist (Pramipexole or ropinirole) are used to control leg movements

5.   HUNTINGTON DISEASE

Huntington disease is progressive neurodegenerative disorder that causes **movement, cognitive and psychiatric disorders.**

Cause: Autosomal dominant disorder; genetic defect in chromosome 4, which results CAG repeats

Si/Sx: Choreiform movements, unsteady gait, personality change, dementia, behavioral disturbance, **hallucinations, irritability**

Diagnosis: Huntington disease is a clinical diagnosis. CT or MRI of the head may show cerebral atrophy (caudate and putamen). Genetic testing may also be done to determine the CAG repeats.

Treatment: there is no treatment to cure Huntington disease. Most of the patients die within 15-20 years after the diagnosis

Tetrabenazine is used to treat **involuntary movements** and **haloperidol** is used to treat **psychosis**

Genetic testing should be offered to young family members

NEUROMUSCULAR DISORDERS

1.   MYASTHENIA GRAVIS (MG)

Myasthenia gravis is a neuromuscular disorder that causes muscle weakness

Cause: Autoantibodies against **postsynaptic acetylcholine receptor**

Si/Sx: muscle weakness **after repetitive use**, dysphagia, diplopia, and ptosis (ptosis is pathognomonic for MG)

Diagnosis:
- **Best initial test** is **acetylcholine receptor antibody**
- Edrophonium test is performed when other tests are inconclusive. In this test patient shows sudden improvement in muscle strength after edrophonium injection
- **Electromyography (EMG) is the most accurate test.** In this test patient shows decreased muscle strength with repetitive nerve stimulation
- Chest CT to check for thymoma and other abnormality in thymus
- Pulmonary function test (PFTs) to evaluate breathing

Treatment:
- If patient's **PFTs are affected**, then give **IVIG and plasmapheresis.** It is also the best treatment in acute myasthenia crisis
- Best **initial treatment is pyridostigmine or neostigmine.** If it is ineffective and the patient is a **postpubertal, but < 60 years** to age, then do **thymectomy.** However if patient is **> 60 years** of age, then give **oral prednisone**
- If symptoms still continues, then give azathioprine, cyclosporine and cyclophosphamide

2. LAMBERT-EATON SYNDROME
Lambert-Eaton syndrome is neuromuscular disorder that causes muscle weakness after **period of inactivity**, but patient **regains** the muscle **strength after the use of that muscle**
Cause: autoantibodies against presynaptic Calcium channel blocker, it is most often seen in patients with small cell cancer of lungs
Si/Sx: muscle weakness with rest, dry mouth, impotence
Diagnosis:
- Blood test to check for antibodies against voltage-gated calcium channel blockers
- EMG shows increased muscle strength with repetitive stimulation
- Chest CT to identify tumor

Treatment: Treat the underlying cancer. Anticholinesterase (pyridostigmine) can be used to improve for muscle strength

DEMENTIA

Dementia is a term used to describe a group of symptoms affecting memory, thinking and social ability.

Cause: there is no specific cause of dementia, but it is seen in conditions such as Alzheimer disease vascular dementia, picks disease, normal pressure hydrocephalus, Lewy body dementia, Creutzfeldt-Jakob disease

1. ALZHEIMER DISEASE

Alzheimer disease is the **most common cause of dementia** in patients over 70 years of age

Si/Sx: Slow progressive memory loss particularly short-term memory, mild personality change, but as the disease progress patients become irritated, quarrelsome, and may even experience hallucinations, delusions

Diagnosis:
- Clinical diagnosis
- CT head shows **diffuse atrophy of the brain**
- Definitive diagnosis is only possible at autopsy

Treatment:
- Supportive therapy for patient and family members
- **First-line treatment** is anticholinesterase inhibitors (Donepezil, rivastigmine, or galantamine) these can slow dementia
- Vitamin E (alpha–tocopherol) can also be given, it slows the cognitive decline
- Antipsychotics and antidepressants, if needed

2. VASCULAR DEMENTIA

Vascular dementia is also known as multi-infarct dementia, which is caused by **impaired blood supply to the brain**

Risk factors: Atherosclerosis, hypertension, stroke, smoking, diabetes

Si/Sx: acute stepwise decline in memory loss, multiple focal deficits, personality change and cognitive changes

Diagnosis: CT head

Treatment: Treat the underlying cause

3. PICKS DISEAE

Picks disease is a neurodegenerative disease that causes **progressive dementia** that is similar to Alzheimer disease, except that it tends to affects frontal and temporal lobes

Si/Sx: Memory loss, aphasia, **abrupt mood swings, violent behavior**
Diagnosis: MRI of head shows frontal and temporal lobe atrophy
Treatment: There is not treatment for picks disease. Symptomatic treatment as **per Alzheimer's disease**

4.   CREUTZFELDT-JAKOB DISEASE (CJD)
Creutzfeldt-Jakob disease is a progressive **neurodegenerative disease** that **causes dementia and, ultimately, death**
Si/Sx: progressive dementia, **jerky movements (myoclonus), seizure,** personality change, anxiety
Diagnosis:
- CT head
- Lumbar puncture: spinal fluid is drawn to check for **14-3-3 protein**
- Brain biopsy is the most accurate test

Treatment: there is no treatment for CJD. **Clonazepam and valproate may help relieve myoclonus seizures**
Prognosis: patients usually die within 6 months after the diagnosis

HEADACHE
Headache is a pain anywhere in the region of head or neck. Headache may be a sharp, throbbing, and dull. Headache may be on certain location or all overhead.

1.   MIGRAINE HEADACHE
Si/Sx: Unilateral or bilateral headache, pulsating and lasts between **4- 72 hours**. Associated with nausea, vomiting, photophobia, and noise sensitivity. 15-20 % of the patients get migraines with visual auras (blind spots, flashing lights, temporary vision loss and jagged lines)
Triggers: Emotional stress, food (aged cheeses, alcoholic beverage), menstrual periods, tensions, tension and change in normal sleep pattern.
Diagnosis: clinical diagnosis

Treatment:
- Avoid known trigger
- **Mild migraine** is treated with **NSAIDs**
- **Acute migraine** attacks are treated with **abortive medications-** sumatriptan or ergotamine.

- **Prophylactic medicine:** propranolol, valproic acid, or verapamil. It is given to a patient, who **has 4 or more migraine headaches per month.**

2. CLUSTER HEADACHE

Cluster headache is characterized by **unilateral headache mostly around eyes**
Si/Sx: Multiple recurrent unilateral headaches, **tearing or watering of the eye, rhinorrhea, stuffy nose, and changes in pupil size**
Diagnosis: clinical diagnosis
Treatment: Acute therapy is 100% oxygen and or sumatriptan

3. TENSION HEADACHE

Tension headache is **the most common cause of headache**
Cause: Inadequate rest, anxiety, fatigue, hunger, emotional stress
Si/Sx: Vise-like bilateral headaches, tenderness on scalp, neck and shoulder muscles
Diagnosis: diagnosis of exclusion
Treatment: relaxation techniques and hot baths. NSIADs or acetaminophen is first-line abortive therapy

4. PSEUDOTUMOR CEREBRI

Pseudotumor cerebri is characterized by **increased fluid pressure around the brain and spinal cord**
Si/Sx: headache **that gets worse** with increased intracranial pressure such as **during coughing, sneezing or leaning forward.** Other symptoms include blurred vision, double vision, nausea, vomiting
Cause: overweight, tetracyclines, vitamin A toxicity, oral contraceptives
Diagnosis:
- CT head
- Most accurate test is lumber puncture

Treatment: Best initial treatment is to remove the offending agent, weight loss and acetazolamide. If it is ineffective, then do **recurrent lumber puncture** to lower the intracranial pressure. If patient counties to experience symptoms after repeated lumber puncture, then do **ventricular peritoneal shunt.**

5. TEMPORAL ARTERITIS

Temporal arteritis (TA) is a condition in which temporal arteries of the head become inflamed and damaged

Si/Sx: headache and tenderness in temple area, jaw claudication, fever, vision impairment

Diagnosis:

- Erythrocytes sedimentations rate (ESR) higher than 60mm/hour, but it is usually >100 mm/hour in TA
- Most accurate test is temporal artery biopsy

Treatment: high dose prednisone, which should be started immediately following ESR test results, otherwise patient may develop irreversible blindness

VERTIGO

Vertigo is characterized by sudden sensation that a person is spinning

Differential diagnosis of vertigo

Condition	Hearing loss and tinnitus	Special characteristic	Treatment
Benign positional vertigo (BPV)	No hearing loss and tinnitus	Vertigo related to **head movement**	Meclizine
Vestibular neuritis	No hearing loss and tinnitus	Vertigo **not related** to head movement	Meclizine
Labyrinthitis	Hearing loss and tinnitus both are present	Symptoms (vertigo) started **following URI**	Meclizine
Meniere's disease	Hearing loss and tinnitus both are present	**Episodic vertigo**	Surgery

DEMYELINATING DISEASES

1. MULTIPLE SCLEROSIS (MS)

Multiple sclerosis is an autoimmune disease that affects the myelin sheath of white matter of central nervous system (brain and spinal cord)

Si/Sx: Optic neuritis, tremor, slurred speech, fatigue, muscle weakness, urine incontinence, sexual dysfunction

Diagnosis:

- **MRI** is the **best initial and most accurate test**. MRI shows multiple, asymmetric, periventricular white matter plaque
- If MRI is inconclusive, then do **lumbar puncture (LP)**. LP shows mild increase in proteins, WBC< 100, increased IgG oligoclonal band (nonspecific for MS)

Treatment: discussed below

Conditions in MS	Treatment
Acute exacerbation	IV steroids, if steroids are ineffective do plasma exchange
Relapsing- remitting disease	Interferon-β1a Interferon-β1b Glatiramer
Secondary progression	Interferon-β1b
Muscle spasticity	**Baclofen** is for **daytime**, and **Tizanidine** is for **nighttime**. Tizanidine is not recommended for daytime use because it cause dizziness
Fatigue	Amantadine
Urinary retention	Bethanechol
Urinary incontinence	Oxybutynin

2. GUILLAIN- BARRÉ SYNDOMRE

Guillain-barré syndrome is an autoimmune disorder that affects the peripheral nerves

Si/Sx: muscle weakness and paralysis that **starts in legs and spreads to upper body**, bladder or bowel incontinence, and autonomic symptoms

Cause: Recent infection with campylobacter jejuni, mycoplasma, or virus

Diagnosis:
- Pulmonary functions tests (PFTs)
- Best initial test is lumbar puncture (LP), which shows increased protein and normal WBC (albuminocytologic dissociation)
- EMG is used to confirm the diagnosis. It shows diffuse demyelinating

Treatment:
- If patient's PFTs are affected, then do intubation and mechanical ventilation.
- IVIG or plasmapheresis is the first-line of treatment

AMYOTROPHIC LATERAL SCLEROSIS
Amyotrophic lateral sclerosis (ALS) is a progressive neurodegenerative disease that affects nerve cells in the brain and the spinal cord

Si/Sx:
- Asymmetric, slow progressive muscle weakens and coordination
- Breathing and swallowing muscles may be affected
- Upper motor neuron (UMN) signs and lower motor neuron (LMN) signs, are discussed below

Sign	UMN sign	LMN sign
Weakness	+	+
Atrophy	-	+
Fasciculation	-	+
Muscle Tone	Increased	Decreased
Muscle reflexes	Increased	Decreased

Note: sexual functions are not affected in ALS

Diagnosis:
- Pulmonary functions tests (PFTs)
- EMG is **best initial diagnostic** test

Treatment:
- If patient's PFTs are affected, then do intubation and mechanical ventilation
- There **is no cure** for ALS. **Riluzole** is given **slowdown the symptoms**

BRAIN LESIONS AREA AND SYMPTOMS

Si/Sx	Brain area
Broca's aphasia = Patients have difficulty with speech	Dominant frontal lobe
Wernicke's aphasia = Patient have difficulty with comprehending language	Dominant temporal lobe
Personality change, labile affect	Frontal lobe
Hemineglect (ignoring one side of the body)	Nondominant parietal lobe (Neglect of contralateral side)
Inability to read and write or do math	Dominant parietal lobe
Visual hallucination	Occipital lobe
Wernicke-Korsakoff encephalopathy	Mammillary body
Cranial nerves III and IV	Midbrain
Cranial nerves V, VI, VII, and VIII	Pons
Cranial nerves IX, X, XI and XII	Medulla

SEIZURES

Seizure is a physical finding or change in behavior that occurs after disorganized and sudden electrical activity in the brain

Cause: Etiology includes: **Mnemonic: VITAMIN C**

      Vascular (stroke, bleed, AV malformation)

      Infection (meningitis, encephalitis)

      Trauma

      Autoimmune disease

      Metabolic (sodium, calcium, magnesium, glucose)

      Idiopathic

      Neoplasm

      PsyChiatric

Types: Seizures can be divided into two main types partial seizure (also called focal seizures) or generalized seizures

- Partial seizure is generated and affects one part of the brain. Symptoms depends on that affected part of the brain
- General seizures are produced by disorganized electrical impulse throughout the brain

DIFFERENTIAL DIAGNOSIS OF SEIZURES

Type	Characteristic	Treatment
Partial seizures		
Simple partial seizure	Consciousness is **maintained.** Symptoms are depends on affected brain area	Carbamazepine or phenytoin is the first choice. Valproic acid or lamotrigine is the 2nd choice
Complex partial seizure	Consciousness is **impaired.** Lip smacking, involuntary but coordinated movements	Same as simple partial seizure
Generalized seizures		
Tonic- clonic seizure	**Rhythmic sudden stiffness and violent jerking of muscles.** Marked by urinary incontinence and tongue biting. EEG will show 10-Hz	Valproic acid is the 1st choice. Lamotrigine, or Carbamazepine or phenytoin is 2nd choice.
Tonic seizures	**Stiffening of muscles**	Same as tonic-clonic seizure
Clonic seizures	**Repetitive, rhythmic jerks of both sides of the body at the same time**	Same as tonic-clonic seizure
Myoclonic seizures	**Isolated, jerking movements**	Valproic acid is 1st choice. Clonazepam is 2nd choice
Atonic seizures	**Sudden and generalized loss of muscle tone**	Same as tonic-clonic seizure
Absence seizure	**Short (5 -10 seconds) loss of consciousness** with few or no symptoms. A patient appears **daydreaming or staring blankly.** EEG will show 3-Hz spike-and-wave	Ethosuximide

Diagnosis:
- CT Head
- Check sodium, calcium, magnesium, creatinine, glucose, oxygen and urine toxicology
- EEG

Treatment:
- Maintain ABCs
- Treat the underlying cause
- It is not necessary to start the patient on antiepileptic medicine after single episode of treatment. However, treatment should be started after single episode of seizure if:
  - Patient has family history of seizure
  - Patient has status epilepticus
  - Patient has abnormal neurological exam
  - Abnormal EEG

STATUS EPILEPTICUS

Status epilepticus is a life-threatening conditioning in which patient have repeated epileptic seizures without gaining consciousness between them

Management: is as follow

Step 1 – Maintain ABCs		
Step 2 - IV Lorazepam		
Step 3 –Patient is still seizing after 10-20 minutes then give **phenytoin or fosphenytoin** Step 4 - Patient is still seizing after 10-20 minutes, then **add 5-10 mg/kg IV phenytoin or fosphenytoin** Step 5 - Patient is still seizing after 10-20 minutes, then **give IV Phenobarbital** Step 6 - Patient is still seizing after 10-20 minutes, then **add 5-10 mg/kg IV phenobarbital** Step 7 - Patient is still seizing, then **intubate the patient plus give propofol or midazolam**	OR	Step 3 - if patient develops status epilepticus in ICU, has comorbid condition or seizure lasting > 60 minute, then **intubate the patient plus give propofol or midazolam**

BRAIN TUMOR

Brain tumors can be classified as primary brain tumor (originate within the brain) and secondary brain tumors (metastatic tumor)

Most **common types of brain** tumors are **secondary brain tumors** (metastatic tumor) that often arise from lungs, breast, kidney, and GI tract.

Si/Sx: headaches, nausea, vomiting, seizures, memory problem, mood and personality change

Diagnosis:

- Contrast CT or MRI to localize the tumor
- CT or MRI guided needle biopsy

Primary brain tumors differential diagnosis

Type	Characteristic	Treatment
Astrocytoma	• Arises from astrocytes • **Most occur in the cerebrum** • Grade III astrocytoma is called anaplastic astrocytoma • Grade IV astrocytoma is called glioblastoma multiforme	Grade III – surgical resection or radiation Grade IV – surgical resection, radiation and chemotherapy
Ependymomas	• Most common in children • **Arise from ependymoma cells** in ventricle or spinal cord and may lead to hydrocephalus	Surgical resection and Radiation
Medulloblastoma	• Most common in children • Arises **from the 4th ventricle** and leads to obstructive hydrocephalus	Radiation and chemotherapy
Meningioma	• Benign slow growing tumors • Arise **from meninges**	Surgical resection. Radiation for unresectable tumor
Schwannomas (Acoustic neuromas)	• Arises from Schwann cells • Affects women as twice as men • Cause **ipsilateral hearing loss**	Surgical resection

SPINE DISORDERS

1. BACK SPRAIN

Back sprain is the most common type of back injury

Cause: improper lifting, overstressing back muscles

Si/Sx: pain that worsens with movement, muscle cramping, decreased range of motion, difficulty walking, bending forwards or sideways and standing

Diagnosis: clinical diagnosis, spine X-ray may be required to rule out fracture

Treatment: NSAIDs and physical therapy

2. SYRINGOMYELIA

Syringomyelia is defined as development of a cavity in the spinal cord. It is mostly seen between T8- C1

Si/Sx: loss of **bilateral pain and temperature in a cape-like distribution across neck and arms**

Note: position, vibration and tactile sensation are spared

Diagnosis: Spine MRI

Treatment: Surgery

3. SPINAL STENOSIS

Spinal stenosis is an abnormal narrowing of spinal canal that can put pressure on spinal cord and nerves that travel through the spine

Cause: overgrowth of bone, herniated disks, thickened ligament, tumor and spinal injuries

Si/Sx: (pseudoclaudication) back pain that exacerbates when walking downhill and **relives with walking uphill, bending forward**

Diagnosis: Spine MRI

Treatment: surgery

4.   CAUDA EQUINA SYNDROME

Cauda equina syndrome is a serious neurological condition in which nerve roots of cauda equina are damaged

Cause: trauma, tumors, lesions, spinal stenosis, and inflammatory conditions

Si/Sx: acute urinary retention, saddle anesthesia (Loss of sensations in buttocks and perineum), decreased anal tone that leads to fecal incontinence, sexual dysfunction, weakness and loss of reflexes in lower extremity

Diagnosis: Spine MRI

Treatment: Corticosteroids and emergent surgical decompression

5.   SPINAL TUMOR

Spinal tumor is a benign or malignant tumor that gowns near or within the spinal cord.

Si/Sx: Pain that is **worse at night or in supine position**, constitutional symptoms (Fever, chills, night sweat, weight loss)

Diagnosis: Spine MRI

Treatment: corticosteroids, surgery and/or radiation therapy

6.   ANTERIOR SPINAL ARTERY SYNDROME

Anterior spinal artery syndrome is condition in which blood supply to the anterior part of the spine is interrupted

Si/Sx: Flaccid paralysis below the level of occlusion, loss of pain and temperature

Note: Proprioception and vibration are spared

Treatment: Supportive

7.   BROWN-SÉQUARD SYNDORME

Brown-séquard syndrome is a condition that results from a lesion in lateral half of the spine

Cause: most common cause is traumatic penetrating injury such as stab or gunshot. Other causes includes tumor, disk herniation, radiation and cervical spondylosis

Si/Sx: Ipsilateral spastic paralysis, Ipsilateral loss of position, vibration and tactile discrimination, **contralateral loss of pain and temperature starting 2-3 segments below the lesion**

Diagnosis: Spine MRI

Treatment: treat the underlying cause

8.   SUBACUTE COMBINED DEGENERATION

Subacute combined degeneration is a neurological condition in which **dorsal and lateral corticospinal tracts** of spine are affected

Si/Sx: Distal paresthesia and weakness, loss of proprioception and vibration

Cause: Vitamin B12

Diagnosis: Serum Vitamin B 12 level, Spine MRI

Treatment: Vitamin B 12 replacement

Notes:

NEUROLOGY INFECTIOUS DISEASES

MENINGITIS

Meningitis is inflammation of meninges of brain and spinal cords

Cause: infection with bacteria, viral, fungus, HSV, TB

Si/Sx: Fever, nausea, vomiting, neck stiffness, photophobia, change in mental status, **positive Kernig's sign and Brudzinski's sign**

Diagnosis:

- Blood culture
- CT or MRI of head
- LP: gram stain, culture, opening pressure, WBC with differential (see table below)
- RBC, glucose and protein (see table below)

CSF finding and differential diagnosis of meningitis

Organism	Opening Pressure (Nml 50–180 mmH$_2$O)	WBC CELL TYPE	Glucose (Nml 40–85 mg/dL)	Protein (Nml 15–45 mg/dL)	RBC
Bacteria	**High**	**Neutrophil**	Low	High	None
Viral	Nml	Lymphocytes	**Nml**	**Nml**	**None**
Fungal	Nml	**Lymphocytes**	Low	**High**	None
HSV	Nml	Lymphocytes	Nml	Nml	**Present**
TB	Nml	**Monocytes**	Low	**High**	None

Treatment: Empiric treatment is given until culture and sensitivity is available (see table on the next page)

Empiric treatment by age

Age	Most common cause	Empiric antibiotics
Neonate (≤ 1 month)	Group B. Strep E.coli Listeria	For neonates < 7 days of age neonate **ampicillin** and **gentamycin** **For neonates > 7 days of age neonate ampicillin** and **Cefotaxime**
Children, teens	N.meningitidis Pneumonia	**Cefotaxime** and **vancomycin**
Adults < 60 years of age	S.pneumonia	Cefotaxime and vancomycin
Adults > 60 years of age	S.pneumonia, Listeria Meningococci gram-negative bacilli	Ampicillin and cefotaxime and vancomycin

1.   NEISSERIA MENINGITIS

Neisseria meningitis is caused by Neisseria meningitides

Transmission: it is transmitted from person-to person via respiratory droplets or throat secretions

Population at risk: infants, adolescents, college freshmen living in dorms, military recruits, asplenia and terminal complement pathway deficiency

Si/Sx: Fever, nausea, vomiting, neck stiffness, photophobia, change in mental status, positive Kernig's sign and Brudzinski's sign. Other less common sign are petechiae on trunk, and legs

Diagnosis:

- LP: as mentioned in bacterial section of CSF finding and differential diagnosis of meningitis table
- Confirmed with blood culture

Treatment: Respiratory isolation and IV ceftriaxone

Neisseria meningitis prophylaxes
A Neisseria meningitis prophylaxis is the primary method to prevent transmission of disease from infected person to **close contacts or health care workers**

- Close contacts are defined as household members and anyone exposed to patient's saliva (kissing, sharing utensil).
- Recommended to **health care workers,** who had **unprotected direct contact with patients' oral or nasal secretion or intubated** the patient

Prophylaxis medicine: Rifampin, ciprofloxacin or ceftriaxone

2. FUNGAL MENINGITIS
Fungal meningitis is a rare form of meningitis; the most common cause of fungal meningitis is **Cryptococcus**
Risk factors: immunocompromised patients such as AIDS, cancer
Si/Sx: Fever, nausea/vomiting, neck stiffness, photophobia, change in mental status, positive Kernig's sign and Brudzinski's sign
Diagnosis: Lumber puncture's findings as follow:

- CSF finding as mentioned as mentioned in fungal section of CSF finding and differential diagnosis of meningitis table
- Cerebrospinal fluid (CSF) culture with **Indian ink** stain shows Cryptococcus
- **Most accurate test is cryptococcal antigen test**

Treatment: Amphotericin B plus flucytosine

3. TUBERCULOSIS MENINGITIS
Tuberculosis meningitis is caused by mycobacterium tuberculosis
Si/Sx: Look for a patient TB with symptoms of meningitis
Diagnosis: LP- as mentioned in TB section of CSF finding and differential diagnosis of meningitis table
Treatment: Same as **pulmonary TB medications plus steroids for 12 months**

ENCEPHALITIS

Encephalitis is an acute **irritation and inflammation** of the brain

Cause: most common causes of encephalitis are HSV and arbovirus. Other causes may include CMV, Toxoplasmosis, poliovirus, coxsackievirus, West-Nile virus, tick-borne viruses (Borrelia, rickettsia), Measles, mumps, and rubella

Si/Sx: confusion, altered consciousness, seizures, fever, headaches, and focal neurological deficits

Diagnosis and treatment: discussed below with cause

1. HERPES SIMPLEX VIRUS (HSV)

HSV is the **most common cause of viral encephalitis**

Si/Sx: olfactory hallucination, confusion, altered consciousness, seizures, fever, headaches, and focal neurological deficits

Diagnosis:

- **Best initial test is CT head**
- Lumber puncture: normal opening pressure, glucose and protein, lymphocytes and RBC.
- Most **accurate test is CSF PCR-DNA**

Treatment: Acyclovir. If a patient is resistant to acyclovir, then give foscarnet

2. TOXOPLASMOSIS ENCEPHALITIS

Toxoplasmosis encephalitis is caused by toxoplasma gondii. It is the most common cause of encephalitis in **HIV-positive patient with CD 4 count < 200 cells/µL**

Si/Sx: confusion, altered consciousness, seizures, fever, headaches, and focal neurological deficits

Diagnosis:

- CT head shows **multiple ring enhancing lesions**
- Toxoplasmosis antibody test is **sensitive test**

Treatment:

Standard care of toxoplasmosis encephalitis is **pyrimethamine plus sulfadiazine for 2 weeks, and then repeat CT of the** head. If CT head shows that ring-enhancing lesion are resolving, then **continue treating the patient** with pyrimethamine plus sulfadiazine. However, if CT head shows no improvement in ring-enhancing lesions, then **order brain biopsy**

Exam TIP

Ring enhancing lesions in the head are caused by number of different things, but standard management for ring enhancing lesion is as follow:

- If the patient is **HIV-negative,** then order brain biopsy
- If the patient is HIV-positive, then treat the patient with **pyrimethamine plus sulfadiazine for 2 weeks, and then repeat CT of the head.** If CT head shows that ring-enhancing lesion are resolving, then **continue treating the patient** with pyrimethamine plus sulfadiazine. However, if CT head shows no improvement of ring-enhancing lesions, then **order brain biopsy.**

BRAIN ABSCESS

Brain abscess is an abscess caused by inflammation and infection material, usually from bacterial or fungal infection

Cause: direct infection or germs that can reach brain via blood

Risk factors: weak immune system, infection, cancer, immunosuppressive medicines (corticosteroids or chemotherapy), and Right-to-left shunt.

Symptoms: headaches, fever, change in mental status, increased intracranial pressure, focal neurological findings

Diagnosis:

- Blood culture
- Best initial test is head CT or MRI
- Needle biopsy is done to identify the cause of infection

Treatment: surgical drainage and antibiotics

NEUROCYSTICERCOSIS

Neurocysticercosis is the most common parasitic disease of the nervous system

Cause: accidental ingestion of food contaminated with eggs of *Taenia solium* (pork tapeworm)

Si/Sx: signs and symptoms of encephalitis in Latin American is neurocysticercosis until proven otherwise.

Diagnosis:

- Best initial test is head CT, which shows multiple cystic lesions
- Diagnosis is confirmed with serology

Treatment: Albendazole plus steroids

Notes:

NEUROSURGERY

ACUTE EPIDURAL HEMATOMA

Acute epidural hematoma is a medical emergency in which traumatic injury to the head leads to blood buildup between the dura mater and the skull.

Blood vessel involved: middle meningeal artery

Si/Sx: lucid interval followed by unconsciousness, contralateral hemiparesis, fixed dilated headache, vomiting

Diagnosis: CT head shows **biconvex lens shaped hematoma**

Treatment: Surgical evacuation of hematoma

ACUTE SUBDURAL HEMATOMA

Acute epidural hematoma is a medical emergency in which traumatic injury to the head leads to blood buildup between the dura mater and the arachnoid mater.

Blood vessel involved: bridging vein

Si/Sx: Gradually increasing headache and confusion

Diagnosis: CT head shows **Crescent- shaped hematoma**

Treatment: Surgical evacuation of hematoma

PARENCHYMAL HEMORRHAGE

Parenchymal hemorrhage is accumulation of blood within brain parenchyma

Cause: hypertension, arteriovenous malformation, intracranial neoplasm, amyloid angiopathy, vasculitis, and trauma

Bleeding Site: Internal capsule, basal ganglia, thalamus

Si/Sx: altered level of consciousness, nausea, vomiting, headache, seizures, and focal neurological deficits

Diagnosis: Non-contrast head CT shows focal edema

Treatment: lower intracranial pressure to prevent further damage: elevate head, hyperventilation to keep pCO2 between 25- 30 mmHG and mannitol. Surgical evacuation of hematoma is necessary if signs of mass effect are present.

SUBARACHNOID HEMORRAHGE

Subarachnoid hemorrhage (SAH) is a medical emergency in which blood buildup in the subarachnoid space, the between the arachnoid membrane and pia mater.

Cause: bleeding from a cerebral aneurysm, bleeding from an arteriovenous malformation, head injury, and bleeding disorder

Si/Sx: sudden onset of the worst headache of life, vomiting, confusion, pupil size difference, stiff neck, altered consciousness

Diagnosis:

- Non-contrast head CT
- Non-contrast head CT is usually normal. In that case, get **lumbar puncture (LP)**; CSF sample is collected, and then centrifuged and analyzed; CSF gives **yellow appearance** (xanthochromia) in **SAH**.
- Angiography is also done to locate the bleeding vessel

Note: Occasionally, there may be blood in the CSF sample that came from the spinal tap itself. If CSF sample remains **clear after centrifusion**, then it means the patient did not have SAH. Blood on the sample was from the spinal tab (LP procedure)

Treatment:

- Surgical clipping of the bleeding blood vessel
- Calcium channel blocker (nimodipine) –is given to prevent ischemic stroke.
- Seizure prophylaxis

POSTOPERATIVE FEVER

MALIGNANT HYPERTHERMIA

Malignant hyperthermia is a life-threatening condition that is triggered by certain anesthesia or drugs. Patient usually develops a high fever (>104°F) **soon after exposure of anesthesia or drugs.**

Treatment: IV dantrolene, discontinue the known trigger, and supportive therapy such as 100% oxygen, correcting acidosis, hyperthermia and cooling measures

Complications: rhabdomyolysis, DIC, kidney failure, arrhythmia

BACTEREMIA

Bacteriemia is the presence of bacteria in the bloodstream. Bacteria can enter the blood during surgery, IV drug abuse. Patient usually develops high fever (>104°F) **30-45 minutes after procedure**

Diagnosis: blood culture

Treatment: empiric antibiotics until culture and sensitivity results are available

POSTOPERATIVE FEVER (101° - 103°F)

Most common causes of postoperative fever are known as mnemonic 5W's. Which stands for wind, water, walking, wound, and wonder (drug or abscess). These tend to occur at particular days after surgery

1. Wind

Fever presents **1-2 days** postoperatively. It is possibly caused by **lungs** condition such as atelectasis, pneumonia, or aspiration.

Diagnosis: chest x-ray followed by sputum culture

Treatment: antibiotic

Prevention: deep breathing, coughing, incentive spirometry or postural drainage after the surgery

2. Water

Fever presents **3-5 days** postoperatively. It is possibly caused by **urinary tract infection**

Diagnosis: urinalysis, urine culture and sensitivity

Treatment: antibiotics based on culture and sensitivity

3. Walking

Fever presents **4-6 days** postoperatively. It is possibly caused by **deep vein thrombosis**
Diagnosis: ultrasound of leg and pelvic veins
Treatment: Heparin and warfarin

4.   Wound

Fever presents **5-7 days** postoperatively. It is possibly caused by **wound infection or cellulitis**
Diagnosis: physical exam shows erythema and tenderness at surgical site
Treatment: Incision and drainage followed by antibiotics

5.   **Wonder** (drug or abscess)

Fever presents **8-15 days** postoperatively. It is possibly caused by **drug fever or infection from intravenous line**
Diagnosis: CT
Treatment: CT-guided percutaneous drainage

PSYCHIATRY

PSYCHOTIC DISORDERS
Psychotic disorders are the mental disorders that cause abnormal thinking and perception. Two main characteristics of psychotic disorders are delusions and hallucinations
Types: there are many psychotic disorders, but the most common psychotic disorders are **schizophrenia, schizophreniform, brief psychotic disorder, and schizoaffective disorder**

SCHIZOPHRENIA
Schizophrenia is a psychotic disorder. Approximately 1% of the world has schizophrenia. Common age of onset in males is 18-25 and female 25-35, but male to female ratio is 1:1.
Si/Sx: Most common symptoms include delusion, hallucination, disorganized speech, behavior disturbance and impaired social function. However, it is often described in terms of positive symptoms and negative symptoms

- **Positive symptoms** include delusion, hallucination (more auditory than visual), agitation, and disorganized speech or behavior
- **Negative symptoms** include flat affect, apathy, anhedonia, poor attention, and apathy

Subtypes of schizophrenia:

- **Paranoid type** is characterized by **hallucination and delusion,** but normal cognitive function
- **Disorganized type** is characterized by disorganized speech and behavior, and flat affects. It is associated with worst prognosis
- **Residual type** is characterized by lack of positive symptoms
- **Catatonic type** is characterized by extreme distribution, which may include stupor, rigidity, negativity, mania
- **Undifferentiated type** is characterized by presence of symptoms seen in all of above subtype, but not enough to have pin-point to one particular subtype

Treatment:

- Acutely psychotic patients may need to be hospitalized
- Antipsychotic and psychotherapy is the best treatment for schizophrenia. **Antipsychotics are given based on side effects, not the efficacy**
- Patients with negative symptoms responds better to atypical antipsychotics

Antipsychotics Medicines

	High potency conventional antipsychotic	**Low potency** conventional antipsychotic	**Atypical** antipsychotics
Medicine	• Haloperidol • Fluphenazine	• Chlorpromazine	• Clozapine • Olanzapine • Risperidone • Ziprasidone • Aripiprazole
EPS* side effects	• **More** EPS side effects	• **Less** EPS side effects	• **Less** EPS side effects
ANS * side effects	• **Low** incidence of ANS side effects	• **High** incidence of ANS side effects	• **Medium** incidence of ANS side effects

*EPS = Extrapyramidal side effects, *ANS= Anticholinergic side effects

*ANS side effects include dry mouth, urinary retention, blurry vision, orthostatic hypotension, and sedation

Side effects of atypical antipsychotic

Medicine	Side effects
Aripiprazole	Minimal weight gain,
Clozapine	Agranulocytosis, decreases seizure threshold
Olanzapine	Increases weight gain, glucose intolerance
Ziprasidone	Increases QT interval, minimal weight gain
Risperidone	Increases prolactin,
Quetiapine	Very sedating

EPS side effects of Antipsychotics

Condition	Time of onset	Symptoms	Treatment
Acute dystonia	• Within hour or first week of treatment	• Muscle spasms • Difficulty swallowing • Tongue protrusion • Twisting of head	• Lower the dose of antipsychotic and give antihistamines (diphenhydramine) or anticholinergics (benztropine or trihexyphenidyl)
Akathisia	• With first few days of treatment	• Feeling of restlessness • Pacing constantly • Alternating sitting and standing • Unable to sit or stand still	• Lower the antipsychotic dose, plus add beta-blockers or benzodiazepine
Parkinsonism	• Within a first few months of treatment	• Parkinson's like symptoms (resting tremor, rigidity, akathisia, postural instability)	• Lower the dose of antipsychotic and give antihistamines (diphenhydramine) or anticholinergics (benztropine or trihexyphenidyl)
Tardive dyskinesia	• Occurs months to years of treatment	• Choreoathetosis movement of head limbs and trunk • Frog like tongue movement	• Stop the antipsychotics and start atypical antipsychotics
Neuroleptic malignant syndrome	• Can occur at anytime during the treatment	• High fever • Altered metal status • Rigidity • Bradykinesia • Tachycardia • Rhabdomyolysis	• Stop offending drugs, and give IV fluids bromocriptine, and lastly dantrolene

Prognosis: prognosis depends on the following
- **Good prognosis:** presence of positive symptoms, late onset, known precipitating factor, married, good premorbid symptoms and family history of mood disorders
- **Poor prognosis:** presence of negative symptoms, early onset, no known precipitating factor, single, poor premorbid symptoms and family history of schizophrenia

Suicide rate: 10 % of the patients with schizophrenia commit suicide

PSYCHOTIC DISORDERS AND TIME FRAME
It is necessary to look at the time duration of the symptoms because **symptoms** of brief psychotic disorder, schizophreniform or schizophrenia **are the same,** but the **diagnosis is given based** on the duration of **symptoms**

- **Brief psychotic disorder** is characterized by symptoms present for **more than 1 day, but less than 1 month.** Treatment is same as schizophrenia
- **Schizophreniform disorder** is characterized by symptoms for **more than a month but less than 6 months.** It is treated same as schizophrenia
- **Schizophrenia** is characterized by duration of the symptoms present for **more than 6 months** (treatment disused on page 218)
- **Schizoaffective disorder** is characterized by combination of symptoms of **schizophrenia and depression or mania.** It is treated with antipsychotics and mood stabilizers. Generally **worst symptoms are treated first**

MOOD DISORDERS

MAJOR DEPRESSION DISORDER
Major depression disorder is a mood disorder characterized by persistence-depressed mood that is accompanied by **low self-esteem** and **loss of interest or pleasure**
Diagnosis: diagnosis require depressed mood or loss of interest or pleasure and presence of 5 or more symptoms from mnemonic SIG E CAPS for almost every day for at least 2-week period

- Change in **S**leep pattern   Mnemonic: **SIGECAPS**
- Loss of **I**nterest or pleasure
- Feeling of worthless or **G**uilt
- Loss of **E**nergy
- Difficulty in **C**oncentration
- Change in **A**ppetite &/or weight
- Change in **P**sychomotor activity
- Thoughts of **S**uicide or death

Treatment:

- Before initiating treatment is important to inquire about the **suicidal thoughts**. If a patient is at increased risk of suicide, then hospitalized the patient, even if it is against patient's will.
- **Psychotherapy** (Cognitive, behavioral therapy) with **pharmacotherapy** is the most the effective treatment. Psychotherapy teaches patient to identify the concern and or problems and develop a solution to bring satisfactory results.

Important: Patients are at high risk of committing suicide when antidepressants being to work because the patient gets little more energy to carry out a suicide plan

Indications and side effects of antidepressant treatment

Medication	Indications	Side effects
Serotonin selective reuptake inhibitor (SSRIs) (Fluoxetine, sertraline, paroxetine, citalopram, escitalopram)	• First-line medicine for depression	• Weight gain • GI disturbance • Sexual dysfunction
Serotonin selective reuptake inhibitor (Venlafaxine, duloxetine, desvenlafaxine)	• Preferred in chronic pain	• Hypertension • Blurry vision • Sexual dysfunction
Bupropion	• When **sexual dysfunction or weight gain is a concern.** (It causes modest weight loss)	• Lowers seizure threshold
Mirtazapine	• Preferred in **anorexic patients** with depression because one of its side effect is weight gain	• Agranulocytosis • Weight gain
Trazodone	• Preferred in patient with **insomnia** because one of its effect is sedation	• Priapism • Sedation
Tricyclic anti-depressant (TCAs) Nortriptyline, amitriptyline, imipramine)	• Are **not given to elderly** due to their side effects	• Dry mouth, urinary retention, constipation, blurry vision, and confusion
Monoamine oxidase inhibitors (MAIOs) (Phenelzine, tranylcypromine)	• No special indications	• Sexual side effects • Hypertensive crisis if taken with food high in tyramine (cheese, red wine)
Electroconvulsive therapy (ECT)	• Acutely suicidal • Other medicines are ineffective	• Headaches • Anterograde and retrograde amnesia

SEROTONIN SYNDROME

Serotonin syndrome is a potentially life-threatening reaction that may occur when there is high level of serotonin in the body

Cause: SSRIs, SNRIs, MAOIs, lithium, St. John's wort

Si/Sx: fever, altered mental status, muscle spasms (myoclonus), hyperreflexia

Diagnosis: Clinical diagnosis, but rule out others with blood test, urine test

Treatment: stop offending drug, give benzodiazepine and cyproheptadine

DIFFERENTIAL DIAGNOSIS OF DEPRESSION

1. DYSTHYMIA

Dysthymia is characterized by **mild form of depression** that lasts most of the days for **more than 2 years**

Treatment: **insight-oriented psychotherapy**; SSRIs is the second choice therapy

2. SEASONAL DEPRESSIVE DISORDER

Seasonal depressive disorder is a depression that occurs at the same time every year. It is more common in **fall and winter seasons**

Treatment: **light therapy** (phototherapy, sunlight)

3. BEREAVEMENT

Normal bereavement (grief) usually begins **after the death of loved ones** and **resolves in 1 year**. Patients experience similar symptoms of depression. However, lack of self-esteem, feeling worthlessness, suicidal ideation, and psychomotor retardation are symptoms of depression, not of bereavement. Usually requires **supportive treatment**.

4. ATYPICAL DEPRESSION

Atypical depression is a depression in which patient experience **increased appetite, increased sleep**, and trouble maintaining a long-term relationship due to the sensitivity to the rejection. **Depression temporarily goes away** in response to good news or positive events, but returns later. Patients also complain of heavy feeling in extremities

Treatment: SSRIs (first choice) or MAOIs

BIPOLAR DISORDER

Bipolar disorder is a mood disorder characterized by episodes of **mania** that alternates with episodes of **depression**. It is seen in 1% of the population and male to female ratio is 1:1.

Symptoms of **mania**:   Mnemonic: **DIG FAST**

- **D**istractibility
- **I**nsomnia
- **G**randiosity (increased self-esteem)
- **F**light of ideas
- **I**ncreased activities
- **H**ypersexuality
- **T**alkativeness

Mania is characterized by presence of above listed symptoms for at least 1 week that affects the quality of life or symptoms severe enough to require hospitalization. **Hypomania** is lower state of mania, in which symptoms of mania are present, but not severe enough to affect quality of life or require hospitalization

Subtypes of bipolar disorder
1. **Bipolar disorder type I** is an episode of **mania and depression**
2. **Bipolar disorder type II** is **depression** episodes with **hypomania**
3. **Rapid cycling bipolar disorder** is **4 or more episodes** (depression, mania or mixed) in 12 months
4. **Cyclothymia** is alternating episodes of **hypomania and depression** for ≥ **2 years**

Treatment of bipolar disorder is as follow:

Medicine	Indications	Adverse affects
Lithium	First line treatment for bipolar disorder	Tremors, weight gain, nephrotoxicity, diabetes insipidus, confusion, teratogenic **(Ebstein anomaly)**
Carbamazepine	2nd line treatment	Agranulocytosis, respiratory depression, Stevens-Johnson syndrome
Valproic acid	No special indications	GI disturbance, alopecia, teratogenic, weight gain
Lamotrigine	Refractory patients, pregnant women in 2nd or 3rd trimester	Stevens-Johnson syndrome

Note: Pregnant women with bipolar disorders are given ECT in the 1st trimester and lamotrigine in 2nd or 3rd trimester

DELUSIONAL DISORDER

Delusional disorder is characterized by presence of non-bizarre delusions for more than 1 month in the absence of mood disorders or schizophrenia. Level of function is intact.

Treatment: antipsychotics

ANXIETY DISORDERS

1. ACUTE STRESS DISORDER

Acute stress disorder is a psychological condition that develops **after a traumatic event, symptoms last for ≥ 2 days and maximum of 1 month, and occurs within 1 month of the event**

Si/Sx: common symptoms include numbness, detachment, hypervigilance, nightmare (re-experience event), flashbacks

Diagnosis: Clinical diagnosis

Treatment: Relaxation therapy with cognitive therapy is proven to be helpful.

2. POST-TRAUMATIC STRESS DISORDER (PTSD)

Symptoms of PTSD are same as acute stress disorder, but when symptoms are **present for more than 1 month**, and then it is diagnosed a PTSD Depression and substance must be ruled out.

Treatment:

- SSRIs are the first-line of treatment. Short treatment (up to 4 weeks) with benzodiazepine may be given for anxiety
- Relaxation therapy with cognitive therapy is also been proven to be helpful

3. PANIC DISORDER

Panic disorder is **recurrent** attacks of intense fear along with feeling of impending doom. It is accompanied by 4 of the autonomic symptoms often peaks within 10 -20 minutes: chest discomfort, palpitation, shortness of breath, sweating, trembling, fear of dying, numbing or tingling in the hands or feet, nausea, fear of choking, fear of dying, dizziness

Note: panic attack is a **single attack** with the similar symptoms of panic disorder. Panic attack is often mistaken for heart attack

Diagnosis: clinical diagnosis. But it is important to rule out organic causes such as MI, drug abuse

Treatment:
- Cognitive behavioral therapy
- SSRIs are **first line-treatment**, moreover, SSRIs are also used as a long-term treatment to prevent the future attacks
- Benzodiazepines may be used to relieve immediate symptoms, but are not used for a long-term treatment because of high risk of abuse

4. PHOBIA

Phobia is defined as the fear of an object or situation, and person goes to great length to avoid it

Types: common types of phobias include:
- Specific phobia is a fear of a specific object, animal, or heights
- Social phobia is a fear of social situation such as public speaking, public restroom, or public speaking

Treatment:
- Exposure desensitization, beta-blockers and benzodiazepine may be given prior to the exposure
- Relaxation technique

5. GENERALIZED ANXIETY DISORDER

Generalized anxiety disorder is a condition in which a person is worried and anxious about many things, for > 6 months and finds it hard to control anxiety. Patient may experience fatigue, irritability, trouble sleeping or falling asleep, muscle tension, and restless while awake

Association: it often coexists with depression, panic disorder and phobia

Treatment:
- SSRIs are the first-line of treatment. SNRIs or benzodiazepines may also be used
- Cognitive behavioral therapy

6. OBSESSIVE-COMPLUSIVE DISORDER (OCD)

Obsessive-compulsive disorder is characterized by **unreasonable thought** (obsession) that produces uneasiness, fear or anxiety, which leads a person to **do repetitive act** (compulsion), and that relieves the anxiety. Patient is **aware that this behavior is irrational.**

Associated conditions: depression and substance abuse often co-exists with OCD

Treatment:
- SSRIs or TCAs (particularly clomipramine) is the treatment of choice
- Behavioral therapy may help, it involves learning to tolerate the anxiety

Note: patients with **obsessive-compulsive personality disorder (OCPD)** are not aware that their behavior is irrational.

ADJUSTMENT DISORDER

Adjustment disorder is a group of symptoms that include anxious, hopeless, feeling sad and stressed. It usually starts within 3 months of stressful event and alleviates within 6 months of the event such as divorce or breakup. Symptoms are usually severe enough to cause functional impairment.

Treatment: Psychotherapy. SSRI or SNRIs may be used

SOMATOFORM DISORDERS

Somatoform disorders are characterized by symptoms that indicate physical injury or illness **but no physical cause** can be found

Types of somatoform disorders:
1. **Somatization disorder** is defined as distressing physical symptoms, which must include 1 sexual, 2 GI and 1 neurological symptom

2. **Conversion disorder** usually occurs **after an identifiable stress** such as divorce or breakup. Patient suffers from neurological symptoms, such as blindness, numbness or paralysis that are psychological.
3. **Hypochondriasis,** in which a person worries excessively that he has a **specific disease despite constant reassurance** or extensive normal medical work-up
4. **Body dysmorphic disorder,** in which a patient worries excessively that he has a flaw in his appearance, a flaw that is imagined
5. **Pain disorder** refers to pain that is severe enough to **affect person's daily** life, but **no physical cause is found**. It may be associated with depression

Treatment:

-   Brief monthly visits and individual psychotherapy
-   Depression may co-exist in a patient with somatoform disorder, if it does, then SSRIs may help

FACTITIOUS DISORDER

Factious disorder is a condition in which a person **fakes an illness,** in order to get a reward or secondary gain such as hospital admission, attention or sympathy. For example, a nurse is injecting herself insulin shots to induce hypoglycemia to get medical attention.

Diagnosis: clinical diagnosis, but it is important to rule out medical conditions with similar symptoms such as causes of hypoglycemia

FACTITIOUS DISORDER BY PROXY

Factitious disorder by proxy is a condition in which a **person fakes an illness in another person** (usually a child) who is under their care, in order to assume the caretaker role

Diagnosis: clinical diagnosis

Treatment for factitious disorders & factitious disorders by proxy:

-   Psychotherapy. However, if a child is involved in factitious disorders by proxy, then child protective service may needed to be involved

Note: Factitious disorders are not produced to gain money, if patient is faking symptoms for **financial gain, then it is diagnosed as malingering disorder**

MALINGERING DISORDER

Malingering disorder is a condition in which a person fakes an illness for secondary gain such as money or housing. Patients are usually not co-operative

Treatment: psychotherapy

IMPULSE-CONTROL DISORDERS

Impulse control disorder is characterized by difficulty controlling owns emotions and behavior, which may be harmful to one-self or others. Individual feel **anxiety before the act and gratification afterwards.** Common impulse-control disorders are:

1. **Intermittent explosive disorder** is an extreme expression of anger to a stressor that leads to an assault or property damage
2. **Pyromania** is intentionally setting fire, on ≥ 2 occasions
3. **Kleptomania is** an urge to steal items that are not needed for personal use. Person usually feels guilt after stealing and often returns stolen item
4. **Trichotillomania** is an urge to pull hair that results in irregular patchy hair loss

PERSONALITY DISORDERS

Personality disorder (PD) is characterized by lifelong unhealthy pattern of behavior, emotions and thoughts, which affects person's ability to interact with others. Common personality disorders are:

1. **Paranoid PD:** Patient is **suspicious and distrusts** everything. He or she think everyone is a threat to them
2. **Schizotypal** PD: Patient has **odd and eccentric** beliefs, they often feels **discomfort in social relationships**
3. **Schizoid PD:** Patient has no interest in social relationship, emotionally restricted and **do not want** any friends
4. **Avoidant PD:** Patient **wants friend,** but **do not have friends** because they avoids other out of **fear of criticism**
5. **Dependent PD:** Patients are **very submissive and clingy.** They always need someone to meet their emotional and physical needs. They cannot do anything alone because they do not trust their ability to make decisions

6. **Obsessive-compulsive PD:** Patients are very **inflexible and stubborn.** They are **preoccupied** with **orderliness, perfectionism and control.** They do not think that their behavior is irrational

7. **Narcissistic PD:** Patients are **egocentric,** have a **sense of entitlement.** They lack empathy and get angry when criticized

8. **Borderline PD:** Patients (mostly females) have **unstable mood, behavior and relationships;** they have fear of abandonment, and usually have a history of **multiple suicidal attempts.** They view others as either all good or all bad **(Splitting)**

9. **Antisocial PD:** persistence **violation of social rules.** They lack remorse; torture animals or set fires. There is a strong association of alcoholism ,drug abuse and somatization disorder.

Treatment: Personality disorders are treated with psychotherapy and mood stabilizers, as needed

EATING DISORDERS

1. ANOREXIA

Anorexia is an eating disorder in which the patient has an irrational fear of weight gain even though the **patient is 85 % below their ideal weight.** They lose weight by excessive exercise, purging, fasting, laxatives or diuretics abuse

Diagnosis: measure height and weight, CBC, electrolyte, endocrine and ECG. Psychiatry evaluation to check for comorbid conditions

Treatment:

- Hospitalize patient for IV nutrients, fluid and electrolyte replacement
- Psychotherapy, SSRIs may be used to promote weight
- Treat any comorbid condition

2. BULIMIA

Bulimia is characterized by binge eating followed by purging. Patients have **normal body weight.** They usually have **abrasion on dorsal hands** surface, **parotid swelling, and dental enamel erosion.**

Diagnosis: clinical diagnosis

Treatment:

- Patient usually don't require hospitalization unless there is electrolytes imbalance

- Behavioral psychotherapy
- SSRIs may be needed to prevent bulimia relapse

SUBSTANCE ABUSE

Substance	Intoxication symptoms & treatment	Withdrawal symptoms & treatment
Amphetamine & cocaine	• Agitation, decreased appetite, arrhythmia, MI, HTN, stroke, seizure, nosebleed, dilated pupil • Treatment: Antipsychotics	• Increased appetite, depressed, suicidal, anxiety, tremor • Treatment: Antidepressants
Opiates	• Constricted pupils, constipations, slurred speech, impaired memory, coma, death • Treatment: Naloxone	• Yawning, lacrimation, runny nose, abdominal cramps, muscle spams • Treatment: Clonidine or methadone. Clonidine, if patient has hypertension
Benzodiazepine & barbiturates	• Respiratory and cardiac depression • Treatment: Flumazenil	• Anxiety, seizure, tremors, cardiovascular collapse • Treatment: Long-acting benzodiazepines
LSD & hallucinogens	• Hallucination, dilated pupils, impaired judgment, incoordination • Treatment: Supportive, antipsychotics and benzodiazepines as needed	None
PCP	• Hallucination, horizontal/vertical nystagmus, assaultive, HTN, seizure, coma • Treatment: Supportive, benzodiazepines and antipsychotics	None
Inhalants	• Impaired judgment, blurred vision, assaultive, respiratory depression • Treatment: Antipsychotics	None
Marijuana	• Mostly teenager with red conjunctiva, dry mouth, socially withdrawn, amotivational, impaired time perception • Treatment: None	None

ALCOHOL

ALCOHOL SCREENING
CAGE questionnaire is used to screen person for alcohol
C: ever felt the need to **cut** down
A: feel **annoyed** when asked about drinking
G: feel **guilty** after drinking
E: need drink in the morning (**eye**-opener)

ALCOHOL INTOXICATION
Alcohol intoxication symptoms include emotional lability, slurred speech, ataxia, aggression, hypoglycemia
Treatment: usually no treatment is required. Mechanical ventilation if needed

ALCOHOL WITHDRAWLS
Alcohol withdrawal symptoms are as follow:
1. **Tremor** begins within **5-10 hours** after the last drink. Symptoms include **tremors, irritability, insomnia, increased** blood pressure
2. **Alcohol hallucinosis** begins within **12 – 24 hours** after the last drink. Symptoms include **visual, auditory** and **tactile hallucination.**
3. **Alcohol withdrawal seizure** are **tonic-clonic seizure**, which usually begins within **6-48 hours** after the last drink
4. **Delirium tremens** begins within **2 -3 days** after the last drink. Symptoms includes **hallucinations, confusion, disorientation,** autonomic lability

Management of alcohol withdrawals:
- Benzodiazepines can lessen alcohol withdrawal symptoms. Long- acting benzodiazepine such **chlordiazepoxide** (Librium) or **diazepam is the first-line of treatment**. Short-acting benzodiazepine such as Lorazepam or oxazepam, are preferred in a patient with liver disease
- Give Vitamin B 12, folate, thiamine, magnesium, phosphate, glucose

Note: give thiamine before glucose to prevent Wernicke-Korsakoff

GENDER IDENTITY

- **Sexual identity** is based on person's secondary sexual characteristics
- **Sexual orientation** is defined by whom he or she is sexually attracted to
- **Gender identity** is person's own sense of male or female
- **Gender role** is a public image of a person, a male or female

GENDER IDENTITY DISORDER

Gender identity disorder is a person's inner conflict between his or her physical gender and the gender person identifies himself or herself as. Person is not happy with the gender he or she was born.

Treatment

- Psychotherapy
- Gender reassignment, if surgery is approved

SEXUAL PARAPHILIA

Sexual paraphilia is characterized by sexual fantasies or activities that involve nonhuman objects, a non-consenting partner or in certain situations. Some of the paraphilias are mentioned below:

Paraphilia	Manifestations
Exhibitionism	Sexual arousal from showing one's genital to strangers
Fetishism	Sexual arousal from non-living objects
Pedophilia	Sexual urges towards children
Frotteurism	Rubbing against non-consenting partner for sexual gratification
Masochism	Sexual arousal from being humiliated, hurt
Sadism	Sexual arousal from inflicting pain one someone

SUICIDE

Risk factors for suicide are: Mnemonic: **SAD PERSONS**
- Male **S**ex (more females attempt, but more males succeed)
- **A**ge < 20 or > 40
- **D**epression
- **P**revious suicide attempt
- **E**thanol abuse
- **R**ational thinking loss
- **S**ocial support lacking
- **O**rganized plan
- **N**o spouse (divorced, separated or single)
- **S**ickness (chronic, severe)

Treatment: Hospitalization

SLEEP DISORDERS

1. **Night terrors** are common in children between 3- 7 years of age, they occur during **stage 3 & 4 of sleep.** In night terrors, child wakes up from sleep terrified and often go back to sleep. Children often have **no memory about the event** when they wake up next day.
2. **Nightmares** usually begin before 10 years of age and are a normal part of childhood. They usually occur during **REM sleep**. In nightmares, child wakes up from sleep terrified and can often recall dream when they wake up next day.
3. **Sleepwalking** is a disorder in which people walk or do other activities during sleep. It usually occurs during **3 and 4th stage of** sleep. It is usually **treated with benzodiazepines**.
4. **Narcolepsy** is characterized by excessive daytime sleep patterns, even after adequate nighttime sleep. Patient **goes to REM sleep** within 5 minutes of sleep. Other symptoms may include **cataplexy** (sudden loss of muscles tone), **hypnagogic** (hallucinations while falling asleep), **hypnopompic** (hallucination while awakening from sleep) and **sleep paralysis** (temporary inability to talk or move when waking, it usually lasts few seconds to minutes)
   Treatment: methylphenidate or pemoline

Notes:

PEDIATRIC PSYCHIATRY

PERVASIVE DEVELOPMENT DISORDERS

Pervasive development disorders are a group of disorders characterized by development delay in social interaction, behavior and language, before the age of 3.

Type: four common types of pervasive development disorders are

1. **Autism is characterized by impair social interaction; impair non-verbal communication, impair verbal (speech) communications and purposeless repetitive movements.** It has a higher incidence in males than females

2. **Asperger syndrome is characterized by impair social interaction; impair non-verbal communication, purposeless repetitive movements, but verbal (speech) communication is preserved.** It has a higher incidence in males than females

3. **Childhood disintegrative disorder** is a condition in which all the development milestones are normal till 2 years of age, **but between 2 -10 years of age all the skill are lost;** social skills and self care skills, motor skills, play skills, bowel and bladder control, and language. It has a higher incidence in males than females.

4. **Rett syndrome:** is a neurodevelopment disorder of the gray matter of the brain with **progressive impairment** such as verbal, and motor. Clinical features include small hands, feet and deceleration of head growth. It has a higher incidence in females than males

Treatment: family support, counseling, behavior modification, and antipsychotic, if the patient is aggressive.

ATTENTION DEFICIT HYPERACTIVITY DISORDER (ADHD)

ADHD is characterized by easy **distractibility, fidgety, inability to focus,** inability to complete tasks, **d**eclining school performance

Diagnosis: based on the followings:

- Patient must be < 7 years old
- Symptoms must last > 6 months
- Symptoms must be present in two or more settings (school, home)
- Symptoms must interfere with daily function

Management:
- **Behavioral modification and medication** (methylphenidate or dextroamphetamine)
- **Atomoxetine** is a SNRIs that may be used if a patient is **> 6 years of age and** is at high **risk of methylphenidate abuse**

DISRUPTIVE BEHAVIOR
Two main disruptive behaviors in children are:
1. **Conduct disorder;** in which a child **bully others, start fights, cruel to animals**, and steals. It may **progress to antisocial personality disorder**
2. **Oppositional defiant disorder**, in which a child displays **disrespect and opposition to adults or authority position.** They tend to be angry and resentful of others, blame others for their mistakes.

Treatment: individual and family therapy

TOURETTE'S SYNDROME
Tourette's syndrome is characterized by **multiple repetitive tics, which start before the age of 18 and last more than 1 year.** Vocal tics (e.g. grunting, coprolalia, throat clearing) and motor tics involve the muscles of head and neck (e.g. blinking, head shaking). It is associated with ADHD, OCD and learning disorders.

Treatment: no treatment needed for mild symptoms, but **severe symptoms can be treated with haloperidol, pimozide or clonidine.**

MENTAL RETARDATION
Mental retardation is characterized by impaired intellectual and social function. It is more common in males than females. It is associated with chromosomal abnormalities, inborn error of metabolism, congenital infective, malnutrition and exposure to certain types of toxin or infection

Types and effect on life of mental retardation is as follow:
- Person with **mild mental retardation** (IQ range 50- 70) can live independently, but will need assistant in stressful situation
- Person with **moderate mental retardation** (IQ range 35-49) may work under supervision

- Person with **severe mental retardation** (IQ range 20-34) has limited abilities to take care of him or herself
- Person with **profound mental retardation** (IQ range below 20) needs constant care

Treatment: family counseling, speech and language therapy, behavior therapy, and special education

Notes:

PEDIATRICS

NEWBORN SCREENING

All newborns should be screened for

- Hypothyroidism
- Phenylketonuria (PKU)
- Galactosemia

APGAR SCORE

APGAR score is a simple method to quickly access the health of a newborn immediately after birth. The scores range from 0 to 10; score 7 and above is normal, 4 to 6 is fairly low, and 3 to 0 is critical.

If 1 minute APGAR score is < 7 then do 5 minutes APGAR score

	Score 0	Score 1	Score 2
Appearance	Whole body blue or pale	Pink body and blue extremities	Whole body is pink
Pulse rate	Absent	<100	> 100
Reflex *	No response	Grimace or feeble cry	Strong cry, pull away with stimulated
Activity	None	Some flexion	Active motion
Respiratory	None	Weak, irregular gasping	Good, Strong cry

* Reflex is measured response to stimulation of the sole of the foot or when a catheter inserted into the nose of a baby

NEWBORN EYE DISCHARGE

Cause	Characteristics	Treatment
Chemical conjunctivitis	• **Serous eye** discharge presents within first 24 hours of life	Supportive
Gonococcal conjunctivitis	• **Purulent eye** discharge presents **within 1st week** of birth	Saline irrigation and IV or IM ceftriaxone
Chlamydia conjunctivitis	• **Purulent eye** discharge presents **after 1st week** of birth	Saline irrigation and oral erythromycin

NEWBORN SKIN CONDITIONS

1. PORT-WINE STAIN
Port–wine stain is a pink, dark red or purple color mark. It often occurs on face but may occur anywhere on the body
Cause: capillary malformation of the skin
Treatment: Pulse laser
Complication: it is associated with Sturge-weber syndrome, glaucoma

2. HEMANGIOMA
Hemangioma is an abnormal buildup of blood vessels in the skin or internal organs. When it occurs in the upper layer of the skin it is called capillary hemangioma and when it occurs in the deeper layer of the skin it is called cavernous hemangioma
Si/Sx: Bright red lesion that usually **appears around 2 months** of age and **regresses by 9 years of age**
Treatment: Pulse laser, and steroids if needed

3.   Differential diagnosis of newborn skin conditions

Condition	Characteristics	Treatment
Erythema toxicum	• Yellow-white papules and pustules (with erythematous base	No treatment
Neonate acne	• Acneiform rash on nose and cheeks, which occurs due to maternal androgen	No treatment
Mongolian spots	• Blue/gray macules on the presacral area *(don't this confuse with child abuse)*	No treatment
Milia	• White papules	No treatment
Cutis marmorata	• Lacy reticular pattern	No treatment

4.   DIAPER RASH

Diaper rash is a common term refers to any skin irritation that occurs in the diaper-covered area.

Types and causes: two main types:

4a. IRRITANT DIAPER DERMATITIS

Irritant diaper dermatitis is caused by **prolong exposure to urine or feces** that irritates the skin. It causes erythema and papules in the area of contact and usually **spares intergluteal folds**

Treatment: Topical petrolatum or topical zinc oxide and diaper holidays

4b. CANDIDA DIAPER DERMATITIS

Candida diaper dermatitis affects the skin under diaper area and **intergluteal skin folds**

Treatment: topical nystatin or clotrimazole

DEVELOPMENT MILESTONES

Age	Social/cognition	Language	Fine motor	Gross motor
2 months	Social Smile	Coos	Swipe at objects, eyes follow object past midline	Holds head up
4 months	Laughs	Orient to voice	Grasp objects	Rolls over supine to prone
6 months	Stranger anxiety	Babbles	Transfer objects hand to hands	Rolls over prone to supine, sits unsupported
9 months	Waves bye-bye, plays peek-a-boo	Says mama, dada (nonspecific), says bye-bye	Pincer grasp	Pulls to stand, crawls
12 months	Separation anxiety	Says mama dada (specific)	Mature grasp	**Stands**, plays with ball
15 months	Temper tantrum	Knows 4-6 words	Uses cup, Stacks 3 cube	**Walks** alone
18 months	Imitate parents at task	Knows 10 words, name common objects	Use spoon for solid food, Stacks 4 cubes	Walks downstairs
2 years	Follows 2 step command	Says 2-3 words sentence	Use spoon for semisolid food, Stacks 6 cubes **Copies a line**	Walks up and down stairs
3 years	Knows first and last name	Use 3 word sentence	Use utensils to eat, Stacks 9 cubes **Copies a circle**	Walks down stairs with alternating feet
4years	**Participates in group play**	Counts to 10	Grooms self, **Copies a cross**	Rides tricycle

- Moro reflex disappears by 3-4 months of age
- Rooting and grasp reflex disappear by 4-6 months of age
- Parachute reflex disappears by 6-8 months of age

CARDIOLOGY

CONGENITAL HEART DISEASE

Cyanotic congenital heart disease present at birth and has right-to-left that usually results in low levels of oxygen in the blood. Most common cyanotic disease that present during neonatal period are referred as 5 T's, are:

1. Tetralogy of Fallot (TOF)
2. Tricuspid atresia
3. Truncus arteriosus
4. Transposition of the great arteries (TGA)
5. Total anomalous pulmonary venous connection

MOST COMMOMON CONGENITAL HEART DISEASES

1. TRANSPOSITION OF THE GREAT VESSELS

In this condition aortic and pulmonary veins and arteries have switched their positions

Risk factors: it is associated with infant of diabetic mother

Si/Sx: neonates present with severe **cyanosis** immediately **after delivery**

Diagnosis:

- Murmur: may or may not have single loud S2 murmur
- **Chest X-ray** shows "**egg on string**" appearance

Treatment: Surgery correction is the definitive treatment, but prostaglandin E1 is given to keep ductus arteriosus patent (PDA). PDA may prolong neonate's life until surgical correction is possible.

- TGA is the most common cyanotic condition of infancy
- TOF is most common cyanotic condition in children

---

2. TETRALOGY OF FALLOT

Tetralogy of Fallot is the most common cyanotic heart disease that presents later in life. It is a combination of four different defects: pulmonary stenosis, right ventricle hypertrophy, overriding aorta, and VSD.

Si/Sx: patient usually present with irritability, cyanosis that occurs during exertion and **relives with squatting**

Diagnosis:
- Systolic thrill heard along the left sternal border
- Chest x-ray shows decreased pulmonary marking and" **boot-shaped heart**" appearance of the heart

Treatment: Surgical repair at 4- 12 months of age

3. VENTRICULAR SEPTAL DEFECT (VSD)

Ventricular septal defect is the most common congenital heart defect. It is defined as one or more hole in the ventricle septum that separates right and left ventricle

Risk factor: it is associated with fetal alcohol syndrome, TORCH syndrome, and trisomy 13, 18, and 21

Si/Sx: some babies may not have any symptoms, but symptoms may include shortness of breath, failure to thrive, cyanosis, edema

Diagnosis:
- Physical exam shows harsh holosystolic murmur over left lower sternal border, loud pulmonic S2 murmur
- Chest x-ray shows increased vascular marking
- Echocardiogram shows normal heart with small VSD defects and RVH or large VSD defects with LVH

Treatment:
- Small VSD **closes spontaneously** within 6 months of age
- Large VSDs require surgical repair
- Preexisting CHF is treated with diuretics and digoxin

Complication: CHF, infective endocarditis, pulmonary hypertension, failure to thrive

4. ATRIAL SEPTAL DEFECT (ASD)

ASD is defined as one or more hole in the atrial septum that separates right and left atria

Types:
- Ostium primary
- Ostium secundum (most common)

Si/Sx: patients with small defects may not have any symptoms, or symptoms may not occur until middle age or later. Symptoms includes shortness of breath, fatigue, edema, heart palpitations, cyanosis

Diagnosis:
- Physical exam shows loud S1, wide fixed-split S2 with systolic murmur
- Chest x-ray shows increased pulmonary marking and cardiomegaly
- Echocardiograph with color Doppler shows blood flow between atria

Treatment: Majority of ASD **closes spontaneously** by age 4. Larger ASD or symptomatic ASD are **surgical repaired**

Complications: Pulmonary HTN, MVP, dysrhythmia

5. COARCTATION OF THE AORTA

Coarctation of the aorta is narrowing of the aorta. Almost in all cases it occurs at the origin of left subclavian artery

Risk factors: Turner syndrome, bicuspid aortic valve, patent ductus arteriosus

Si/SX: depends on the severity of the condition. Babies with the severe condition usually are symptomatic soon after birth. Symptoms may include irritability, heavy sweating, difficulty breathing

Diagnosis:
- Physical exam shows **pink upper body and blue lower body, and blood pressure that is higher in arms than legs**
- Chest X-ray shows rib notching and narrowing of aorta at the site of the coarctation giving number **"3" appearance**
- Cardiac catheterization is the definitive diagnosis

Treatment: Surgical correction is the **definitive treatment, but** prostaglandin E1 is given to **keep ductus arteriosus patent** (PDA). PDA may prolong neonate's life until surgical correction is possible.

6. PATENT DUCTUS ARTERIOSUS (PDA)

Ductus arteriosus is a blood vessel that connects the left pulmonary artery to aorta, which allow blood to bypass the fetus' lungs. Soon after birth ductus closes, but when the ductus fails to close, then this condition is called patent ductus arteriosus.

Risk factor: female gender, congenital rubella, prematurity

Si/Sx: Patient with small PDA may not have any symptoms, but symptoms may include poor feeding habits, shortness of breath, poor growth, rapid pulse

Diagnosis:
- Physical exam shows " **Machinery" like, to-and-fro murmur**, wide pulse pressure and bounding arterial pulses
- Diagnosis is confirmed with echocardiography or cardiac catheterization

Treatment:
- **Indomethacin** is given to block prostaglandin production and close the patent ductus
- If indomethacin is ineffective or if the patient is more than 6-8 months old, then do **surgery** to close PDA.

GASTROENTEROLOGY

1. NECROTIZING ENTERCOLITIS

Necrotizing enterocolitis is a medical condition seen mostly in **premature infants**, in which portion of bowel undergoes inflammation and necrosis. If it is not treated promptly, then it can be life-threatening

Si/Sx: symptoms usually develops within first 2 weeks of life, and may include apnea, abdominal distention, bloody stool, fever, lethargy

Diagnosis:
- Based on symptoms and abdominal X-ray, which shows **pneumatosis intestinalis** (air bubbles in the bowel)

Treatment: Stop feeding; decompress the gut by inserting small tube in the stomach, IV antibiotics and surgical removal of necrotic bowel

2. MECONIUM ILIUM

Meconium is the first stool that a newborn has, it is usually very thick and stick. When meconium gets even thicker and stickier than the normal meconium, it blocks the small intestine (ileum), and it is called meconium ilium. Meconium ilium is associated with cystic fibrosis

Si/Sx: abdominal distention, **bilious vomit**, and no passage of the first stool (meconium)

Diagnosis: best initial test is abdominal x-ray

Treatment: Gastrografin enema

3. HIRSCHSPRUNG DISEASE

Hirschsprung disease is a congenital defect in never fiber of distal bowel that results in improper peristalsis and obstruction in the bowel.

Si/Sx: failure to pass meconium shortly after birth, failure to pass stool is first 48 hours of life

Diagnosis:

- Rectal exam shows **patent anus**
- Abdominal X-ray shows distended bowel loop with no air in rectum
- **Barium enema** shows **megacolon** proximal to the obstruction
- Most accurate test is **rectal suction biopsy**

Treatment: Surgical resection of **aganglionic colon**

4. IMPERFORATE ANUS

Imperforate anus is congenital defect in which opening of anus is blocked or missing

Si/Sx: failure to pass meconium shortly after birth, failure to pass stool is first 48 hours of life

Diagnosis: Rectal exam shows **imperforate anus**

Treatment: surgery

5. DUODENAL ATRESIA

Duodenal atresia is a congenital condition in which first part of small intestine (duodenum) is partially or completely blocked

Si/Sx: bilious (greenish) vomiting, upper abdominal swelling, absent of bowel movement after few meconium stool

Diagnosis: Abdominal **X-ray** shows air in the stomach and in the first part of the duodenum, which is known as **double bubble sign**

Treatment: Nasogastric tube is placed to decompress the stomach, IV fluid and electrolytes replacement to correct the fluids and electrolyte imbalance. Definitive treatment is **surgical correction**

6. INTUSSUSCEPTION

Intussusception is a medical condition in which one part of the small intestine slides into another and leads to bowel obstruction

Si/Sx: crying and **drawing knees up to the chest, "Currant jelly stool"** in diaper, lethargy, fever

Risk factors: previous infection with rotavirus, Meckle's diverticulum, intestinal lymphoma, Henoch-Schonlein purpura,

Diagnosis:
- Physical exam shows **sausage shaped mass in RLQ**
- Ultrasound may be helpful
- **Air enema** is diagnostic and therapeutic

Treatment: IV fluids and electrolytes to correct the fluids and electrolytes imbalance. **Air enema** is diagnostic and therapeutic

7.   INTESTINAL MALROTATION

Intestinal malrotation is a congenital anomaly in which intestine is incompletely rotated around the superior mesentery artery

Si/Sx: bilious vomiting, bloody diarrhea, poor appetite, fever, lethargy

Diagnosis:
- Abdominal X-ray may show intestinal obstruction
- Ultrasound is the best initial diagnostic test

Treatment: IV **fluids and electrolytes** to correct the fluids and electrolytes imbalance. **Surgery is the definitive** treatment and it should be done immediately after fluid and electrolytes replacement.

8.   PYLORUS STENOSIS

Pylorus stenosis is narrowing of the pylorus, the opening of the stomach into the small intestine. This prevents the stomach from emptying into the small intestine

Cause: hypertrophy of pylorus sphincter

Si/Sx: **non-bilious projectile vomiting** after feeding presents 2 weeks to 4 months after birth, persistent hunger, dehydration

Diagnosis:
- Physical exam shows **olive -shaped epigastric mass**
- Labs may show hypochloremic hypokalemic metabolic acidosis due to persistent vomiting
- Ultrasound of abdomen shows **"target- like"** cross-section

Treatment: IV **fluids and electrolytes** to correct the fluids and electrolytes imbalance. **Pylorotomy** is the definitive care

9. MECKEL'S DIVERTICULUM

Meckel's diverticulum is the only true congenital diverticulum in the small intestine and is remnant of the omphalomesenteric duct (also known as vitelline duct or yolk stalk).

Rule of 2s of Meckel's diverticulum is:

- It seen in 2% of the population
- Normally found 2 feet proximal to ileocecal valve
- 2 inches in length
- Contains 2 types of ectopic tissue (gastric and pancreatic)
- Commonly seen in less than 2 years of age
- Male to female ratio is 2:1

Si/Sx: most of the patients are asymptomatic, but the most common presenting symptom is **painless rectal bleeding** (melena, hematochezia)
Diagnosis: Tc-99 pertechnetate scan (also known as radionucleotide scan)
Treatment: Surgical resection of diverticulum

10. NEWBORN ABDOMINAL MALFORMATION

Diagnosis	Characteristic	Treatment
Omphalocele	• Intestine and abdominal organs **protrudes through the umbilicus** (belly buttons), • Intestine is covered with a thin layer of tissue • Associated with trisomy 13, 18 and 21	Surgical repair
Gastroschisis	• Intestine and abdominal organs **protrudes from lateral to midline,** • Intestine is not covered with a layer of tissue	Surgical repair
Umbilical hernia	• Outward **bulging of abdominal** organs through trough the area **around the belly button** • Associated with congenital hypothyroidism.	None, most closes spontaneously

PULMONOLOGY

1.   RESPIRATORY DISTRESS SYNDROME (RSD)

Respiratory distress syndrome is seen in infants **born before 32 weeks of gestation.** It is due to **insufficient surfactant**

Si/Sx: tachypnea, nasal grunting, intercostal retractions

Diagnosis:

- **Best initial test is chest X-ray**, which shows ground-glass lung appearance
- **Most accurate test is lecithin-sphingomyelin ratio** (<2:1 in RSD)

Treatment: oxygen and inhaled exogenous surfactant

Prevention: give IM betamethasone to the mother going under labor before 32 weeks of gestation

2.   TRANSIENT TACHYPNEA OF NEWBORN

Transient tachypnea of newborn is a respiratory disorder seen shortly after birth in **full-term or near-term babies**.

Cause: decreased absorption of fluids in lungs

Diagnosis: Chest X-ray shows fluids in fissure, air trapping, perihilar streaking

Treatment: no treatment is required, it usually resolves within 24-48 hours after delivery

3.   TRACHEOESOPHAGEAL FISTULA (TEF)

Tracheoesophageal fistula is condition in which there is an abnormal connection between esophagus and trachea

Type: there are 4 types of TEF, but the most common type is proximal esophageal atresia and distal tracheoesophageal fistula

Si/Sx: coughing, choking, gagging and cyanosis that coincide with feeding

Diagnosis:

- Chest X-ray with nasogastric tube shows **nasogastric tube coils in the chest, rather than going to the stomach**
- Abdominal X-ray shows air in the stomach

Treatment: Surgery

Complications: Tracheoesophageal fistula is associated with other anomalies, most commonly described as **VACTERL** syndrome. It is important to rule out these disorders, as well.

- Vertebral defect
- Anal atresia
- Cardiac abnormality
- TEF
- Renal and radial anomaly
- Limb syndrome

4.   CHOANAL ATRESIA

Choanal atresia is a congenital condition in which there is an abnormal blockage of nasal passage (choana)

Si/Sx: classic symptom that a newborn turns **blue** when **trying to breathe through nose** and **pink when crying,** inability to feed and breath at the same time

Diagnoses: Inability to pass nasogastric tube through nasopharynx

Treatment: establish the airway and then surgical resection of obstruction

Complications: Choanal atresia is associated with other anomalies, most commonly described as **CHARGE syndrome**. It is important to rule out these disorders, as well.

- Coloboma
- Heart defects
- Atresia of nasal choana
- Growth Retardation
- Genitourinary abnormalities
- Ear abnormality

5.   PERTUSSIS

Pertussis (also known as whooping cough) is highly contagious respiratory disease caused by *Bordetella pertussis*

Stages: Pertussis presents in three stages:

- **Catarrhal stage**, which usually lasts from 1-2 weeks. It begins as "cold-like" symptoms such as rhinorrhea, sneezing, but later in phase, cough develops and symptoms become worse
- **Paroxysmal stage**, which lasts 2-4 weeks. It usually begins as harsh and dry cough, but later in phase, it becomes "whooping" cough

- **Convalescent stage**, which lasts for 1-2 weeks, and patient usually recovers in this period, frequency of cough decreases

Diagnosis:
- Clinical diagnosis, patient often have history of **incomplete immunization**
- Initial test is **PCR of nasopharyngeal** aspiration
- Accurate: **Culture**

Treatment: Oral **erythromycin** to **patient** and all **close contacts**

6. CROUP

Croup also known as laryngotracheobronchitis is an **acute inflammatory condition around the larynx (vocal cord)**, mostly in the subglottic space. It is usually seen in fall and winter seasons, in 3 months to 3 years of age children

Cause: most common cause is **parainfluenza virus type 1 and 2**; other causes include influenza A and B, RSV, adenovirus, measles and mycoplasma pneumonia

Si/Sx: barking cough, inspiratory stridor, hoarseness and difficulty breathing which is **worse at night**

Diagnosis:
- Clinical diagnosis
- Anterior-posterior neck x-ray shows **steeple sign (rarely done)**

Treatment: treatment depends on the symptoms
- Patients with **mild** symptoms are managed **outpatient with cool mist therapy**
- Patient with **moderate or severe** symptoms may need **corticosteroids and racemic epinephrine** to reduce airway inflammation
- Unstable patient or patients with severe symptoms may need **intubation**

7. EPIGLOTTITIS

Epiglottitis is a life-threatening condition characterized by inflammation of epiglottis

Cause: Strep. Pyogenes, S. Pneumonia, S. aureus, Mycoplasma, H. Influenza type B (less common cause)

Si/Sx: sudden onset of **dysphagia, drooling in tripod-sitting position**, high fever, stridor, **"hot potato"** voice

Diagnosis:
- Clinical diagnosis
- **Lateral neck** x-ray shows the **thumbprint sign,** but is rarely needed and negative X-ray does not rule out epiglottitis

Treatment: Epiglottitis is a **medical emergency**; do not waste time in doing neck X-ray, immediately **transfer the patient to OR** and treat patient with intubation or tracheostomy and antibiotic such as ceftriaxone or 3rd generation cephalosporin's)

Complication: H. Influenza type B is the rare cause of epiglottitis, but it is very contagious. If it is the known cause of epiglottitis, then **all close contacts should be receive rifampin prophylaxis**

8.   BACTERIAL TRACHEITIS

Bacterial tracheitis is a secondary bacterial infection of trachea and it can cause airway obstruction

Cause: S. aureus is the most common cause

Si/Sx: brassy cough, high fever, toxic appearance, respiratory distress, stridor

Diagnosis:
- Clinical diagnosis
- Labs show leukocytosis
- Neck X-ray shows **ragged tracheal air column and subglottic narrowing**

Treatment: nafcillin or ceftriaxone

9.   FOREIGN BODY ASPIRATION

Foreign body aspiration is a life-threatening condition caused by aspiration of an object that may lodge in the larynx or trachea.

Si/Sx: sudden onset of **respiratory distress, choking coughing** and **wheezing**

Diagnosis:
- Chest X-ray, but it may not show some objects because radiolucent objects do not appear on X-ray
- Bronchoscopy is diagnostic

Treatment: rigid bronchoscopy

10. BRONCHIOLITIS

Bronchiolitis is characterized by inflammation and mucus plugs in the smallest airway (bronchioles)

Si/Sx: mild upper respiratory tract infection symptoms (fever, rhinorrhea, cough fever), that soon progress to dyspnea, tachypnea, apnea, intercostal retractions

Cause: RSV (most common cause), parainfluenza, adenovirus

Diagnosis:

- **Chest X-rays** shows intestinal infiltrate, atelectasis, **hyperinflation** of lungs
- Most specific test is **ELISA** of nasopharyngeal swab

Treatment:

- Patient with mild symptoms is managed outpatient with fluids, nebulizer and oxygen, if needed
- Patient with respiratory distress is hospitalized and may require IV fluids, oxygen and nebulized beta-2 agonist

Prevention: high-risk patients should receive RSV IVIG or RSV monoclonal antibodies to prevent bronchiolitis

11. CYSTIC FIBROSIS

Cystic fibrosis is genetic disorder characterized by formations of cyst and fibrosis of exocrine glands

Cause: autosomal recessive defect in CFTR gene on chromosome 7

Si/Sx: multiple respiratory tract infections, failure to thrive, greasy stools, salty sweat. Most common symptom in newborn is meconium ileus

Diagnosis:

- Best initial test is sweat chloride concentration of >60 mEq/L, simultaneously taken from **two different body sites**, on **two separate days**

Treatment:

- Encourage adequate fluid intake
- Oral replacement of pancreatic enzymes and fat-soluble vitamins (A, D, E, and K)
- Nutritional counseling
- Chest physiotherapy, nebulized albuterol or saline
- Long-term ibuprofen to slow the disease progression
- Pneumococcal and influenza vaccine
- Antibiotics, as needed

- Lung transplant for advance disease

12. PNEUMONIA

Differential diagnosis of pneumonia

Age group	Most common cause of pneumonia
Newborn	Streptococcus agalactia, Gram negative rod Chlamydia trachomatis
Infants	Streptococcus agalactia, Gram negative rod Chlamydia
Preschool	RSV, Mycoplasma
Adolescent	Mycoplasma, Chlamydia S. Pneumonia

13. CHLAMYDIA TRACHOMATIS

Chlamydia trachomatis is the common cause of pneumonia in infants of **1-3 months of age.** Patient may have history of chlamydia conjunctivitis
Si/Sx: staccato cough, no fever and no wheezing
Diagnosis:
- CBC with peripheral smear shows **eosinophilia**
- Chest X-ray shows mild interstitial disease

Treatment: erythromycin or other macrolides

14. VIRAL PNEUMONIA

Viral pneumonia is a common in children **less than 5 years of age.** RSV is the most common cause
Si/Sx: low-grade fever, tachypnea and symptoms is upper respiratory tract infection
Diagnosis
- Labs shows WBCs < 20,000 **predominantly lymphocytes**
- Chest X-ray shows hyperinflammation with bilateral interstitial infiltrate and peribronchial cuffing

Treatment: patient with mild pneumonia or no respiratory symptoms usually require **no treatment**. Antibiotics may be given to a patient with worsening symptoms

15. BACTERIAL PNEUMONIA

Bacterial pneumonia is common in children **more than 5 years of age**.
Streptococcus pneumonia is the most common cause of bacterial
pneumonia

Si/Sx: high fevers, chills, cough

Diagnosis

- Chest exam shows rhonchi, diminished breath sounds and
  dullness to percussion
- Labs show WBCs between 15,000 to 40,000 **predominantly
  granulocytes**
- Chest X-ray shows lobar consolidation

Treatment: patient with **mild symptoms** can be managed **outpatient** with
amoxicillin or cefuroxime. Patient with **severe pneumonia** may require
inpatient treatment with **cefuroxime**

16. MYCOPLASMA PNEUMONIA

Mycoplasma pneumonia is most common in adolescents **more than 15
years of age**

Si/Sx: mild symptoms appear over the period of 1-3 weeks. Symptoms
may include fever, chest pain, dry cough, sore throat, rash

Diagnosis:

- CBC may show anemia
- Sputum culture
- IgM viral titer
- Chest x-ray shows lower lobe interstitial pneumonia

Treatment: Erythromycin or other macrolides

MUSCULOSKELETAL DISORDER

1. NEWBORN BRACHIAL NERVES INJURIES

Disorder	Characteristics	Management
Erb-Duchenne palsy	• Injury to C5-C6 • Unable to abduct the shoulder, external rotation and supination of forearm, • **"Waiters tip"** appearance of the arm	Most cases resolve spontaneously but if it does not resolve in first 6 months of life, then patient may have permanent damage
Klumpke paralysis	• Injury to C7-T1 • Hand paralysis with Horner syndrome • **"Claw hand"** appearance of the hand	Same as above

2. CLAVICULAR FRACTURE

Clavicular fracture in a newborn is common during vaginal delivery. X-ray is the best diagnostic test. Clavicular fracture often self-resolves and requires no treatment other than **immobilization of the arm**

3. CLEFT LIP

Cleft lip is a birth defect caused by **failure of fusion of the maxillary and medial nasal processes.** It is surgically treated at 3 months of age

4. CLEFT PALATE

Cleft palate is a birth defect caused by **failure of fusion of the lateral palatine processes, nasal septum, and median palatine processes**. It is surgically treated between 9- 18 months of age.

5.   CONGENITAL HIP DYSPLASIA

Congenital hip dysplasia is dislocation of the hip in infants

Diagnosis

- Physical exam shows positive **Barlow maneuver and Ortolani maneuver. Barlow maneuver;** mild adduction of the hip while applying pressure on the knee causes hip dislocation. Ortolani maneuver moves the dislocated hip back into the socket. **Ortolani maneuver** in which index and middle finger are placed along the greater trochanter of femur and thumb along the inner thigh. Place the infant with hip and leg at 90 degrees and gently abduct the hip while lifting forward on the femur.
- Ultrasound of the hip

Treatment: Pavlik harness

6.   LEGG-CAVLÉ-PERTHES (AVASCULAR NECROSIS OF FEMORAL HEAD)

Legg-cavlé-perthes is childhood hip disorder caused by the disruption of blood flow to the head of the femur. Lack of blood supply leads to bone death (avascular necrosis). It is common in children between 2 to 8 years of age

Si/Sx: hip, knee or groin pain that may exacerbate with hip or leg movement, painful limp

Diagnosis

- Labs show **normal WBS and ESR**
- X-ray shows femoral head sclerosis and femoral head widening

Treatment: goal of management is to reduce pain and prevent permanent damage; casting, **rest, NSAIDs and get surgical consult**

7.   SLIPPED CAPITAL FEMORAL EPIPHYSIS

Slipped capital femoral epiphysis refers to the separation of the ball of the hip joint from the femur. It is often seen in obese adolescence males

Si/Sx: knee pain, hip pain, **painful limp, externally rotated leg**

Diagnosis: X-ray shows widening of joint space, slippage of acetabulum of femoral neck gives " **ice-cream cone sign**"

Treatment: surgical pinning

8.   TRANSIENT SYNOVITIS

Transient synovitis of the hip is a **self-limited inflammatory condition**. It is common in children between 5-10 years of age. It occurs following **viral infection** (most commonly an URI) or **trauma**

Si/Sx: low-grade fever, insidious onset of hip pain

Diagnosis:

- Transient synovitis is a **diagnosis of exclusion**
- WBC, ESR and x-ray are all normal

Treatment: Bed rest and NSAIDs

COLLAGEN VASCULAR DISEASE

1.   JUVENILE RHEUMATOID ARTHRITIS (JRA)

Juvenile rheumatoid arthritis is the most common type of arthritis in children between 6 months to 16 years of age

Cause: Autoimmune

Types: three most common are of JRA are:

- **Systemic still's disease,** which causes joint pain, **daily spiking fever that returns to normal daily,** salmon colored rash, generalized lymphadenopathy
- **Polyarticular arthritis,** which involves > 5 joints, causes low-onset fever and lethargy. It may progress to rheumatoid arthritis
- **Pauciarticular arthritis,** which involves < 4 joints, primarily knee, ankle and elbows

Diagnosis:

- Rheumatoid factor (RF)
- ESR
- ANA
- X-ray of joints

Treatment: NSAIDs is best initial therapy. If NSAIDs are ineffective, then use methotrexate

Prognosis: positive RF signifies poor prognosis, whereas positive ANA signifies good prognosis

2. KAWASAKI DISEASE

Kawasaki disease is an autoimmune disorder that affects the mucus membrane, lymph nodes, large and medium size blood vessels and heart. It is common in children < 5years of age, mainly Japanese children
Diagnosis: fever> 104°F for > 5 days, not responding to any antibiotics, plus 4 out of 5 criteria: (mnemonic CRASH)

1. Conjunctivitis
2. Nonvascular **Rash**
3. Coronary **A**rtery aneurysm
4. **S**trawberry tongue, oropharyngeal erythema, dry & cracked lips
5. **H**and and feet swelling, desquamation of fingertips

Treatment:

- Immediate **IVIG and high dose aspirin**
- Get baseline **2D echocardiogram**; follow **up 2D echo in 2-3 weeks** and **again at 6-8 weeks**

Complications of Kawasaki diseases are coronary artery aneurysm, myocarditis MI, CHF

Note: Kawasaki disease is the only exception in which aspirin is given to the children.

3. HENOCH-SCHÖNLEIN PURPURA (HSP)

Henoch-Schönlein purpura is an immunoglobulin (IgA) mediated vascular damage that causes the inflammation and bleeding in the small blood vessels in skin, joints, intestines and kidney
Si/Sx: abdominal pain, **petechiae and purpura on legs and buttocks,** hematuria
Diagnosis:

- Urinalysis may show RBC casts
- Blood test shows increased platelet
- Increased WBC and ESR
- Increased IgA and IgM immunoglobulins

Treatment: symptomatic treatment for mild disease. Patient with severe disease may require steroids

NEUROLOGY

1. NEWBORN HEAD CONDITIONS

Condition	Characteristics	Treatment
Caput Succedaneum	• **Diffuse swelling** of the scalp that crosses **the midline suture**	No treatment, **resolves itself in days**
Cephalohematoma	• **Subperiosteal hematoma** that **does not cross** the midline suture • May need do CT head to rule out fracture	No treatment, **resolve itself in weeks to months**

Anterior fontanelle usually closes by 18 months of age. Delayed closure or abnormally large fontanelle usually suggests IUGR, rickets, hydrocephalus or hypothyroidism

2. SPINA BIFIDA
Spina bifida is the congenital disorder of spinal cord, which is caused by incomplete closure of the embryonic neural tube. Three types of spina bifida are as follow:

2a. **Spina bifida occulta** (occulta means hidden) is often **hidden by newborn's skin.** In some patients, it is found incidentally during x-ray or other imaging. However, in some cases classic clues may be helpful such as abnormal tufts of hair on the back, dimple on the skin, collection of fat or skin discoloration on the skin above spinal defect.

2b. **Meningocele** is a rare form, in this condition **meninges** (membrane of the spinal cord) **comes out of the vertebral opening**

2c. **Myelomeningocele** is a severe form, in this **condition meninges** and **spinal cord** comes out of the vertebral defect.

Prevention: neural tube defects can be prevented; if a pregnant woman **without risk factors** takes **1mg folic acid** per day or pregnant woman **with risk factors** takes **4 mg folic** acid per day

3.   NEUROFIBROMATOSIS
Neurofibromatosis is a genetic disorder of the nervous system. Two main types of neurofibromatosis are:

  3a. Type 1 neurofibromatosis is an autosomal dominant defect in **chromosome 7**. Patients usually present with **café-au-lait spot, axillary freckles, pigmented Lisch nodules**

  3b. **Type 2 neurofibromatosis** is an autosomal dominant defect in **chromosome 22.** Patient usually present with bilateral acoustic neuroma (**bilateral hearing loss**), gait disturbance

4.   FEBRILE SEIZURE
Febrile seizure is characterized by seizure lasting < 15 minutes, which is triggered by a fever (> 102° F). It is common in otherwise healthy children between 9 months to 5 years of age
Diagnosis:
  • Physical exam is usually normal
  • No labs work or imaging is needed
Treatment: Acetaminophen is given to control fever

5.   ABSENCE SEIZURE
Absence seizure also knows as petit mal seizure, characterized by brief loss and return of consciousness without post-ictal state.
Diagnosis: EEG shows 3 seconds spike and waves
Treatment: Ethosuximide

HEMATOLOGY

1.   LEAD POISONING
Lead poisoning screening is usually done in children at 12 months of age,
but it is done at 6 months of age in children with high risk factors
High risk factors: living in building built before 1960's or painted before
1978, eating paint, live near battery recycling plant
Si/Sx: **change in behavior, stomach pain, constipation, lead lines on
gums**
Diagnosis:
- Labs: MCV< 90, hypochromic anemia, basophilic stippling,
  increased free erythrocyte porphyrin
- Best initial test **is blood lead level**
- Confirmatory test is **venous blood level**
- **X-ray** of the long bone shows dense lead lines

Treatment: usually depends on blood lead level (discussed below)

Blood lead level (BLL) g/dl	Management
10 – 14	Educate patient and family, repeat BLL **in 3 months**
15 - 19	Educate patient and family, repeat BLL **in 2 months**
20 - 44	Educate patient and family, repeat BLL **in 1 month**
45 - 70	Remove patient from source, and give **EDTA*** or DMSA*
≥ 70	Hospitalization + 2 medicines • If a patient has **encephalop**athy, then give EDTA*+ **BAL*** • If a patient has **no encephal**opathy, then give **EDTA*+ BAL* or DMSA***

*EDTA = Ethylenediaminetetraacetic acid
*BAL = Dimercaprol or British anti-lewisite
*DMSA= Succimer or 2,3-dimercaptosuccinic acid

RENAL AND URINARY TRACT MALFORMATION

1. HYPOSPADIAS
Hypospadias is a congenital defect in which there is an **abnormal opening on the ventral (underside) side of the penis.** In this condition parents of the patients are advised to **not to have circumcision in newborn** because the foreskin of the penis is used to close the hypospadias

2. EPISPADIAS
Epispadias is a congenital defect in which urethra ends in an abnormal opening on the **dorsal (upper) side of the penis**. This condition is often associated with exstrophy of the bladder. Therefore, it is essential to get an urologist consult before repairing the epispadias

3. CRYPTORCHIDISM
Cryptorchidism or undescended testes is a condition in which **one or both testes fail to descend** in the scrotum. Normally testes are fully descended in the scrotum by 1year of life. Patient is **observed until 1 year of age** and if tests **do not descend by that time, then surgery is performed**. Cryptorchidism is associated with **testicular cancer; higher the testes are found higher the risk**. Moreover, risk of testicular cancer **does not decrease after the surgery.**

4. HYDROCELE
Hydrocele is fluid-filled sac in the scrotum. It is common is newborn infants. However, in some cases it may occur with an inguinal hernia.
Diagnosis:
   * Physical exam: **scrotum** may **light up** with transillumination test (shine a light through scrotum)
   * Ultrasound can confirm the diagnosis
Treatment: Hydroceles usually resolves within 6 months. However, if hydrocele is caused by inguinal hernia, then it should be surgically corrected

5. VARICOCELE
Varicocele is an abnormal **dilation of the pampiniform venous plexus** in the scrotum
Si/Sx: aching pain in the scrotum, feeling of heaviness in the testicles

Diagnosis:
- Scrotum exam shows visibly enlarged veins " **bag of worms**"
- Most accurate test is ultrasound

Treatment: treatment may not be necessary, but it is surgically repaired if it is causing severe pain, testicular atrophy or infertility

6. WILMS' TUMOR

Wilms' tumor is a rare tumor that may affect one or both kidneys. Usually seen in children between 2-4 years of age

Risk factors: Wilms tumor associated with aniridia, hemihypertrophy, hypospadias, undescended testes, Beckwith-Wiedemann syndrome, WAGR syndrome: Wilms tumor, aniridia, genitourinary abnormalities, and mental retardation

Symptoms: painless abdominal or flank mass that **does not cross the midline**, fever, nausea, vomiting, hematuria, hypertension

Diagnosis:
- Abdominal ultrasound or CT shows intrarenal mass
- Biopsy is usually not done because of high risk abdominal seeding with malignant cells

Treatment: Total nephrectomy, chemotherapy and radiation. Partial nephrectomy if both kidneys are involved

7. NEUROBLASTOMA

Neuroblastoma is a malignant tumor of the neural crest cell. It is usually seen in infants and children less than 2 years of age.

Location: most Neuroblastoma begins in adrenal gland, but they may occurs next to spinal cords or chest and spread to bones, face, skull, pelvic, shoulder, arms, legs, bone marrow, lymph node, eyes and skin

Si/Sx: opsoclonus-myoclonus syndrome also know as " **dancing eyes and dancing feet syndrome**", bone pain, flushed skin, tachycardia, profuse sweating

Diagnosis
- CBC, ESR, coagulation studies
- Urinary VMA and HMA
- Imaging: Abdominal and chest CT, bone scan
- BUN/Cr, LFTs

Treatment: localized tumors are surgically resected. Chemotherapy and radiation for metastatic tumors

8. TESTICULAR TORSION

Testicular torsion is the twisting of the spermatic cord, which blocks the testicle's blood supply

Si/Sx: sudden onset of testicular pain, nausea, vomiting, lightheadedness

Diagnosis:

- Physical exam shows **tender and high riding testes, and absent cremasteric reflex**
- Diagnoses can be confirmed with ultrasound, but it is rarely needed

Treatment: immediate surgical intervention

9. EPIDIDYMITIS

Epididymitis is characterized by inflammation of epididymis. It is common in young men between 19-35 years of age

Causes: gonorrhea and chlamydia are the most common cause, but other causes may include regular use of a urethral catheter, recent surgery of urinary tract

Si/Sx: testicular pain with fever, pyuria, painful scrotal swelling

Diagnosis:

- Physical exam shows **tests at normal position**, tenderness around epididymis
- Urinalysis and urine culture

Treatment: bed rest and antibiotics

CHILDHOOD IMMUNODEFICIENCY

1. HEREDITARY ANGIOEDEMA

Hereditary angioedema is a serious condition caused by hereditary deficiency of **C1 esterase inhibitor**

Si/Sx: **diffuse swelling** of face and airway, and abdominal cramping

Diagnosis: C1 inhibitor level, C1 inhibitor function , C2 and C4 compliment pathway

Treatment:

- **Acute attack treatment: Fresh frozen plasma, it contains C1 inhibitor**
- Chronic treatment: androgen medication (danazol, or stanzol), these increasing the liver production of C1 esterase inhibitor, which reduces the frequency and severity of the attacks.

CHILDHOOD IMMUNODEFICIENCY continued.

Condition	Characteristics	Treatment
Wiskott-Aldrich syndrome	• X-linked disease • Newborn with nonstop bleeding after circumcision • Triad consists of: **eczema, thrombocytopenia and recurrent infection** • Diagnosis: clinical + genetics	Bone marrow transplant
Chediak-Higashi syndrome	• Increased bleeding time, recurrent infection, albinism • Diagnosis: giant granules in leukocytosis	Bone marrow transplant
DiGeorge's syndrome	• New born with **tetany and seizure** (due to hypocalcemia) **within 24-48 hours of life** • Physical exam: wide set eyes and low set ears • Cause: congenital absent of 3rd and 4th pharyngeal pouch results in absent thymus and parathyroid • Diagnosis: clinical	Bone marrow transplant or thymus transplant
IgA deficiency	• Recurrent respiratory, **skin, GI, GU infection** • Anaphylaxis reaction during blood transfusion	Supportive care
Burton agammaglo-bulinemia	• Recurrent **sinopulmonary infection** starting around 6 months of age • **Small or absent lymph nodes, thymus and spleen** • Diagnosis: **B-cells are missing** and other **immunoglobulins are decreased**	IVIG
Severe combined immune deficiency	• Multiple viral, fungal and bacterial infections • Diagnosis: **Absence lymph nodes, thymus** and **spleen**	Bone marrow transplant
Chronic granulomatosis disease	• Recurrent **pneumonia, abscess formation** • Diagnostic test is **NBT or DHR test**	Bone marrow transplant

CHILDHOOD VIRAL ILLNESS

Virus	Characteristics	Treatment
Measles	• Maculopapular rash that starts on the face, then spreads down the body, and it fades in the similar pattern • **Cough, coryza, conjunctivitis** and **Koplik spots** (gray white spots on buccal mucosa) • Diagnosis: Clinical	Supportive and oral vitamin A supplement
Rubella	• Maculopapular rash that starts on the face, then spread down the body, and it fades in the similar pattern • **Retroauricular, posterior and occipital lymphadenitis, arthralgia** • Diagnosis: clinical	Supportive
Roseola (HHV-6)	• High fever, up to 106°F or 41°C and occipital lymphadenopathy. When **fever resolves** generalized **rose-colored** popular **rash appears** • Diagnosis: Clinical	Supportive
Varicella	• **Pruritic rash** in **various stages**: macules, papules, vesicle and pustules • Diagnosis: Tzanck test, most accurate test is viral culture	Supportive and topical ointment
Erythema infectiosum (Parvovirus 19, fifth's disease)	• Fever, headache, malaise, **arthritis, lacy reticular rash** on extremities and over trunk, **"slapped cheek"** appearance on the face • Diagnosis: Clinical	Supportive
Mumps	• Fever, headache, malaise **swelling of parotids** (unilateral or bilateral), **orchitis** • Diagnosis: Clinical	Supportive

EAR INFECTION

1. OTITIS EXTERNA

Otitis Externa also know as swimmer's ear, is inflammation of the outer ear and ear canal

Si/Sx: severe pain with **manipulations of outer ear**

Cause: Excessive dryness, wetting

Diagnosis:
- Clinical diagnosis
- Ear exam may show thick otorrhea, edema, and erythema

Treatment:
- Combination of topical antibiotics neomycin, polymyxin and topical steroids
- If there is marked ear edema to the point that the ear canal is blocked and topical antibiotics may not penetrates far enough into the ear canal to be effective. Carefully place a **soaked wick** with **topical drops 3 times daily for 2 days to open the ear canal**, so that topical medicines will penetrate the canal

2. OTITIS MEDIA

Otitis Media is an inflammation of the middle ear. It is common in children following upper respiratory infection (URI)

Cause: Eustachian tube drain fluid from the middle ear. Blockage of eustachian tube can lead to fluid buildup, which can cause ear infection

Risk factors: children between 6 months to 2 years are high risk due to short and straight eustachian tube, air pollution

Si/Sx: decreased hearing, ear pain, irritability fever, otorrhea

Diagnosis:
- Otoscope shows **loss of light reflex and decreased mobility of tympanic membrane** (most sensitive and specific factor)

Treatment: Amoxicillin is the best initial treatment. If amoxicillin is ineffective, then give oral amoxicillin-clavulanate or IM ceftriaxone

Complication: Mastoiditis, meningitis

ENDOCRINOLOGY

1. CONGENITAL HYPOTHYROIDISM
Congenital hypothyroidism is caused by decreased thyroid hormone production or agenesis of thyroid

Si/Sx: most infant have few or no symptoms, but infant with severe hypothyroidism may have **large tongue, hypotonia,** edema, mental retardation, umbilical hernia, widened anterior and posterior fontanels

Diagnosis: low T4 and increased TSH

Treatment: levothyroxine

Complications: Untreated or delayed treatment may lead to mental retardation and growth problems.

Note: it is mandate by law to screen all newborn for hypothyroidism

2. CONGENITAL ADRENAL HYPERPLASIA (CAH)
Congenital adrenal hyperplasia is group of autosomal recessive disorders of adrenal gland

Types: three main types of CAH are: discussed below

Type	Characteristics	Treatment
21 - hydroxylase CAH	• **Hypotension and virilization** • **Diagnosis:** labs show **increased** K, ATCH and 17-hydroxyprogestrone, and **decreased** Na, aldosterone and cortisol	Prednisone, fluid and electrolytes replacement as needed
11-beta-hydroxylase CAH	• **Hypertension and virilization** • **Diagnosis: increased serum 11 -deoxycortisol**	Same as above
17alpha-hydroxylase CAH	• **Hypertension** • **Diagnosis:** labs shows **hypokalemia and metabolic alkalosis**	Same as above

NEWBORN JAUNDICE
Type: two main types of newborn jaundices are **physiologic** and
pathologic jaundice (discussed in below)

1. PHYSIOLOGIC JAUNDICE
Physiologic jaundice usually appears **2-4 days** after birth.
Mechanism: Before the baby is born and is growing inside the mother's
womb, placenta removes the bilirubin. After the baby is born, baby's liver
removes the bilirubin from the body via enzyme **glucuronosyltransferase.**
However, after birth it takes some time for the liver to gain its function, as
a result, unconjugated **bilirubin** increases, which results in jaundice.
Cause:
- Relative **glucuronosyltransferase** deficiency in newborn
- Increased bilirubin production (In full-term newborn RBCs life
  span is 80-90 days, compare to adults 100-120 days)

Risk factors: factors that increase the risk of physiologic jaundice are
prematurity, polycythemia, breast feeding
Treatment: no treatment needed, physiologic jaundice usually clears on its
own

2. PATHOLOGIC JAUNDICE
Pathologic jaundice is caused by the factors that alter the bilirubin
metabolism in the liver
Characteristics of pathologic jaundice
- If it appears in first 24 hours of life or after 14 days of life
- Direct bilirubin> 2mg/dl/day
- Total bilirubin increases > 5mg/dl/day
- Total bilirubin > 12mg/dl/day in terms infant

Cause: Causes pathologic jaundice can be divided into conjugated and
unconjugated hyperbilirubinemia
Conjugated hyperbilirubinemia is caused by the followings:
- **Infection:** TORCH infection, sepsis, hepatitis A & B, syphilis,
- **Metabolic cause:** galactosemia, alpha -1 antitrypsin deficiency
- **Heredity cause:** Rotor syndrome, Dubin-Johnson syndrome
- **Other cause:** cystic fibrosis, hypothyroidism, **breastfeeding
  jaundice**

Unconjugated hyperbilirubinemia is caused by the followings:

- **Hemolytic** such as sickle cell disease, G6PD deficiency, Rh incompatibility, alpha-thalassemia
- **Congenital causes:** Crigler-Najjar syndrome, Gilbert syndrome
- **Other causes:** jaundice, polycythemia, hypothyroidism, **breast milk**

Complication: elevated unconjugated (indirect bilirubin) can cross the blood brain barrier and cause kernicterus (bilirubin encephalopathy)

Treatment:

- Treat the underlying cause
- When **unconjugated** bilirubin is **10-15 mg/dl**, start **phototherapy** to break down the bilirubin pigment
- If **phototherapy is ineffective** or patient has developed **bilirubin encephalopathy,** then do **exchange transfusion**

What is the difference between breastfeeding jaundice and breast milk jaundice?

Breastfeeding jaundice occurs in the **first week of life**. It is caused by insufficient breast milk intake, which results in dehydration or low caloric intake. Treatment: **Increase breastfeeding sessions to 8-10 time a day**

Breast milk jaundice occurs around **10-14 days of life**. There is no clear cause of breast milk jaundice. Substances in the maternal milk such as beta-glucuronidase and nonesterified fatty acid may inhibit the normal bilirubin metabolism, which increases the level of **unconjugated bilirubin**. Treatment: **phototherapy or exchange transfusion**. Breastfeeding it continued.

LYSOSOMAL STORAGE DISEASE

Lysosomal storage disease is caused by deficiency of lysosomal enzymes that usually eliminates unwanted substance from the cells of the body. Substance builds up in the cells of organs and causes organ damage

Mode of inheritance: all the below mentioned lysosomal disease are **autosomal recessive** disease, other than **Fabry's disease** and **Hunter's syndrome both of which are X-linked recessive**

Disease	Characteristics
Gaucher disease	• Deficiency of Beta-glucocerebrosidase enzyme leads to glucocerebroside accumulation in brain, liver, spleen, and bone marrow. • Gaucher cells are characterized as " **crinkle paper"**
Niemann-Pick disease	• Deficiency of sphingomyelinase enzyme leads to accumulation of sphingomyelin and cholesterol to in reticuloendothelial system and causes hepatosplenomegaly
Tay-Sachs disease	• Deficiency of hexosaminidase A leads to ganglioside GM2 to build up in cells, especially nerve cells in the brain. • Patient usually die by age 4 or 5 • Eye exam usually shows **cherry-red** spot in the macula
Metachromatic leukodystrophy	• Deficiency of arylsulfatase A leads to sulfatide accumulation in brain, kidneys, gallbladder and peripheral nerves
Krabbe's disease	• Deficiency of galactocerebroside beta-galactosidase leads to glucocerebroside in brain, which causes myelin breakdown in nerves and optic nerve. • Patient usually die before age 2
Fabry's syndrome	• Deficiency of alpha-galactosidase leads to ceramide trihexoside in kidney, heart, and skin. • It usually leads to renal failure
Hurler's syndrome	• Deficiency of alpha-L-iduronidase leads to mucopolysaccharides build up and cause corneal clouding, mental retardation, joint disease
Hunter's syndrome	• This is a milder form of hurler's syndrome. It is caused by deficiency of iduronate sulfatase. There is no corneal clouding in Hunter's syndrome

GENETIC DISORDERS

1. DOWN SYNDOMRE

Cause: Down syndrome also known as trisomy 21, caused by presence of three copies of chromosome 21, instead of normal two copies

Characteristics: metal retardation (Down syndrome is the most common cause of mental retardation), **slanted palpebral fissure, epicanthal folds, transverse palmar crease**

Associated with endocardial cushion defect, VSD, ASD, duodenal atresia, hypothyroidism, increased risk of acute lymphocytic leukemia, Alzheimer's disease

2. EDWARDS' SYNDROME

Cause: Edwards' syndrome also known as trisomy 18, caused by presence of three copies of chromosome 18, instead of normal two copies

Characteristics: clenched fist with index finger **overlapping 3rd and** 4th fingers, **rocker bottom feet**, hammer toe, low set ears, hypoplastic mandible

Associated with VSD, ASD, Polycystic kidney disease

Life expectancy: patient usually dies within first year of life

3. PATAU'S SYNDROME

Cause: Patau's syndrome also known as trisomy 13, caused by presence of three copy of chromosome 13, instead of normal two copies

Characteristics: cleft lip, cleft palate, holoprosencephaly, small head, small eyes, polydactyly

Associated with VSD, ASD, Polycystic kidney disease

Life expectancy: patient usually dies within first year of life

4. FRAGILE X SYNDROME

Cause: X-linked disorder associated with CGG trinucleotide repeats, affecting methylation and expression of Fragile X mental retardation protein (FMRP), which is required for normal neural development

Characteristics: elongated face with large jaw, large or everted ears, low muscle tone, hyperextensible ear, double-jointed thumbs, autism

5. DOUBLE Y MALES

Cause: genetic defect in which a male has an extra Y chromosome (XYY)
Characteristics: very tall height, nodulocystic acne, **antisocial behavior, aggressive**

6. KLINEFELTER SYNDROME

Cause: Genetic defect in which a male has an extra X chromosome (XXY)
Characteristic: tall height, **eunuchoid body shape** (long extremities, short trunk, shoulder equal to hip size), **small testicles, gynecomastia, female type hair distribution**

7. TURNER SYNDROME

Cause: genetic defect in **females in which** one of the X chromosomes is missing (X0)
Characteristics: short stature, broad and flat chest, **wide spread nipples, sparse pubic hair, webbed neck, puffy hand and feet**

8. MARFAN SYNDROME

Cause: Autosomal dominant disorder, defect in folding of Fibrillin -1 protein
Characteristics: very tall height, slender limbs with long fingers and toes, flexible joints, **subluxation of lens in one or both eyes, scoliosis**

9. EHLERS-DANLOS SYNDROME

Cause: autosomal dominant defect in elastin gene
Characteristics: Hyperextensible skin, **blue sclera, easy scarring, poor** wound healing, increased joint mobility

10. PHENYLKETONURIA

Cause: autosomal recessive defect in phenylalanine hydroxylase, which is necessary to metabolize phenylalanine. Phenylalanine builds up and converts to phenylpyruvate
Characteristics: mental retardation, **fair skin, fair hair, eczema, fruity smell urine**
Treatment: diet modification, low phenylalanine and high tyrosine

11. GLACTOSEMIA

Cause: Galactose-1 phosphate uridyltransferase deficiency (most common types) impairs galactose metabolism

Characteristic: infant develops symptoms within few days after drinking formula or breast milk that contains lactose. Symptoms include irritability, lethargy, poor feeding, poor weight gain,

Treatment: lactose free milk

12. ANGELMAN SYNDROME

Cause: deletion of **maternal gene located on 15q13q11**

Characteristics: puppet-like movement, ataxia, inappropriate laughter and lack of speech

13. PRADER-WILLI SYNDROME

Cause: deletion of **paternal gene located on 15q13q11**

Characteristics: obese, **hyperphagia, short stature, small genitals,** small hands and feet

FAILURE TO THRIVE (FTT)

Failure to thrive as defined as **height and weight less than 5th percentile** for the age

Cause: FTT can be divided into three main types:
- **Organic factors:** when there is a mental or physical issue with the child himself. Such as GI disorders, inborn error of metabolism, cystic fibrosis, parasites, UTI
- **Inorganic factor:** when a caregiver is providing inadequate or improper feeding
- **Mixed** condition is caused when both organic and inorganic factors are present

Diagnosis:
- Plot height, weight and head circumference on growth chart
- Look for underlying condition
- Dietary history

Treatment: depends on cause
- Treat the underlying cause, if any
- Educate the parents about feeding infant and educate them about formula, food and liquids

TORCH INFECTION

1.   TOXOPLASMOSIS
Presentation: newborn with intracranial calcification, chorioretinitis, hydrocephalus
Cause: if during pregnancy mother consumes infected food (raw meat, drinking raw goat milk) or handles infected cat feces
Diagnosis: IgM serology,
Treatment: Pyrimethamine and sulfadiazine to mother
Prevention
- Mother should avoid above mention risk factor during pregnancy
- Spiramycin given to mother to prevent vertical transmission

2.   VARICELLA-ZOSTER
Presentation: newborn with limb hypoplasia, " zigzag" skin lesions
Risk: Fetus or newborn is at risk of acquiring infection, if rash appears on mother 5 days before the delivery or 2 days after the delivery
Treatment: VariZIG to mother and neonate
Prevention: VZIG within 96 hours after exposure, but VZIG only decreases the effects of virus, it doesn't cures infection
Complication: Maternal pneumonia during varicella zoster infection is the leading cause of maternal death

3.   SYPHILIS
Presentation: depends on time
- **Large edematous placenta** at birth
- Early (<2 years of age) presentation includes snuffles, failure to thrive, maculopapular rash
- Late (>2 years of age) presentation includes Mulberry molars, Hutchinson teeth, saber shins, saddle nose

Diagnosis:
- Best initial test is VDRL or RPR
- Most accurate test is FTA ABS or dark field microscope

Treatment: none
Prevention: Penicillin is only the medicine given to the pregnant mother with positive syphilis to prevent fetal transmission

4. RUBELLA
Presentation: newborn with deafness (most common presentation), congenital heart disease (e.g. PDA), **blueberry muffin rash, cataract**
Diagnosis: IgM serology
Treatment: None

5. CYTOMEGALOVIRUS (CMV)
Presentation: Newborn presents with **periventricular calcification, sensorineural hearing loss**
Diagnosis:
- Best initial test is neonate's urine or saliva titer
- Most accurate is urine or saliva PCR

Treatment: Ganciclovir. Advise parents that ganciclovir doesn't cure the infection; it prevents viral shedding and hearing loss

6. HERPES SYMPLEX VIRUS
Presentation: Newborn with **pneumonia, shock, petechiae on skin, eye and mucous membrane**
Diagnosis:
- Best initial test is Tzanck smear
- Most Accurate is PCR

Treatment: Acyclovir (to mother)
Prevention: If **active lesions** are present on mother genitals **during L&D,** then perform C-section

SCARLET FEVER
Scarlet fever is a bacterial illness caused by group A Streptococcus bacteria. It is common in children between 2 -10 years of age
Si/Sx: 5 main characteristic of scarlet fever are:
1. Strawberry tongue
2. Sandpaper like rash on the trunk
3. Cervical adenopathy
4. Pharyngitis
5. Fever

Diagnosis:
- Throat culture for group A strep
- Rapid antigen test

Treatment: penicillin, azithromycin or cephalosporin. Antibiotic is given to treat infection and **prevent rheumatic fever.**

RHEUMATIC FEVER

Rheumatic fever is an inflammatory disease that can affect heart, joints, skin and brain. It is common in children between 5-15 years of age

Cause: it usually develops 14-28 days after infection with groups A streptococcus bacteria such as strep throat or scarlet fever

Si/Sx: Sydenham chorea (uncoordinated jerky movements of face, hands and feet), chest pain, joint pain, joint swelling, skin rash, skin nodules, fever

Diagnosis: diagnosis of rheumatic fever depends on **two factors:**

1. Jones criteria (2 major and 1 minor)

Major criteria	• Migratory arthritis • Carditis • Subcutaneous skin nodules • Skin rash (Erythema marginatum) • Sydenham's chorea
Minor criteria	• Fever • High ESR • Arthralgia • Prolong PR interval on EKG

2. In addition, evidence of prior group A streptococcus infection by either a culture or positive antistreptolysin O (ASO) antibody titer

Treatment: Penicillin

2013 Recommended Immunizations for Children from Birth Through 6 Years Old

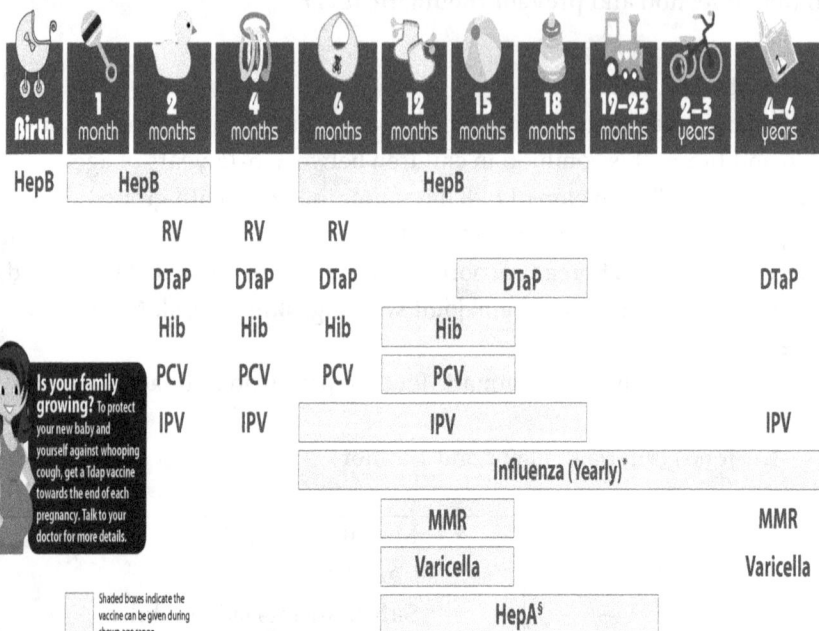

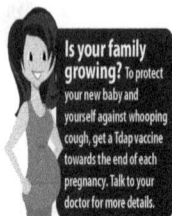

Birth	1 month	2 months	4 months	6 months	12 months	15 months	18 months	19–23 months	2–3 years	4–6 years
HepB	HepB			HepB						
		RV	RV	RV						
		DTaP	DTaP	DTaP		DTaP				DTaP
		Hib	Hib	Hib	Hib					
		PCV	PCV	PCV	PCV					
		IPV	IPV	IPV						IPV
				Influenza (Yearly)*						
					MMR					MMR
					Varicella					Varicella
					HepA§					

Is your family growing? To protect your new baby and yourself against whooping cough, get a Tdap vaccine towards the end of each pregnancy. Talk to your doctor for more details.

Shaded boxes indicate the vaccine can be given during shown age range.

NOTE: If your child misses a shot, you don't need to start over, just go back to your child's doctor for the next shot. Talk with your child's doctor if you have questions about vaccines.

FOOTNOTES:
* Two doses given at least four weeks apart are recommended for children aged 6 months through 8 years of age who are getting a flu vaccine for the first time and for some other children in this age group.

§ Two doses of HepA vaccine are needed for lasting protection. The first dose of HepA vaccine should be given between 12 months and 23 months of age. The second dose should be given 6 to 18 months later. HepA vaccination may be given to any child 12 months and older to protect against HepA. Children and adolescents who did not receive the HepA vaccine and are at high-risk, should be vaccinated against HepA.

If your child has any medical conditions that put him at risk for infection or is traveling outside the United States, talk to your child's doctor about additional vaccines that he may need.

SEE BACK PAGE FOR MORE INFORMATION ON VACCINE-PREVENTABLE DISEASES AND THE VACCINES THAT PREVENT THEM.

For more information, call toll free
1-800-CDC-INFO (1-800-232-4636)
or visit
http://www.cdc.gov/vaccines

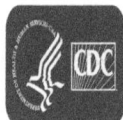

U.S. Department of Health and Human Services
Centers for Disease Control and Prevention

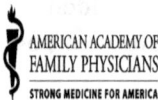

AMERICAN ACADEMY OF **FAMILY PHYSICIANS**
STRONG MEDICINE FOR AMERICA

American Academy of Pediatrics
DEDICATED TO THE HEALTH OF ALL CHILDREN

Vaccine-Preventable Diseases and the Vaccines that Prevent Them

Disease	Vaccine	Disease spread by	Disease symptoms	Disease complications
Chickenpox	Varicella vaccine protects against chickenpox.	Air, direct contact	Rash, tiredness, headache, fever	Infected blisters, bleeding disorders, encephalitis (brain swelling), pneumonia (infection in the lungs)
Diphtheria	DTaP* vaccine protects against diphtheria.	Air, direct contact	Sore throat, mild fever, weakness, swollen glands in neck	Swelling of the heart muscle, heart failure, coma, paralysis, death
Hib	Hib vaccine protects against *Haemophilus influenzae* type b.	Air, direct contact	May be no symptoms unless bacteria enter the blood	Meningitis (infection of the covering around the brain and spinal cord), intellectual disability, epiglottitis (life-threatening infection that can block the windpipe and lead to serious breathing problems), pneumonia (infection in the lungs), death
Hepatitis A	HepA vaccine protects against hepatitis A.	Direct contact, contaminated food or water	May be no symptoms, fever, stomach pain, loss of appetite, fatigue, vomiting, jaundice (yellowing of skin and eyes), dark urine	Liver failure, arthralgia (joint pain), kidney, pancreatic, and blood disorders
Hepatitis B	HepB vaccine protects against hepatitis B.	Contact with blood or body fluids	May be no symptoms, fever, headache, weakness, vomiting, jaundice (yellowing of skin and eyes), joint pain	Chronic liver infection, liver failure, liver cancer
Flu	Flu vaccine protects against influenza.	Air, direct contact	Fever, muscle pain, sore throat, cough, extreme fatigue	Pneumonia (infection in the lungs)
Measles	MMR** vaccine protects against measles.	Air, direct contact	Rash, fever, cough, runny nose, pinkeye	Encephalitis (brain swelling), pneumonia (infection in the lungs), death
Mumps	MMR** vaccine protects against mumps.	Air, direct contact	Swollen salivary glands (under the jaw), fever, headache, tiredness, muscle pain	Meningitis (infection of the covering around the brain and spinal cord), encephalitis (brain swelling), inflammation of testicles or ovaries, deafness
Pertussis	DTaP* vaccine protects against pertussis (whooping cough).	Air, direct contact	Severe cough, runny nose, apnea (a pause in breathing in infants)	Pneumonia (infection in the lungs), death
Polio	IPV vaccine protects against polio.	Air, direct contact, through the mouth	May be no symptoms, sore throat, fever, nausea, headache	Paralysis, death
Pneumococcal	PCV vaccine protects against pneumococcus.	Air, direct contact	May be no symptoms, pneumonia (infection in the lungs)	Bacteremia (blood infection), meningitis (infection of the covering around the brain and spinal cord), death
Rotavirus	RV vaccine protects against rotavirus.	Through the mouth	Diarrhea, fever, vomiting	Severe diarrhea, dehydration
Rubella	MMR** vaccine protects against rubella.	Air, direct contact	Children infected with rubella virus sometimes have a rash, fever, swollen lymph nodes	Very serious in pregnant women—can lead to miscarriage, stillbirth, premature delivery, birth defects
Tetanus	DTaP* vaccine protects against tetanus.	Exposure through cuts in skin	Stiffness in neck and abdominal muscles, difficulty swallowing, muscle spasms, fever	Broken bones, breathing difficulty, death

* DTaP combines protection against diphtheria, tetanus, and pertussis.
** MMR combines protection against measles, mumps, and rubella.

Last updated on 03/20/2013 • CS239274-A

2013 Recommended Immunizations for Children from 7 Through 18 Years Old

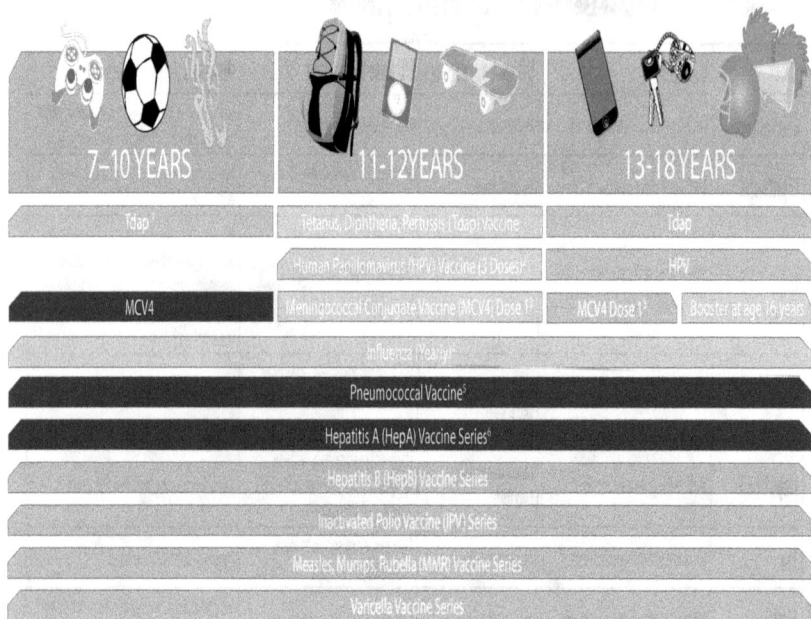

7-10 YEARS	11-12 YEARS	13-18 YEARS
Tdap [1]	Tetanus, Diphtheria, Pertussis (Tdap) Vaccine [1]	Tdap
	Human Papillomavirus (HPV) Vaccine (3 Doses) [2]	HPV
MCV4	Meningococcal Conjugate Vaccine (MCV4) Dose 1 [3]	MCV4 Dose 1 [3] / Booster at age 16 years
	Influenza (Yearly) [4]	
	Pneumococcal Vaccine [5]	
	Hepatitis A (HepA) Vaccine Series [6]	
	Hepatitis B (HepB) Vaccine Series	
	Inactivated Polio Vaccine (IPV) Series	
	Measles, Mumps, Rubella (MMR) Vaccine Series	
	Varicella Vaccine Series	

These shaded boxes indicate when the vaccine is recommended for all children unless your doctor tells you that your child cannot safely receive the vaccine.

These shaded boxes indicate the vaccine should be given if a child is catching-up on missed vaccines.

These shaded boxes indicate the vaccine is recommended for children with certain health conditions that put them at high risk for serious diseases. Note that healthy children **can** get the HepA series [6]. See vaccine-specific recommendations at www.cdc.gov/vaccines/pubs/ACIP-list.htm.

FOOTNOTES

[1] Tdap vaccine is combination vaccine that is recommended at age 11 or 12 to protect against tetanus, diphtheria and pertussis. If your child has not received any or all of the DTaP vaccine series, or if you don't know if your child has received these shots, your child needs a single dose of Tdap when they are 7-10 years old. Talk to your child's health care provider to find out if they need additional catch-up vaccines.

[2] All 11 or 12 year olds – both girls *and* boys – should receive 3 doses of HPV vaccine to protect against HPV-related disease. Either HPV vaccine (Cervarix® or Gardasil®) can be given to girls and young women; only one HPV vaccine (Gardasil®) can be given to boys and young men.

[3] Meningococcal conjugate vaccine (MCV) is recommended at age 11 or 12. A booster shot is recommended at age 16. Teens who received MCV for the first time at age 13 through 15 years will need a one-time booster dose between the ages of 16 and 18 years. If your teenager missed getting the vaccine altogether, ask their health care provider about getting it now, especially if your teenager is about to move into a college dorm or military barracks.

[4] Everyone 6 months of age and older—including preteens and teens—should get a flu vaccine every year. Children under the age of 9 years may require more than one dose. Talk to your child's health care provider to find out if they need more than one dose.

[5] A single dose of Pneumococcal Conjugate Vaccine (PCV13) is recommended for children who are 6 - 18 years old with certain medical conditions that place them at high risk. Talk to your healthcare provider about pneumococcal vaccine and what factors may place your child at high risk for pneumococcal disease.

[6] Hepatitis A vaccination is recommended for older children with certain medical conditions that place them at high risk. HepA vaccine is licensed, safe, and effective for all children of all ages. Even if your child is not at high risk, you may decide you want your child protected against HepA. Talk to your healthcare provider about HepA vaccine and what factors may place your child at high risk for HepA.

For more information, call toll free 1-800-CDC-INFO (1-800-232-4636) or visit http://www.cdc.gov/vaccines/teens

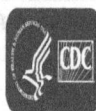

U.S. Department of Health and Human Services
Centers for Disease Control and Prevention

American Academy of Pediatrics
DEDICATED TO THE HEALTH OF ALL CHILDREN™

AMERICAN ACADEMY OF FAMILY PHYSICIANS
STRONG MEDICINE FOR AMERICA

Vaccine-Preventable Diseases and the Vaccines that Prevent Them

Diphtheria (Can be prevented by Tdap vaccine)

Diphtheria is a very contagious bacterial disease that affects the respiratory system, including the lungs. Diphtheria bacteria can be passed from person to person by direct contact with droplets from an infected person's cough or sneeze. When people are infected, the diphtheria bacteria produce a toxin (poison) in the body that can cause weakness, sore throat, low-grade fever, and swollen glands in the neck. Effects from this toxin can also lead to swelling of the heart muscle and, in some cases, heart failure. In severe cases, the illness can cause coma, paralysis, and even death.

Hepatitis A (Can be prevented by HepA vaccine)

Hepatitis A is an infection in the liver caused by hepatitis A virus. The virus is spread primarily person-to-person through the fecal-oral route. In other words, the virus is taken in by mouth from contact with objects, food, or drinks contaminated by the feces (stool) of an infected person. Symptoms include fever, tiredness, loss of appetite, nausea, abdominal discomfort, dark urine, and jaundice (yellowing of the skin and eyes). An infected person may have no symptoms, may have mild illness for a week or two, or may have severe illness for several months that requires hospitalization. In the U.S., about 100 people a year die from hepatitis A.

Hepatitis B (Can be prevented by HepB vaccine)

Hepatitis B is an infection of the liver caused by hepatitis B virus. The virus spreads through exchange of blood or other body fluids, for example, from sharing personal items, such as razors or during sex. Hepatitis B causes a flu-like illness with loss of appetite, nausea, vomiting, rashes, joint pain, and jaundice. The virus stays in the liver of some people for the rest of their lives and can result in severe liver diseases, including fatal cancer.

Human Papillomavirus (Can be prevented by HPV vaccine)

Human papillomavirus is a common virus. HPV is most common in people in their teens and early 20s. It is the major cause of cervical cancer in women and genital warts in women and men. The strains of HPV that cause cervical cancer and genital warts are spread during sex.

Influenza (Can be prevented by annual flu vaccine)

Influenza is a highly contagious viral infection of the nose, throat, and lungs. The virus spreads easily through droplets when an infected person coughs or sneezes and can cause mild to severe illness. Typical symptoms include a sudden high fever, chills, a dry cough, headache, runny nose, sore throat, and muscle and joint pain. Extreme fatigue can last from several days to weeks. Influenza may lead to hospitalization or even death, even among previously healthy children.

Measles (Can be prevented by MMR vaccine)

Measles is one of the most contagious viral diseases. Measles virus is spread by direct contact with the airborne respiratory droplets of an infected person. Measles is so contagious that just being in the same room after a person who has measles has already left can result in infection. Symptoms usually include a rash, fever, cough, and red, watery eyes. Fever can persist, rash can last for up to a week, and coughing can last about 10 days. Measles can also cause pneumonia, seizures, brain damage, or death.

Meningococcal Disease (Can be prevented by MCV vaccine)

Meningococcal disease is caused by bacteria and is a leading cause of bacterial meningitis (infection around the brain and spinal cord) in children. The bacteria are spread through the exchange of nose and throat droplets, such as when coughing, sneezing or kissing. Symptoms include nausea, vomiting, sensitivity to light, confusion and sleepiness. Meningococcal disease also causes blood infections. About one of every ten people who get the disease dies from it. Survivors of meningococcal disease may lose their arms or legs, become deaf, have problems with their nervous systems, become developmentally disabled, or suffer seizures or strokes.

Mumps (Can be prevented by MMR vaccine)

Mumps is an infectious disease caused by the mumps virus, which is spread in the air by a cough or sneeze from an infected person. A child can also get infected with mumps by coming in contact with a contaminated object, like a toy. The mumps virus causes fever, headaches, painful swelling of the salivary glands under the jaw, fever, muscle aches, tiredness, and loss of appetite. Severe complications for children who get mumps are uncommon, but can include meningitis (infection of the covering of the brain and spinal cord), encephalitis (inflammation of the brain), permanent hearing loss, or swelling of the testes, which rarely can lead to sterility in men.

Pertussis (Whooping Cough) (Can be prevented by Tdap vaccine)

Pertussis is caused by bacteria spread through direct contact with respiratory droplets when an infected person coughs or sneezes. In the beginning, symptoms of pertussis are similar to the common cold, including runny nose, sneezing, and cough. After 1-2 weeks, pertussis can cause spells of violent coughing and choking, making it hard to breathe, drink, or eat. This cough can last for weeks. Pertussis is most serious for babies, who can get pneumonia, have seizures, become brain damaged, or even die. About two-thirds of children under 1 year of age who get pertussis must be hospitalized.

Pneumococcal Disease

(Can be prevented by Pneumococcal vaccine)

Pneumonia is an infection of the lungs that can be caused by the bacteria called pneumococcus. This bacteria can cause other types of infections too, such as ear infections, sinus infections, meningitis (infection of the covering around the brain and spinal cord), bacteremia and sepsis (blood stream infection). Sinus and ear infections are usually mild and are much more common than the more severe forms of pneumococcal disease. However, in some cases pneumococcal disease can be fatal or result in long-term problems, like brain damage, hearing loss and limb loss. Pneumococcal disease spreads when people cough or sneeze. Many people have the bacteria in their nose or throat at one time or another without being ill—this is known as being a carrier.

Polio (Can be prevented by IPV vaccine)

Polio is caused by a virus that lives in an infected person's throat and intestines. It spreads through contact with the feces (stool) of an infected person and through droplets from a sneeze or cough. Symptoms typically include sudden fever, sore throat, headache, muscle weakness, and pain. In about 1% of cases, polio can cause paralysis. Among those who are paralyzed, up to 5% of children may die because they become unable to breathe.

Rubella (German Measles) (Can be prevented by MMR vaccine)

Rubella is caused by a virus that is spread through coughing and sneezing. In children rubella usually causes a mild illness with fever, swollen glands, and a rash that lasts about 3 days. Rubella rarely causes serious illness or complications in children, but can be very serious to a baby in the womb. If a pregnant woman is infected, the result to the baby can be devastating, including miscarriage, serious heart defects, mental retardation and loss of hearing and eye sight.

Tetanus (Lockjaw) (Can be prevented by Tdap vaccine)

Tetanus is caused by bacteria found in soil. The bacteria enters the body through a wound, such as a deep cut. When people are infected, the bacteria produce a toxin (poison) in the body that causes serious, painful spasms and stiffness of all muscles in the body. This can lead to "locking" of the jaw so a person cannot open his or her mouth, swallow, or breathe. Complete recovery from tetanus can take months. Three of ten people who get tetanus die from the disease.

Varicella (Chickenpox) (Can be prevented by varicella vaccine)

Chickenpox is caused by the varicella zoster virus. Chickenpox is very contagious and spreads very easily from infected people. The virus can spread from either a cough, sneeze. It can also spread from the blisters on the skin, either by touching them or by breathing in these viral particles. Typical symptoms of chickenpox include an itchy rash with blisters, tiredness, headache and fever. Chickenpox is usually mild, but it can lead to severe skin infections, pneumonia, encephalitis (brain swelling), or even death.

Last updated on 01/16/2013 • CS237027-A

Notes:

GYNECOLOGY

VAGINITIS

Vaginitis is inflammation of the vagina, which results in the discharge, itching and pain.

Cause: infection or overgrowth of normal vaginal organism

Types of vaginitis: most common types of vaginitis are:

- **Bacterial vaginosis**, which results from overgrowth of normal vaginal bacteria known as Gardnerella
- **Trichomonas**, which results from infection with Trichomonas vaginalis. It is the most common **non-viral sexual transmitted disease (STD)**
- **Candidiasis**, which result from naturally occurring fungus called candida albicans. Candidiasis is usually seen in diabetics, pregnant women, immunocompromised women such as HIV infection

Discharge, diagnosis and treatment of vaginitis

Type	Bacterial vaginosis	Trichomonas	Candida
Discharge	Fishy odor vaginal discharge	Green frothy discharge	Cheesy white discharge
Diagnosis	• Vaginal pH >5 • Microscopy with saline wet mount shows " **clue cells"**	• Vaginal pH >6 • Microscopy with saline wet mount shows **motile organism**	• Vaginal pH <4.5 • Microscopy with KOH prep shows **pseudohyphae**
Treatment	Metronidazole	Metronidazole **to patient and sexual partners**	**Fluconazole**

CERVICITIS

Cervicitis is inflammation of cervix, a lower end of uterus that opens into the vagina

Cause: causes of cervicitis can be divided into two main groups: infectious and non-infections

- **Infectious cause**: most common causes are **chlamydia and gonorrhea,** but other cause may includes trichomoniasis, herpes virus, HPV
- **Non-infectious** cause includes malignancy, systemic inflammation, radiation, local trauma

Si/Sx: most of the patients are asymptomatic, but symptoms may include **yellow-green mucopurulent discharge**, painful urination, pain during intercourse, vaginal bleeding after intercourse

Diagnosis:

- Pelvic exam may show redness of cervix, inflammation of the vaginal walls, discharge from cervix
- **Best initial test** is cervical swab for gram stain
- **Most accurate test** includes urethral culture, DNA probe or nucleic acid amplification test

Treatment: Treat the underlying cause

PELVIC INFLAMMATORY DISEASE (PID)

Pelvic inflammatory disease is an infection of upper reproductive tract organs (uterus lining, fallopian tubes, ovaries). It occurs when bacteria from lower reproductive tract organs (vagina or cervix) moves to upper reproductive tract organs.

Cause: most common causes are gonorrhea, and chlamydia, but bacteria can also enter upper reproductive tract during IUD insertion, childbirth, abortions, endometrial biopsy

Si/Sx: Pain and tenderness of lower abdominal, cervical motion tenderness, fever, chills, purulent cervical discharge

Diagnosis:

- Labs shows WBC > 10,000, ESR> 15mm/hr.
- Endocervical culture for gram stain
- Beta-HCG to **rule out pregnancy**
- Ultrasound to rule out pregnancy, and tubo-ovarian abscess
- **Laparoscopy** is the **most accurate test**

Treatment: treatment should not be delayed while waiting for culture results. All **sexual partners** should be checked and **treated** to prevent passing the infection back and forth.

- **Outpatient treatment:** Ceftriaxone and doxycycline, or ofloxacin and metronidazole
- **Inpatient treatment** with IV cefotetan or cefoxitin + doxycycline or Clindamycin + gentamicin

Inpatient treatment is given, if a patient meets the following criteria:

- Fever>102.2 F
- Nulligravida
- Adolescent
- IUD in place
- Outpatient treatment failure
- Ultrasound shows pelvic abscess
- Pregnant

Complication: PID can cause scarring of pelvic organ, and that can lead to chronic pain, ectopic pregnancy, and infertility

URINE INCONTINENCE

Urine incontinence is involuntary urine loss

Types and causes: the most common types are:

- **Stress incontinence** that is usually caused by **weakness of pelvic floor** muscles that support the bladder and urethra
- **Overflow incontinence** is usually seen patient with nerve denervation such as diabetic neuropathy, multiple sclerosis or patients taking anticholinergic medicine. In this conditions patients **do not sense bladder fullness and, urine leaks** when bladder pressure exceeds the urethral pressure
- **Urge incontinence** is seen patients with **involuntary contractions** of detrusor muscles
- **Bypass fistula is** seen in patients with obstetric and gynecology trauma or injury. Two most common fistulas are vesicovaginal fistula and uterovaginal fistula.

Diagnosis:

- UA and urine culture should be done to exclude UTI
- BUN/Cr, to exclude renal dysfunction
- Specific diagnosis depends on the specific cause, discussed below

Symptoms, diagnosis and treatment of urine incontinence

Diagnosis	Symptoms	Diagnostic tests	Treatment
Stress incontinence	**Small volume** of urine loss during physical movement such as **cough, sneezing exercising**	Q-tip test	Pelvic strengthening exercises and estrogen. Surgery is reserved for refractory cases
Overflow incontinence	**Small volume** of urine loss, pelvic fullness present **during day and night**	Cytometric studies show residual bladder volume > 200 cc	Discontinue offending medicine, intermittent catheterization
Urge incontinence	**Large volume** of urine loss **without any warning,** present during day and night	Cytometric studies show residual bladder volume < 50 cc, and involuntary detrusor muscle contractions	Oxybutynin
Bypass fistula	**Continues** small amount of urine lost during day and at night	Intravenous pyelogram shows dye leaking from the urinary tract fistula	Surgery

ENDOMETRIAL CANCER

Endometrial cancer is a cancer that beings in the endometrium of the uterus. Majority of the endometrial cancers are seen in postmenopausal women

Cause: there is no exact known cause of endometrial cancer, but increased level of estrogen seems to have a significant role. Estrogen stimulates the endometrial lining of the uterus

Risk factors: diabetes, obesity, infertility, polycystic ovarian syndrome, early mensuration (before age 12), and menopause starting after age 50

S/Sx: vaginal bleeding after menopause, bleeding between periods, lower abdominal pain, pelvic pain

Diagnosis:
- Endometrial biopsy
- Vaginal ultrasound to measure the endometrial thickness, in postmenopausal women normal endometrial thickness is < 5mm

Treatment:
- Total abdominal hysterectomy/ bilateral salpingo–oophorectomy (TAH/BSO) and radiation.
- Chemotherapy is added to the treatment if the patient has metastatic disease.

CERVICAL CANCER

Cervical cancer is the cancer of the cervix. It mostly affects women < 40 years of age

Risk factors: Human papillomavirus (HPV) infection, smoking, family history of cervical cancer, sexual activity at an early age, multiple sexual partners

Note: HPV 16, 18, 31, 33, and 35 are associated with **cervical cancer. HPV 6 and 11** are associated with **venereal warts**

Si/Sx: abnormal vaginal bleeding between periods, bleeding after intercourse, pelvic pain and vaginal discharge. Patient with advanced stages may have urine incontinence, fecal incontinence, back pain, bone pain or fractures

Diagnosis:
- Pap smear
- Visible lesion should be followed up with colposcopy and endocervical biopsy

Treatment:
- Localized disease and early stages cancer is treated with hysterectomy and lymph node dissection
- Metastatic cancers are treated with radiation and chemotherapy

Prevention:
- Pap smear screening starting at age 21, or 3 years after first intercourse, whichever comes first
- Safe sex to prevent HPV infection
- HPV vaccine to all females between 9-26 years of age

Note: HPV vaccine does not protects against all HPV strains, it only protects against HPV 6,11,16, and 18

VULVAR CANCER

Vulvar cancer is a cancer that affects outer surface of female genitalia such as labia, skin folds outside the vagina, clitoris, or the glands outside of the vaginal opening

Cause: most common vulvar cancer is squamous cell carcinoma, other causes include adenocarcinoma, basal cell carcinoma, melanoma, sarcoma, Paget's disease, malignant melanoma

Risk factors: HPV infection, obesity, diabetes, hypertension

Si/Sx: Pruritus, irritation, raised lesions

Diagnosis:
- Biopsy
- Staging is surgically done
  - Stage I: Tumor confined to vulva with size < 2 cm
  - Stage II: Tumor confined to vulva with size > 2 cm
  - Stage III: tumor spreads to lower urethra, vagina or anus

Treatment: Local excision for stage I and II cancer, and wide excision for stage III cancer. Radiation for metastatic tumors

OVARIAN TUMOR

Ovarian tumors are tumors that arise from the ovaries. These can be benign or malignant

Types: Three main types of ovarian tumors are:
- **Epithelial cell tumors** arise from the cells on the surface of the ovaries. Epithelial cell tumors account for 70 % of all ovarian tumors. Most common epithelial tumors as serous, mucinous, clear ell and endometrioid
- **Germ cell tumors** arise from the reproductive cells of the ovaries. Germ cell tumors account for < 2% of ovarian tumors. Most common germ cell tumors are dysgerminoma, choriocarcinoma, teratomas, yolk sac tumor

- **Stromal cell tumors** arise from supporting tissues within the ovaries. Stromal cell tumors account for 5-8% of ovarian tumors. Most common stromal cell tumors are granulosa-stromal tumors and Sertoli-Leydig cell tumor

Risk factors: Increased number ovulations, nulliparity, infertility, BRCA 1 gene, family history of ovarian, breast and colorectal cancer
Si/Sx: depends on stage
- Patient in early stages of ovarian cancer may be asymptomatic or may have palpable adnexal mass, vague abdominal symptoms
- Patients in late stages of ovarian cancer usually have palpable abdominal mass, increased abdominal girth, distention and pain

Diagnosis:
- Abdominal ultrasound
- Tumor markers (discussed below)

Tumor markers

Tumor marker	Ovarian tumor
CA-125, CEA	Epithelial tumor
Estrogen	Granulosa-stromal tumor
Testosterone	Sertoli-Leydig tumor
LDH	Dysgerminoma
HCG	Choriocarcinoma
AFP	Endodermal sinus tumor
HCG, AFP	Embryonal carcinoma

Treatment:
- Benign tumors are surgically removed
- Malignant tumor: TAH/BSO plus postoperative chemotherapy

OVARIAN CYSTS
Ovarian cysts are fluid-filled sacs in the ovaries. These are **common in reproductive aged women**
Cause: cysts forms during the menstrual cycle from follicles. These follicles produce estrogen and progesterone hormones and releases egg during the ovulation. Some times follicles keep growing and become functional cysts
Si/Sx: menstrual irregularities, pelvic pain, and pelvic pressure. Ruptured cysts causes sudden severe abdominal or pelvic pain, fever

Diagnosis:
- Beta-HCG to exclude pregnancy or ectopic pregnancy
- Diagnosis is confirmed with ultrasound

Treatment:
- Simple cysts < 7 cm are treated with OCP and follow-up in 6-8 weeks to ensure resolution
- Simple cysts > 7 cm are removed by laparoscopic
- Ruptured cysts require laparotomy

GESTATIONAL TROPHOBLASTIC TUMOR (GTT)

Gestational trophoblastic tumor is a form of tumor that is derived from abnormal placental tissue, inside women's uterus (womb).

Types: Two main types of gestational trophoblastic tumor are hydatidiform mole and choriocarcinoma

1. **Hydatidiform mole** (also known as **molar pregnancy**) accounts for about 80% GTT. It rarely spreads outside of the uterus. Sub-type of hydatidiform moles are:
1a. **Complete molar pregnancy** occurs when **a sperm fertilizes an abnormal egg**. Instead of forming embryo, the cell forms a "grape-like" cysts, it has chromosomal pattern of **46, XX**.
1b. **Partial mole** occurs when **two sperms fertilize an egg**. Some fetal parts are formed, it has chromosomal pattern of **69, XXY**.
2. **Choriocarcinoma** accounts for about 5% of GTT. It can spread outside of the uterus.

Si/Sx: irregular vaginal bleeding that usually occurs in early second trimester, hyperemesis gravidarum, uterus size more than gestational dates

Diagnosis:
- Physical exam shows **uterus size more than gestational dates**, missing fetal heart tone
- Serum Beta-HCG, which is usually markedly high (>100,000 mIU/mL)
- Pelvic ultrasound

Treatment:

- Dilation and curettage (D&C)
- **Non-metastatic tumor** is treated with **methotrexate. OCPs** are given for **a year** to prevent pregnancy, and Beta-HCG is followed for a year to monitor the disease
- Tumor metastasized to **brain or liver** is treated with a combination of three medicines - **methotrexate, actinomycin D, and cyclophosphamide.** OCPs are given for **5 years** and Beta-HCG is checked for 5 years to monitor the disease.

HIRSUTISM AND VIRILIZATION

Hirsutism is excessive body hair. Virilization is a hyperandrogenism state (clitoromegaly, temporal balding, voice deepening, increased muscle mass, and amenorrhea).

Si/Sx: women usually present with excessive hair growth on chest, abdomen, chins, upper lips and virilization

Causes: most common causes of hirsutism and virilization are adrenal tumor, congenital adrenal hyperplasia, ovarian cancer and polycystic ovarian syndrome (disused in table below)

Differential diagnosis of hirsutism and virilization

Disease	Diagnosis	Treatment
Adrenal tumor	• Labs shows **increased DHEAS** • Abdominal CT or ultrasound	Surgery
Congenital adrenal hyperplasia	• Usually due to 21-alpha-hydroxylase defect • Labs shows **increased 17-hydroxyprogestrone,**	Glucocorticoids
Ovarian cancer	• Labs shows very high **testosterone level (> 200 ng/dL)** • Pelvic CT or ultrasound	Surgery
Polycystic ovarian syndrome (PCOS)	• Labs shows **LH: FHS ratio 3:1** • Pelvic ultrasound shows " Pearl necklace sign"	Treatment of PCOS is discussed on the next page

Treatment for PCOS:
- Weight loss may help ovulation and spare the fertility
- Clomiphene citrate to induce ovulation
- Metformin for diabetes
- Spironolactone to treat facial hair growth
- OCPs are given to prevent endometrial hyperplasia and endometrial carcinoma

PRIMARY AMENORRHEA

Primary amenorrhea is a condition in which menstrual bleeding never occurred

Diagnosis: it is diagnosed by presence of one of the following:
- Absence of menses, plus **no signs of secondary sexual** development (growth, breast development, pubic hair and axillary hair) **at age 14**
- Absence of menses, but **presence of secondary sexual development** at age 16

Cause: lots of causes can cause primary amenorrhea, but the primary causes can be divided into three main type based on presence or absence of breast and uterus. Which are as follow:
1. **Both uterus and breasts are present** (discussed on the next page)
2. **Breasts are present, but uterus is absent** (discussed on the next page)
3. **Breasts are absent, but uterus is present** (discussed on the next page)

Note: Pregnancy is the **most common cause of primary amenorrhea.** Therefore, it is necessary to rule out pregnancy first with the urine pregnancy test.

Diagnostic workup:
- Rule out pregnancy
- Physical exam to check for breath development (normal breast development suggest adequate estrogen production)
- Get abdominal ultrasound to check if uterus is present

1. Differential diagnosis of primary amenorrhea, **when both uterus and breasts are present**

Diagnosis	Characteristic	Treatment
Imperforate hymen	• Patients usually complain of cyclic pelvic pain • Genital exam shows **red-purple bulging membrane** at introitus	Surgical opening of imperforate hymen
Transverse vaginal pouch	• Patient usually complain of cyclic pain • Genital exam shows **blind vaginal pouch**	Surgical repair
Physical stress such as anorexic, athletes, Excessive exercise	• Patient's history and physical exam is usually helpful	OCP

2. Differential diagnosis primary amenorrhea, when **breasts are present, but uterus is absent**

Diagnosis	Characteristic	Treatment
Androgen insensitivity syndrome	• Physical exam shows **no pubic and axillary hair** • Karyotype shows **XY** chromosomes • Ultrasound **shows internal testes**	**Surgical removal of internal testes,** otherwise patient may develop testicular cancer. **Estrogen replacement** after the surgery
Müllerian agenesis	• **Normal pubic and axillary hair** • Karyotype show **XX** chromosome • Ultrasound shows **absence of mullerian duct derivatives**: fallopian tube, uterus, and upper vagina.	**Surgical elongation of vagina**

Note: In Müllerian agenesis, ovaries and lower vagina are present because these are not derived from Müllerian duct.

3. **Differential diagnosis** for primary amenorrhea, when **breasts are absent** but **uterus is present**

Diagnosis	Characteristic	Treatment
Turner syndrome	• Physical exam shows **short stature female, broad nipple, no secondary sexual** characters • **Increased FSH** level • Karyotypes shows X0 chromosome • Ultrasound shows streak ovaries	Estrogen and progesterone replacement
Hypothalamic-pituitary failure	• **Low FSH** • Karyotype shows XX chromosome • Heat CT to rule out tumor	Estrogen and progesterone replacement
Kallmann syndrome	• Anosmia **(loss of smell)** • Rest is same as hypothalamic- pituitary failure	Estrogen and progesterone replacement

SECONDARY AMENORRHEA

Secondary amenorrhea is absence of menstruation in a women who has been having normal menstrual cycles before

Diagnosis: it is diagnosed by presence of one of the following:

- Absence of menses for **3 months** if **previous regular menses**
- Absence of menses for **6 months** if **previous irregular menses**

Cause: lots of causes that can cause secondary amenorrhea such as pregnancy, hypothyroidism, elevated prolactin level, outflow obstruction, PCOS, brain tumor, estrogen deficiency, ovarian failure, brain tumors, change in LH and FSH levels

Diagnosis: diagnosing the exact cause of secondary amenorrhea can be challenging. Follow the approach below to narrow down a diagnosis.

1. **Pregnancy test:** pregnancy is the **most common cause of the secondary amenorrhea.** Therefore, it is important to rule out pregnancy before doing further tests

2. **TSH:** after ruling out the pregnancy check TSH. Low TSH level leads to increased TRH, which can further lead to increased prolactin level. Prolactin suppresses the LH and FSH and causes amenorrhea. If patient has **hypothyroidism,** then treat the patient with **levothyroxine**

3. **Prolactin level:** after ruling out hypothyroidism. Check prolactin levels. Anti-psychotics or brain tumors can cause high prolactin. If a patient is taking anti-psychotics, then **switch medicine.** However, if the patient is not taking anti-psychotics, then get CT head to look for a pituitary tumor. **Pituitary tumor less than 1 cm** can be treated with **bromocriptine.** Tumor **more than 1 cm is surgically removed.**

4. **Progesterone challenge test** (PCT) is performed after excluding pregnancy, THS and prolactin level. In this test patient is given one IM progesterone shot or oral 7 days medroxyprogesterone, and then follow-up with patient after 2-7 days to check if patient has withdrawal bleeding

4a. If patient experiences **withdrawal bleeding,** it means she is not ovulating (**anovulation**). Treatment: **Cyclic progesterone** is given to prevent endometrial hyperplasia, and clomiphene if pregnancy is desired

4b. If **no bleeding occurs,** then either this patient has **low estrogen** or there is **outflow obstruction** such as adhesions or cervical stenosis. If an **obstruction** is found, then it is **surgically relieved.** However, if no obstruction is found, then it is likely due to **low estrogen** level and that should be further evaluated with **estrogen progesterone challenge test**

5. **Estrogen progesterone challenge test** is performed after PCT. In this test patient is given estrogen for 21 days followed by progesterone for 7 days, and is checked for withdrawal bleeding

5a. If **no bleeding** occurs, then either this patient has **Asherman syndrome** or there is outflow tract obstruction such as adhesions or cervical stenosis. If an **obstruction** is found, then it is **surgically relieved.** However, if no obstruction is found, then it means the patient has **Asherman syndrome,** which **is** further diagnosed with **hysterosalpingogram,** and treated with **adhesion lysis and estrogen replacement.** Stents are usually left in place to prevent re-adhesion

5b. If the **bleeding occurs, check FSH level.** Low FSH (< 40 mIU/mL) means **gonadal failure**, whereas, FSH > 40 mIU/mL means **hypothalamus-pituitary dysfunction**, get head CT to rule out tumor. Treatment: Regardless of the cause, give patient **estrogen and progesterone.** Estrogen replacement is given to prevent osteoporosis and estrogen deficiency. Cyclic progesterone is also required to prevent endometrial hyperplasia. If the tumor is found, then surgically remove the tumor, and then treat with estrogen and progesterone.

PRECOCIOUS PUBERTY

Precocious puberty refers to the development of secondary sexual characteristics and growth, before age 8 in females and 9 in males.

Normal puberty landmarks

Normal puberty landmarks	Age
Thelarche (Breast development)	9-10 years
Adrenarche (pubic and axillary hair)	10-11 years
Growth spurt	11-12 years
Menarche (onset of first menses)	12-13 years

Cause: there is no known specific cause, but some known causes include, transient hormonal change, CNS tumors, genetic disorder, ovarian tumor
Types: two main types of precocious puberty are **incomplete** and **complete** isosexual precocious puberty

1. **Incomplete isosexual precocious puberty** refers to early development of **one puberty landmark** such as thelarche, adrenarche or menarche. This condition is caused by either transient hormone spike or increased end-organ sensitivity. Treatment: conservative management

2. **Complete isosexual precocious puberty** refers to early development of **all puberty landmarks.** This condition is caused by CNS pathology, McCune-Albert syndrome, granulosa cell tumor or idiopathic (discussed below)

2a. **McCune-Albert syndrome**
   Si/Sx: precocious puberty, **Cafe-au-lait spots,** multiple bone fractures
   Diagnosis: labs show increased aromatase enzyme activity, increased estrogen

Treatment: Aromatase enzyme inhibitor

2b. Granulosa cell tumor
Si/Sx: precocious puberty, pelvic mass
Diagnosis: labs show increased estrogen. Pelvic ultrasound shows a mass
Treatment: Surgery

2c. CNS etiology
Cause: CNS etiology such as tumor, meningitis, encephalitis, hydrocephalus
Si/Sx: complete precious puberty, other symptoms depend on the cause
Diagnosis: labs show increased GnRH and increased FSH
Treatment: treat the underlying cause

2d. Idiopathic
Idiopathic precious precocious puberty accounts for majority of the precocious puberty cases
Si/Sx: no specific symptoms
Diagnosis: diagnosis of exclusion
Treatment: GnRH antagonist

PRIMARY DYSMENORRHEA
Primary dysmenorrhea is characterized by cramping pain in the lower abdomen that occurs just before the periods. It usually begins 2-5 years after the menarche
Cause: Excessive production of **prostaglandin F2- alpha**
Si/Sx: aching pain in the abdomen, feeling of pressure in the abdomen, nausea, vomiting
Treatment: **Best initial treatment is NSAIDs,** which relieves symptom by inhibiting prostaglandin syntheses. **OCPs is the second-line** treatment

ENDOMETRIOSIS
Endometriosis is an abnormal growth of endometrial cells outside of the uterus. It is the **most common cause of infertility in women more than 30 years of age**. Ovaries are the most common location of ectopic endometrial gland.

Endometriosis is most common cause of secondary dysmenorrhea

Cause: there is no known cause

Si/Sx: dysmenorrhea (painful periods), dyspareunia (painful intercourse), dyschezia (painful bowel movement), pelvic or low back pain during menstrual cycle

Diagnosis:
- Pelvic exam may show uterosacral nodularity
- Laparoscopy is used to visualize the ectopic gland

Treatment:
- Best initial treatment is **continuous dose of progesterone or OCPs**. Second-line treatment is testosterone derivatives (danazol or Danocrine) or GnRH analogs (Lupron or leuprolide)
- Surgery is reserved for **refractory cases**; laparoscopy lysis adhesion is done if the patient desires fertility. If the patient does not want to preserve fertility or an older patient, then consider total hysterectomy and bilateral salpingoopherectomy (TAH/BSO)

ADENOMYOSIS

Adenomyosis is an ectopic endometrial gland **within the myometrium** of uterus

Cause: there is no known cause

Si/Sx: most of the patients are asymptomatic, but symptoms may include dysmenorrhea, menorrhagia, dyspareunia

Diagnosis:
- Pelvic exam shows **symmetric and tender uterus**
- Ultrasound shows ectopic endometrial gland and stroma within the myometrium of the uterus

Treatment: intrauterine levonorgestrel

UTERINE LEIOMYOMA

Uterine leiomyoma refers to benign neoplasm that arises from **smooth muscle of the uterus**. Uterine leiomyoma is **estrogen–dependent**, they show rapid growth during pregnancy or with estrogen-progesterone combined OCPs, and shrinks after menopause.

Si/Sx: most of the patients are asymptomatic, but symptoms may include bleeding between periods, menorrhagia (heavy menstrual period), infertility

Diagnosis: Ultrasound

Treatment: If the patient wants to maintain her fertility, then perform **myomectomy**. Hysterectomy is usually considered for older women.

DYSFUNCTIONAL UTERINE BLEEDING (DUB)

Dysfunctional uterine bleeding is abnormal bleeding from the uterus due to change in hormonal level

Cause: anovulatory cycle (unopposed estrogen), estrogen producing tumor, infection, vWF factor deficiency, and endocrine disorder such as thyroid, adrenal

Si/Sx: Menorrhagia (bleeding between periods), menorrhagia (heavy bleeding), oligomenorrhea (period lasting 35- 90 days),

Diagnosis:

- DUB is diagnosis of exclusion
- Rule out bleeding disorder, endocrine disorder, renal disorder, pregnancy
- Rule out anatomic lesions, endometrial cancer, polyps

Treatment:

- If a patient is **unstable,** then put a **Foley catheter to tamponade bleeding, give high dose IV estrogen, and perform D&C.**
- **Stable patient** is usually treated with **iron supplements and OCPs**

INFERTILITY

Infertility is defined as failure to conceive **after 12 months of unprotected** intercourse

Cause: abnormal sperm production accounts for 40 % of the infertility, anovulation 30%, anatomic defect of the female reproductive tracts 20 % and 10 % of cases have no known cause

Diagnosis:

Abnormal sperm factor accounts for most of the cases of infertility, so it necessary to rule out male conditions first

1. **Male workup** usually involves checking semen for any abnormalities. Normal semen has the following characteristics:
   - Ejaculation volume > 2 ml
   - Sperm pH 7.2- 7.8
   - Sperm density > 20 million/ml,
   - Initial sperm forward motility > 50 %
   - Normal sperm morphology > 50%

1a If semen meets the normal **criteria,** then we can move to **female** workup

1b If the semen **does not meet** the normal criteria, then **repeat the semen test** in 2-3 days. If results **come back normal**, then proceed to **female testing.** However, if **results are still abnormal**, then the following treatment options may be tried

Treatment: if the male has semen abnormalities, then treatment **depends** on severity of **semen abnormalities:**

- If **sperm is minimal abnormal,** then **intrauterine insemination** may be tried
- If sperm is **severely abnormal** sperm, then **intracytoplasmic sperm injection with in vitro fertilization** may be tried
- If **sperm is not viable** or if **above discussed options fail,** then the **sperm donor is needed**

2. **Female work-up** should be performed after normal semen test . Do the tests in the following order:

2a. Check the for endocrine disorders such as hypothyroidism, Prolactinoma

2b. Check the for anovulation history (menstrual regularities)

2c. Check uterine cavity with hysterosalpingogram

2d. Laparoscopy

Treatment:

- If any endocrine disorder is found, then treat the disorder
- Anovulation is treated with **clomiphene citrate (**is the first choice) **or HMG.**
- **Laparoscopy** may be tried to fix tubal damage and restore fertility, but if tubal damage is severe, then **In-vitro fertilization** should be planned

PELVIC ORGAN PROLAPSE

Pelvic organ prolapse is a disorder in which muscles and ligaments supporting women's pelvic organs weaken and pelvic organs drop from their normal position.

Cause: Childbirth, heavy lifting, obesity, normal aging, menopause

Si/Sx: pelvic pressure, sensation that something is falling out of vagina, urine incontinence, difficulty with bowel movement,

Types: four main types of pelvic organ prolapse are:

Types of pelvic organ prolapse

Type	Location	Common symptoms
Uterine prolapse	Cervix descends in the **vagina**	Urinary incontinence, urgency and/or frequency
Cystocele	Bladder bulges into the **anterior wall of vagina**	Urine incontinence, urgency and/or frequency
Rectocele	Rectum bulges into the **posterior wall of vagina**	Constipation
Enterocele	Loop of bowel bulges into the **posterior vaginal wall**	Constipation

Treatment:

- **Best initial treatment** is pelvic **strengthening exercises** such as Kegel exercise. However, if symptoms are **affecting patient's** daily living, then **vaginal pessary device** may be used to support uterus, bladder and rectum.
- **Surgery** is a **last resort**. However, it is also the first-line of treatment in patients **with procidentia** (entire uterus outside the introitus).

BREAST MASS

1. **FIBROCYSTIC DISEASE**

Fibrocystic breast disease is a benign breast disease, characterized by painful lump in the breast. It is common in women, in her 30s.

Cause: there is no known cause, but symptoms are **related to woman's hormones levels**, which occur just before and during menstruation

Si/Sx: breast pain, multiple, bilateral cysts that are tender to touch, cysts usually resolve within a few weeks

Diagnosis: usually no work-up is needed, ultrasound is done if cyst does not disappear in few weeks

Treatment: OCPs and **follow-up patient** in 6 weeks

2. FIBROADENOMA

Fibroadenoma is the most common benign tumor of the breast; it is composed of **fibrous and glandular tissue**

Cause: fibroadenoma is estrogen dependent tumors that grows during pregnancy and OCPs use, and gets smaller after the menopause

Si/Sx: lump that may be painless, rubbery, moves easily under the skin

Diagnosis:
- Ultrasound
- Fine needle biopsy

Treatment: Excision

3. MASTITIS

Mastitis is an infection of the breast that causes breast inflammation, erythema, and pain. It is usually seen in **postpartum breastfeeding women**

Cause: S. Aureus that is transferred from infants throat or nose, during breastfeeding

Treatment: anti-staphylococcal medicine such as dicloxacillin or cephalexin and advice the patient to **continue breast feeding** from affected side of the breast to prevent duct blockage, otherwise it will progress to breast abscess

Compilation: Breast abscess – is a painful collection of pus in the breast. Most breast abscesses develop secondary to bacterial infection such as S.Aureus. Patient develops a painful fluctuating mass. Diagnosis is usually confirmed with ultrasound, and treated by **draining the abscess**

BREAST CANCER

1. **Ductal carcinoma in situ** (DCIS) is the most common noninvasive breast cancer, which develops in milk ducts. It may progress to invasive ductal carcinoma

2. **Lobular carcinoma in situ** (LCIS) is the second most common noninvasive breast cancer, which develops in the lobules of the breast. It may progress to invasive lobular carcinoma.

3. **Inflammatory breast disease** is very aggressive form of breast malignancy. In this condition cancer cells blocks the lymph vessels of the skin of the breast, and breast skin appears as skin of an orange " **Peau d' orange"**

4. **Paget disease of breast / nipples** is rare breast malignancy, which affects the nipple and breast. It gives breast **eczema-like appearance**: red, scaly, itchy and inflamed. **Nipples may become inverted and may have straw-colored or bloody discharge.**

Stages of breast cancer

Stage	Area involved
Stage 0	Carcinoma in situ
Stage 1	Tumor size < 2cm
Stage 2	Tumor size > 2 cm but < 5 cm
Stage 3	Tumor > 5 cm plus lymph nodes involvement
Stage 4	Distance metastasis

Risk factors for breast cancer:
- Female gender
- Family history of breast cancer
- Personal history of breast cancer
- BRCA 1 or BRCA 2 gene
- Radiation exposure
- Having first child after age 35
- Nulliparity
- Postmenopausal hormone therapy
- Alcohol
- High fat and low fiber diet

Diagnosis:
- Breast **ultrasound for women < 30 years** of age
- **Mammogram** for women **> 30 years of** age
- Breast lump biopsy
- Lymph node biopsy
- Estrogen and progesterone receptors
- HER2 receptor
- Bone scan, alkaline phosphate, Chest x-ray, CT scan

Treatment:
- Stage 1 and 2 cancers are treated with lumpectomy, axillary lymph node dissection, and radiation therapy.
- Moderate to high risk cancer are treated with chemotherapy followed by radiation therapy

- Women with ER or PR positive receptor should be treated tamoxifen and chemotherapy
- Trastuzumab is given to patient with positive HER2 receptors

CONTRACEPTION

Barrier methods advantages and disadvantages
- Male condoms are protective against STDs
- Female diaphragm needs to insert in vagina an hour prior to planned intercourse. However, they do not provide any protection against STDs

Progestin only contraceptives: three main types of progestin only modalities are:
- Progestin only **oral** pill are called " **minipill"**, it needs to taken **daily and continuously**
- Progestin-only **intramuscular** also known as **Depo-Provera**, has to be administered **every three months**. It is the only **safe contraceptive** to use in patients with **sickle-cell disease, epilepsy or iron deficiency anemia**
- Progestin only **subcutaneous patch** is a slow release and works **continuously for 3 years**

Estrogen- progesterone combined contraceptives: main types of combined contraceptive are:
- Oral form also known as **YAZ**, is 24 days of active pill followed by 7 days of placebos
- Vaginal ring also known as **NuvaRing**, it is inserted into the vagina for 3 weeks, and then removed for 1 week to allow withdrawal bleeding
- Transdermal patch also known as **Ortho Evra** is placed for 3 weeks, and then removed for 1 week to allow for withdrawal bleeding

Intrauterine device (IUD): two main types of IUDs are:
- **Levonorgestrel IUD** also known as **Marina**, it releases hormones **over 5-year period**. It may also **lower the bleeding and cramping**

- **Copper T band** also known as **Paraguard**, it releases hormones over **10-years period**. It may **increase the bleeding and cramping**

Permanent sterilization is permanent and irreversible; it is a best option for those who do not desire any more children
- Vasectomy: it is removal of segment of vas deference in men
- In female, permanent sterilization options include cutting, clipping or ligation of fallopian tubes

MENOPAUSE

Menopause is the cessation of woman's menstrual cycles. In US average age of menopause 51 years
Si/Sx: Menstrual periods that occur less often and eventually stop, hot flashes and sweating, skin flushing, insomnia,
Diagnosis: increased FSH; **FSH to LH ratio 3:1**
Treatment: Hormone replacement therapy (HRT), it is a combination of estrogen and progesterone. Estrogen controls the vasomotor symptoms (e.g. hot flashes, palpitations) and progesterone is added to the treatment because unopposed estrogen can cause endometrial hyperplasia and increase the risk of endometrial cancer.

Risks and benefits of HRT therapy

Benefits of HRTs	Reduces the risk of colorectal cancer and osteoporotic fractures
Risks of HRT	Increases the risk of DVT, heart attack and breast cancer

OSTEOPOROSIS

In osteoporosis bones become fragile, weak and more easily to break
Risk factors: thin white female with family history, smoking, alcohol, sedentary lifestyle, low calcium intake and steroids
Diagnosis:
- Spine x-ray
- Bone density testing with DEXA scan; DEXA ≥ -2.5 signifies osteoporosis

Treatment:

- First-line of treatment is bisphosphonate (alendronate, risedronate), which inhibits the osteoclast cell. Second-line treatment is raloxifene, which increases the bone density.
- Estrogen replacement is the last resort because estrogen increases the hypercoagulable states

Lifestyle modifications

- Vitamin D and calcium supplement
- Weight bearing exercises, as tolerated
- Smoking cessation
- Stop alcohol consumption

OBSTETRICS

Gravida is total number of pregnancies, whether or not they were carried to terms, including the current pregnancy
Parity is total number of pregnancies carried > 20 weeks, including viable and non-viable
Term delivery is delivery of an infant after 37 weeks of gestation
Premature delivery or preterm delivery is delivery of an infant before 37 weeks of gestation

Estimated delivery date by Nagele rule = Last menstrual period (LMN) + 7 days – 3 months + 1 years
For example: if LMP began 04/20/ 2014, delivery date is 01/27/2015

FIRST TRIMESTER SCREENING

First trimester screening includes:
1. PAP smear
2. Complete blood test, to check for blood disorders such as iron deficiency, folic acid deficiency
3. Blood type, rhesus (Rh) type and antibody screening
4. Platelet count
5. Syphilis
6. HIV
7. Rubella IgG antibody
8. Urinalysis and urine culture, to check for asymptomatic bacteriuria
9. Gonorrhea and chlamydia
10. Trichomonas
11. Bacterial vaginosis
12. Tuberculosis
13. Glucose screening is done at first visit only in patients with a risk factor for diabetes, such as obesity, family history, age >30, personal history of diabetes. Otherwise, glucose screening is performed between 24- 28 weeks of gestation

NORMAL WEIGHT GAIN DURING PREGNANCY
- Average weight gain during the pregnancy is approximately 28 lbs.

FETAL HEART TONE
- Between 10-12 weeks of gestation, fetal heart tones can be heard with Doppler ultrasound
- Between 16-20 weeks of gestation, fetal heart tones can be heard with normal stethoscope

UTERUS LOCATION AND SIZE
- Uterus enter the abdomen at 12th week of gestation
- Uterus reaches the umbilicus approximately at 20th week of gestation
- Uterine size is measured in centimeters, from the pubic symphysis to the top of the fundus. Approximately 20-35 weeks of gestation uterus size should be equal to the number of gestation weeks. Any difference more than 2-3 cm, between the uterine size and gestation week is called size and date discrepancy, which should be further evaluated with ultrasound.

Biparietal diameter is measured with ultrasound between 16-20 weeks of gestation. It is the **most accurate way to measure fetal age**

NORMAL PHYSIOLOGIC CHANGES IN WOMEN DURING PREGNANCY

HEMATOLOGY
- During pregnancy, the plasma volume increases by 5% and red blood cell mass increases by 20-30%. Hematocrit and hemoglobin values decrease, which is due to the dilution effect. However, **hemoglobin < 11.0mg/dL is likely due to iron deficiency anemia.**
- Increased liver coagulation factors and decreased ambulation, increases the risk for hypercoagulable state such as DVT, PE
- WBCs count is increased and can increase more than 20mil/mL
- Platelet count is decreased to 100-150 mil/mL

CARDIOVASCULAR

- Heart rate increases by 10-15 bpm, stroke volume increases and cardiac output increases by 30-50 %
- Elevated progesterone causes vasodilation and smooth muscle relaxation, which in turns decreases systemic vascular resistance
- Blood pressure drops in first trimester and hits the lowest point at 24th week of gestation, and it normalizes by 40 weeks
- Heart is displaced to the left and upward. Chest x-ray may show cardiomegaly

PULMONARY

- Tidal volume increases by 30-40 %
- Total lung capacity, functional residual capacity, tidal volume and minute ventilation are decreased, which my lead to **relative dyspnea**

RENAL

- Kidney size increases, right ureter dilates more than left ureter
- GFR increases by 50% and may last until 20 weeks postpartum
- Plasma renin and angiotensin increases which leads to increased aldosterone and water absorption

GASTROINTESTINAL

- Increased beta-hCG leads to nausea and vomiting, which usually resolves by 14-16 weeks
- Prolonged gastric empty time and decreased gastroesophageal sphincter tone leads to acid reflux
- Decreased colonic motility leads to increased water absorption and constipation

ENDOCRINE

- Increased estrogen increases thyroxine-binding globulin, which in turn increases total and bound T3/T4, but **active T3/T4 remains unchanged**
- Increased human placental lactogen (hPL) leads to increased lipolysis, but it also antagonizes insulin to maintain fetal glucose levels

MUSCULOSKELETAL
- Relaxin leads to relaxation of sacroiliac ligament, pubic symphysis and sacrococcygeal joint

DERMATOLOGY
- Melanocyte stimulation hormone (MSH) leads to **hyperpigmentation of nipples, umbilicus, linea nigra, perineum, and face**
- Increased estrogen may also leads to cirrhotic like changes such as spider angiomata, palmar erythema

ORAL GLUCOSE TOLERANCE TEST (OGTT)
Oral glucose tolerance test is performed to screen for gestational diabetes. It is usually performed between **24-28 weeks** of gestation, but in a **high-risk** patient, it should be performed at **first the prenatal visit**.
High risk: obesity, >30 years of age, family history of diabetes mellitus, previous fetal macrosomia, stillbirth or neonatal death.
OGTT test work-up includes two tests, **1-hour 5g OGGT**, and **3-hour 100g.** OGTT is done in a following manner:

1-hour oral 50g OGGT
A patient is given 50 grams of oral glucose, and then blood sample is taken from a **vein of the arm after 60 minutes** and results are interpreted as follow:
- If blood glucose level is < 140 mg/dl: it is considered a **normal response,** no additional glucose testing is required
- If blood glucose level is more than > 185 mg/dl: it is diagnosed as a **gestational diabetes,** and the patient should be **started on insulin,** no additional glucose test is required
- If blood glucose is between 140mg/dl -185 mg/dl: it requires further confirmation with **3-hour 100g glucose tolerance test**

3-hours 100 g OGGT

Overnight fasting is required before this test is performed, and patients fasting blood glucose is checked before the test. If patient's **fasting blood glucose is >126 mg/dl**, then this is considered as **gestational diabetes**. No additional OGGT test is needed, start the patient on **treatment**. However, if patient's **blood sugar is <126 mg/dl, then perform a 3-hour 100g OGTT.** 100 g oral glucose is given to the patient, and blood sample is taken from a vein of the arm at **3-hour intervals**. Results are interpreted as follows:

- Pregnant woman with one abnormal value (see table on the side) is diagnosed with **impaired glucose tolerance**

- Pregnant woman with 2 or more impaired values is diagnosed with **gestational diabetes**

> **Normal person** has following lab values
> o   Fasting glucose < 95 mg/dl
> o   **1-hour** glucose value <180 mg /dl
> o   **2-hour** glucose value < 155 mg/dl
> o   **3-hour** glucose value < 140 mg/dl

Treatment: mother with impaired glucose tolerance and gestational diabetes is treated as follow:
- Tight glucose control
- ADA diet and regular exercise
- Insulin

Fetus monitoring
- Obtain echocardiogram, triple marker screening, NSTs, Amniotic fluids index

Mode of delivery
- Labor may be induced, if fetus is < 4,500 g, but if fetus is > 4,500 g, then a C-section delivery is performed to prevent the vaginal delivery compilations
- During delivery, maternal blood glucose should be maintained between 80- 100 mg/dl with dextrose and insulin

SIGNIFICANCE OF MATERNAL SERUM ALPHA-FETOPROTEIN (MS-AFP)

Purpose: purpose of this test is to determine, if a fetus have trisomy (trisomy21 or trisomy 18), neural tube defect, intrauterine growth retardation (IUGR) or fetal demise

Screening criteria: MS-AFP is offered to all pregnant women, but it is recommended for a pregnant woman with the family history of birth defects, age>35 during the time of pregnancy, use of harmful drugs during pregnancy

Best performed: MS-AFP is most accurate, if it is measured between 16-20 weeks' of gestation (Normal MS-ASP values: .85 -2.5 MoM)

Note: the most common cause of abnormal MS-AFP level is incorrect gestation date. If MS-AFP level is abnormal (lower or higher than normal range), then get an ultrasound to confirm the gestation dates.
 If gestation **date is not correct,** then **repeat the MS-AFP,** but only if pregnancy is within 15-20 weeks of gestation. However, if gestation **date is correct,** then check MS-ASP level:

1.   MS-ASP < .85 MoM signifies trisomy, get **amniocenteses, to check karyotype abnormalities and serum markers** (MS-AFP, estriol, beta-hCG and inhibin-A). Results are as follow:

Karyotype	MS-AFP	Estriol	Beta-HCG	Inhibin-A
Trisomy 21	Low	Low	High	High
Trisomy 18	Low	Low	Low	N/A

2.   **MS-ASP >2.5MoM** usually signifies **neural tube defects, fetal demise or IUGR.** To distinguish between them, get **amniotic fluid-AFP and acetylcholinesterase levels.** Both are increased in **neural tube defects.** Whereas, only acetylcholinesterase is increased in **IUGR and stillbirth.**

GROUP B BETA-HEMOLYTIC STREPTOCOCCI (GBS) SCREENING

All pregnant women should get vaginal swab between 37-38 weeks of gestation to check for GBS. If GBS is present, then give her **penicillin during labor and delivery** to prevent neonatal sepsis and endometritis. Treatment **given before labor and delivery is ineffective** because GBS re-grows during labor and delivery.

PRENATAL DIAGNOSTIC TESTING

1. AMNIOCENTESES
Amniocentesis is a prenatal test in which a small amount of amniotic fluid is removed using ultrasound-guided needle, and then fluid is sent for chromosomal analysis. It is performed after 15 weeks of gestation.
Recommended to woman with the followings:
- Abnormal abdominal ultrasound
- Family history of certain birth defects, previous pregnancy or child with birth defect
- Mothers age 35 or more at the time of delivery

Complications miscarriage risk **0.06 %**, infection, preterm labor

2. CHORIONIC VILLUS SAMPLING (CVS)
Chorionic villus sampling is a prenatal test, which can be done earlier than the amniocentesis, in the first trimester (10-12 weeks of gestation). This test is performed to detect certain birth defects. In this test, ultrasound-guided needle is used to take a tissue sample of chorionic villus.
Compilations: miscarriage risk **1%**, **limb defect** if CVS is performed before 9 weeks of gestation

3. PERCUTANEOUS UMBILICAL BLOOD SAMPLING (PUBS)
PUBS is a prenatal test, in which fetus' blood is drawn from the fetal umbilical cord, and then that blood is used to detect birth defects. It is performed after 17 weeks of gestation
Complication: miscarriage **1-2%**, infection, premature rupture of membrane

NON-STRESS TEST (NST)
Non-stress test is performed in pregnancies over > 28 weeks gestation. This test checks if the fetus is well-being. Doppler is used to monitor fetal heart rate, and how fetal heart rate responds to the fetal movements. Results are interpreted as a **reactive NST or non-reactive NST**
- **A reactive NST** means that the fetus shows at least two heart accelerations 15 bpm above baseline for at least 15-20 seconds within 20 minutes. This indicates that fetus is doing well

- **Nonreactive NST** means that the fetus is not showing result as reactive stress test. It could mean that the fetus is **either sleeping or in jeopardy**. Vibroacoustic stimulation can help if differentiate in them. **Vibroacoustic test** will wake up a sleeping baby and will show reactive stress test. However, if the fetus is still showing nonreactive test, then do the **biophysical profile**.

BIOPHYSICAL PROFILE
Biophysical profile has 5 components and score is assigned based on these components, which are:
1. Fetal movement
2. Fetal breathing
3. Fetal tone
4. Amniotic fluid volume
5. Fetal heart rate

All components are measured with ultrasound. A sore 8-10 means fetus is well, and 0-2 scores worrisome. 0-2 score required future testing with contraction stress test

CONTRACTION STRESS TEST (CST)
In a contraction stress test, oxytocin is given to the mother to induce uterine contractions and fetal heart strip is monitored.

- A positive CST is defined as late deceleration with each contraction, it implies that the fetus is in jeopardy and in most cases C-section is performed.

OLIGOHYDROMONA
Oligohydromona is characterized by amniotic fluid < 500 ml or amniotic fluid index less than 5 cm
Cause: renal agenesis, IUGR, premature rupture of membrane,
Diagnosis: Ultrasound
Treatment: treat the underlying cause
Complication: pulmonary hypoplasia, limb deformity, musculoskeletal abnormalities, cord compression,

POLYHYDRAMNIOS
Polyhydramnios is characterized by amniotic fluid more than 2 L or amniotic fluid index >25 cm

Cause: GI disorders (duodenal atresia, esophageal atresia, gastroschisis and diaphragmatic hernia), CNS disorders (anencephaly and myotonic dystrophy), achondroplasia, maternal causes (DM, intrauterine infection), and Rh incompatibility

Diagnosis: ultrasound, Rh typing, maternal DM

Treatment: treat the underlying cause

Complications: Cord prolapse, placental abruption, premature death, perinatal death

INTRAUTERINE GROWTH RETARDATION (IUGR)

Intrauterine growth retardation characterized as a developing baby weighs less than 90% of other babies of the same gestational cause.

Types: two main types of IUGR are symmetric and asymmetric IUGR, which are based on 4 parameters measured with ultrasound. Results are following:

Parameters	Symmetric	Asymmetric
Abdominal circumference	Decreased	Decreased
Biparietal diameter	Decreased	**Normal**
Head circumference	Decreased	**Normal**
Femur length	Decreased	**Normal**

Cause: maternal (smoking, alcohol, drugs abuse or SLE), **fetal** (TORCH infection, chromosomal abnormalities, congenital abnormalities) and **placental** (preeclampsia, infarction, abruption).

Note: Maternal and placental factors usually give asymmetric IUGR, and fetal factors usually give symmetric IUGR

Diagnosis:
- Ultrasound
- NST, BPP, CST
- Doppler flow of umbilical artery

Treatment: IM betamethasone to enhance lung development and early delivery.

SAFE DRUGS DURING PREGNANCY

Condition	Medicine
Pain, fever, minor aches, headache	Acetaminophen
Heartburn	Antacids
Morning sickness, vomiting	Phenergan, scopolamine, Reglan
Constipation	Stool softener and laxative (Metamucil, Dulcolax, Colace)
Allergies	Antihistamine (Benadryl, Claritin)
Infection	Antibiotics: penicillin, ampicillin, amoxicillin, cephalosporins, erythromycin and nitrofurantoin
Antihypertensive	Hydralazine, methyldopa, labetalol
Diabetes	Insulin
Coagulopathy	Heparin

TERATOGEN DRUGS AND SIDE EFFECTS

DRUG	SIDE EFFECTS
Alcohol	Fetal alcohol syndrome (flat mid face, smooth philtrum, short palpebral fissures, thin vermillion borders of lips)
Angiotensin converting enzyme inhibitors (ACEIs)	**Renal** anomalies, **c**raniofacial abnormalities
Anesthetics	**Respiratory** depression, CNS depression
Aminoglycosides	Deafness
Barbiturates	Respiratory depression, CNS depression
Cigarettes	**Prematurity**, intrauterine growth retardation
Carbamazepine	Neural tube defect
Diethylstilbestrol (DES)	**Adenocarcinoma** of vagina, clear cell vaginal cancer, cervical incompetence
Iodine	Cretinism
Lithium	Cardiac (Ebstein) anomaly
NSAIDs	Premature ductus arteriosus closure
Oral contraceptives (OCPs)	VACTERL syndrome
Phenobarbital	Vitamin K deficiency
Phenytoin	Hypoplastic nails, Intrauterine growth retardation, typical face
Tetracycline	**Yellow** or brown colored teeth
Valproate	Neural tube defect
Warfarin	Craniofacial defect, chondrodysplasia

ABORTION

Spontaneous abortion is also known, as miscarriage is unintentionally loss of pregnancy before 20th week of gestation

Cause:

- Chromosome abnormality (the most common cause of miscarriage)
- Anatomic reproductive organ/tract problems
- Infection (STDs, listeria, or toxoplasmosis)
- Drugs
- Malnutrition
- Exposure to environmental toxins
- Hormone abnormalities
- Rh isoimmunization
- Endocrine abnormalities (diabetes, hypothyroidism)
- Cervical incompetence
- Immunologic abnormalities (SLE, anti-phospholipids)

Diagnosis:

- Beta-hCG
- CBC to determine the need for blood transfusion
- Rh blood type screening
- Pelvic exam
- Doppler ultrasound to check the fetal heartbeat
- Ultrasound to see if **all or some parts of the fetus are present**. This will help determine the type of abortion

Types of abortion and treatment: discussed in table next page

Differential diagnosis of abortion

Types of abortion	Characteristics	Treatment
Threatened abortion	• Vaginal bleeding • Pelvic exam shows **no cervical dilation** • **Fetal heart tones** are present on doppler ultrasound • Ultrasound shows **intact product of conception**	Bed rest, Pelvic rest
Inevitable abortion	• Vaginal bleeding • Pelvic exam shows **cervical dilation** • **Fetal heart tones** are present on doppler ultrasound • Ultrasound shows **intact product of conception**	D& C
Complete abortion	• Vaginal bleeding • Pelvic exam shows no cervical dilation • **No fetal heart tones** are present on doppler ultrasound • Ultrasound shows **no product of conception**	Follow beta-hCG until it becomes zero
Incomplete abortion	• Vaginal bleeding • Pelvic exam shows no cervical dilation • **No fetal heart tones** are present on doppler ultrasound • Ultrasound shows **some** product of conception	D& C
Missed abortion	• Vaginal bleeding • Pelvic exam shows no cervical dilation • **No fetal heart tones** are present on doppler ultrasound • Ultrasound shows **product of conception**	Induce the labor

ECTOPIC PREGNANCY

Ectopic pregnancy is an obstetric condition in which embryo implants outside the uterus. Most of the ectopic pregnancies occurs in fallopian tube (tubal-pregnancy), but can also occur in cervix, ovaries or abdomen

Risk factors: pelvic inflammatory disease, Intrauterine device in place while getting pregnant, tubal surgery, tubal ligation,

Si/Sx: lower abdominal pain, vaginal bleeding

Diagnosis:

- Beta-hCG
- Ultrasound
- Laparoscopy

Treatment:

- If patient is unstable, then do **laparotomy**
- Stable patient can be treated with methotrexate, salpingostomy or salpingectomy. **Methotrexate is given, only if beta-hCG < 6,000 mIU, ectopic mass < 3.5 cm, no fetal heart motion, and no history of folic acid use.** However, if a patient does not meet the criteria for methotrexate, then perform **laparoscopy** to determine the size of ectopic pregnancy. If it is **< 3 cm, then do salpingostomy.** Fallopian tube is left open to heal on its own to maintain fertility. However, If it is **> 3 cm, then do salpingectomy**
- Beta-hCG is followed weekly, until it reaches zero to ensure complete resolution

FETAL HEART RATE

- Normal fetal heart rate is between 110- 160bpm
- Normal fetal heart rate has following characteristics: beat-to-beat variability has accelerations and no decelerations

1. **Early decelerations** are decreased fetal heart rate below the baseline, but soon returns to baseline. These decelerations **coincide with uterine contraction;** means that the decelerations begin and end approximately the same time of the uterine contraction. Early deceleration usually signifies fetal **head compression.** Treatment: no treatment required because these are not harmful

2. **Late decelerations** are gradual decrease in fetal heart rate that occurs **after the uterine contractions.** Late decelerations are worrisome and signify **uteroplacental insufficiency. Treatment:** Place the mother in lateral decubitus position, give oxygen and stop oxytocin, if applicable. Give IV fluids and tocolytic such as ritodrine or magnesium sulfate to relax the uterus. If decelerations are still present, then deliver the baby.

3. **Variable decelerations** have **no relation to uterine contraction.** It often signifies **umbilical cord prolapse.** Treatment: **Place the mother in lateral decubitus position, give oxygen and stop oxytocin, if applicable. Give IV fluids and check out umbilical cord prolapse.**

UMBILICAL CORD PROLAPSE
Umbilical cord prolapse is obstetrics emergency in which umbilical cord comes out of the cervix.
Treatment: put mother in knee-to-chest position, elevate the presenting parts, give terbutaline, and perform urgent C-section

ABRUPTIO PLACENTA
Abruptio placenta is a premature (before the baby is delivered) separation of the placenta from the uterus. It occurs 1 out of 100 deliveries
Risk factors: abdominal trauma (hit to the abdomen, fall, or automobile accidents), cocaine use, HTN, previous abruption placenta, increased uterine distention (multiple pregnancies or large volume of amniotic fluid),
Si/Sx: painful vaginal bleeding, abdominal pain, uterine tenderness, hyperactive uterine contraction
Diagnosis:
- Clinical diagnosis
- Transvaginal or transabdominal ultrasound can be used, but it may not be reliable because ultrasound detects only a small percentage of abruptio placenta

Treatment:
- If the mother or fetus is in **distress,** then stabilize the mother, and do **emergency C-section**
- **Vaginal delivery may be induced,** if bleeding is heavy, but controlled, fetus is dead, or pregnancy is > 36 weeks of gestation with mother and fetus stable

- If pregnancy is far-term with mother and fetus stable or mild abruption, then **managed expectantly**; hospital observation, bed rest, fetal monitoring, IV fluids and blood products, as needed

Complication: DIC, hemorrhagic shock, fetal hypoxia, fetal death

UTERINE RUPTURE

Uterine rupture is a tear in the wall of the uterus. It is a life-threatening condition for the mother and fetus, and may occur before or during the labor

Risk factors: prior classic uterine incision, myomectomy, grand multiparity, excessive oxytocin stimulation

Si/Sx: painful vaginal bleeding, abdomen pain, chest pain, **loss of fetal electronic fetal heart rate signals,** maternal hypotension, **may be able to palpate fetal part in maternal abdomen**

Treatment:

- Immediate **laparotomy** with delivery of the fetus. A C-section is not done because **baby is in abdomen instead of uterus**
- Further management depends on the severity of rupture and condition of the patient. If the patient is unstable or does not desire any more children, then **uterus is removed** (hysterectomy). However, if the patient is stable or desires more pregnancies then uterus is usually **repaired** to preserve fertility.

Compilation: Those patients who have had uterus repair should have C-section delivery at 36 weeks for the subsequent pregnancies to reduce the risk of uterus re-rupture

PLACENTA PREVIA

Placenta Previa is an obstetric condition in which **placenta grows on the lower part of the uterus and covers all or some part of the cervical opening.**

Risk factors: Previous placenta previa, advance maternal age, grand multiparous, multiple gestations, abnormal uterus shape

Si/Sx: Painless vaginal bleeding, which may stop on its own in 1-2 hours and starts again in days or weeks. Fetus is mostly normal

Diagnosis: transabdominal ultrasound

Types: types of placenta previa depend on uterus proximity to cervical os. Discussed in the table on the next page

Types of Placenta Previa

Type	Characteristics
Marginal	Placenta is next to cervix but is not covering internal os
Partial	Placenta is covering some part of internal os
Complete	Placenta is covering all of the cervical os opening

Treatment:
- If the mother or fetus is **unstable**, then do **emergency C-section**
- If the **pregnancy is remote and mother and fetus are stable or mild abruption,** then pregnancy can be **managed expectantly**: hospital observation, bed rest, fetal monitoring, IV fluids and blood products as needed. Corticosteroids (betamethasone) is also given to the mothers, who is < 32 weeks of gestation, to enhance the fetal lung maturity
- Stable mother with term pregnancy should have **C-section delivery. Vaginal delivery** can only be tried **if placenta is > 2 cm away** from cervical os.

Complication: placenta accreta, placenta incerta, and placenta percreta

VASA PREVIA

Vasa previa is an obstetrics condition in which fetal vessels are crossing or running close to inner cervical os. These vessels are at increased risk of rupture when membranes ruptures and can cause fetal death

Risk factors: Multiple gestation, accessory lobe, velamentous insertion of umbilical cord

Si/Sx: classic triad - painless vaginal bleeding, membranes rupture and fetal bradycardia

Diagnosis:
- Clinical diagnosis (classic triad)
- Ultrasound with color-flow Doppler, rarely needed to confirm the diagnosis, it shows fetal vessels crossing the membranes over the internal cervical os

Treatment: immediate c- section otherwise fetal may die

HYPERTENSION

Hypertension is common medical problem, which may also be present during pregnancy. Three main types of hypertension seen during pregnancy are:

1. **Chronic hypertension** is defined as BP > 140/90 mm Hg that is **present before the conception or < 20 weeks of gestation.** Chronic hypertension may progress to pre-eclampsia. **Treatment-** oral methyldopa, labetalol or Nifedipine.

2. **Gestational hypertension** is defined as BP > 140/90 mmHg, which **develops > 20 weeks of gestation.** Gestational hypertension may progress to pre-eclampsia. **Treatment-** close follow-ups and treatment with oral methyldopa, labetalol or Nifedipine

Note: ACEs and ARBs are not used to treat HTN during pregnancy because both of them are teratogen

PRE-ECLAMPSIA

Pre-eclampsia is a characterized by BP > 140/90 mmHG and protein urea developing after 20 weeks of gestation. Pre-eclampsia is subdivided into mild and severe pre-eclampsia. If it is left untreated, it may progress to eclampsia. Discussed in table on next page

Differential diagnosis of pre-eclampsia

Type	Physical symptoms	Lab value
Mild pre-eclampsia	• Edema of hands, feet and face	• BP> 140/90 mmHg • Proteinuria: 1 -2 + on urine dipstick or 300 mg in 24 hours
Severe pre-eclampsia	• Generalized edema • **Headaches** • **Visual changes** • **RUQ epigastric pain**	• BP > 160/100 mmHg • Proteinuria: 3-4 + on urine dipstick or 5 g in 24 hours
Eclampsia	• Same as severe pre-eclampsia • **New onset seizure**	• Same as severe pre-eclampsia

Treatment:

Mild pre-eclampsia:
- If mother is near-term, then stabilize the mother and induce delivery
- If mother is far-term, then lower the BP with hydralazine or labetalol, then maintain the lower blood pressure with methyldopa, bed rest and expectant management

Severe pre-eclampsia and eclampsia
- Stabilize the mother; lower BP (goal: systolic BP 160-110 and diastolic BP 90-100, to maintain fetal blood flow), seizure control and prophylaxis with IV MgSO4, then induce the vaginal delivery regardless of gestation age
- Betamethasone is given to the mother with gestational age < 32 weeks to enhance the fetal lung maturity

HELLP Syndrome
HELLP Syndrome is a life-threatening obstetrics complication. It is usually considered variant of pre-eclampsia. HELLP is the abbreviation of the main features of the condition:
- Hemolysis
- Elevated liver enzymes (AST & ALT)
- Lower platelets

Si/Sx: same as mild or severe pre-eclampsia
Labs: same as mild or severe pre-eclampsia **plus hemolysis, low platelet and high liver enzymes**
Treatment:
- Stabilize the mother; lower BP (goal 160-110/90-100 to maintain fetal blood flow), seizure control and prophylaxis with IV MgSO4, Platelet transfusion if platelets are < 20, 000 or if platelets are < 50,000 mm and C-section is planned, and then deliver the baby regardless of gestational age
- Betamethasone is given to the mother with gestational age < 32 weeks to enhance the fetal lung maturity

FIBRONECTIN TEST
Fibronectin is a protein produced by fetal cells. It begins to break down and can be detected in vaginal discharge after 35 weeks of gestation. However, if it is present between 22-34 weeks of **gestation indicates preterm delivery is likely to occur.**

LABOR
True labor is defined as uterine contraction occurring every 2-3 minutes, lasting 45-60 seconds with the intensity of 50 mmHg

PRETERM LABOR
Preterm labor is defined as labor that occurs between 20-27 weeks of gestation, has at least 3 contraction in 30 minutes, and cervical dilation > 2cm or serial exams show change in cervical dilation or effacement
Risk factors: maternal smoking, previous preterm pregnancy, multiple pregnancy, pyelonephritis, chorioamnionitis, premature rupture of membrane
Symptoms: lower abdominal or backache, abdominal cramping or menstrual-like cramping, fluid leak form vagina, increased pressure in pelvis or vagina
Diagnosis:
- **Pelvic exam shows** at least 3 contraction in 30 minutes, and cervical dilation > 2cm or serial exams show change in cervical dilation or effacement
- **Nitrazine paper** test shows that **paper turns blue** when a small amount of vaginal fluid is placed on it
- **Fern test shows** " fern-like" pattern on a slide, when a small amount of vaginal fluid is placed on a slide and viewed under microscope
- **Ultrasound**

Treatment:
- Place the mother in lateral decubitus position, pelvic rest, bed rest, IV fluids and oxygen. If contraction still persists, then give tocolytic such as beta2 agonists (terbutaline, ritodrine), calcium channel blockers (Nifedipine) or magnesium sulfate
- IM betamethasone to mother < 32 weeks of gestation
- Stable with < 24 weeks gestation can be managed outpatient with tocolytic and bed rest

Contraindication to tocolytic: fetal demise, lethal fetal anomaly, advances cervical dilation; severe preeclampsia, eclampsia, abruption placenta, chorioamnionitis

PREMATURE RUPTURE OF MEMBRANE (PROM)

Premature rupture of membrane is defined as **rupture of membrane rupture of membrane before the onset of labor**
Risk factors: most common cause is ascending infection from lower genital tract, other risk factors includes smoking, STDs, young maternal age
Diagnosis:
PROM is diagnosed by sterile speculum exam to evaluate cervical dilation and effacement and following

- Amniotic fluid pooling in posterior vaginal fornix (most useful and definitive diagnostic test)
- **Nitrazine paper** test shows paper turn blue when small amount of vaginal fluid is placed on it
- **Fern test shows** " fern-like" pattern on slide, when small amount of vaginal fluid is placed on slide and viewed under microscope
- Ultrasound

Treatment:
If **chorioamnionitis is present,** then obtain cervical culture, given broad-spectrum antibiotics and induce delivery
If **chorioamnionitis is not present,** then management depends on the gestational age. Manage the patient as follow:

- Patient with **< 24 of gestation** has poor outcomes. Baby can be delivered or send home and advise bed rest
- Patients between **24- 33 weeks of gestation** should be hospitalized get cervical culture, and give prophylactic ampicillin and erythromycin. Additionally, give IM betamethasone if mother is < 32 week of gestation
- Prompt delivery if patient >**34 weeks** of gestation

Chorioamnionitis is an inflammation of the fetal membranes (chorion and amnion). Ascending bacterial infection from lower genital tract causes it. Chorioamnionitis is a **clinical diagnosis**: based on PROM, uterine tenderness and maternal fever, in the absence of UTI or URI.

LABOR

Order of fetal positions during normal labor and delivery (L&D)
During normal L&D fetus goes through the following 6 step-wise positions:
1. Descent
2. Flexion
3. Internal rotation
4. Extension
5. External rotation
6. Expulsion

STAGES AND DURATION OF LABOR

Stages	Characteristic	Duration
Stage 1 – has two phases: latent and active phase	Divided into two sub-phases; latent and active phase (see below)	
1a. Latent phase	From **0 to 3-4 cm** cervical dilation	Highly variable
1b. Active phase	From **3-4 cm cervical dilation to full dilation** (10 cm)	Cervical dilation >1 cm/hr. in nulligravida and >1.2 cm/hr. in multigravida
Stage 2	From full cervical dilation to **delivery of the baby**	Nulligravida 30 min -3 hr. Multigravida 5- 30 min
Stage 3	From delivery of baby to **delivery of placenta**	30 minutes

DISORDERS OF LABOR
1. **Arrest disorder** refers to **no change in cervical dilation** for over 2 hours or no change in **fetal descent** for 1 hour
2 **Protracted disorder** refers to **slow labor** during **active phase**, which is taking longer than normal time (as mention in stage and duration of labor)

3   Prolonged latent stage refers to **slow labor** during **latent phase**

Cause: the most common causes are:
- Sedation
- Cephalopelvic disproportion
- Malpresentation
- Abnormal uterine contraction

Management: depends on the cause
- **Prolong latent phase** is usually treated with **rest and hydration**
- C-section is performed if there is **cephalopelvic disproportion**
- Breech presentation (see below)
- If mother has **hypertonic contraction**, then give **morphine**. If mother has **hypotonic contraction**, then give **oxytocin**

BREECH PRESENTATION

Breech presentation is defined as fetal lie with the buttocks or feet close to the cervix, opposed to head (cephalic presentation)

Types: Three main types of breech presentations are:
- **Frank breech,** in which fetus' hips are flexed and knees are extended
- **Complete breech,** in which fetus's both hips and knees are flexed
- **Footling or incomplete breech**, in which one or both feet or knees are prolapsed into the maternal vagina

Treatment: external cephalic version is performed in women after 36 weeks of gestation. In this maneuver pressure is applied to mother's abdomen to achieve cephalic (head down) presentation. It is not recommended before 36 week of gestation because sometime fetus maneuver itself into cephalic presentation

SHOULDER DYSTOCIA

Shoulder dystocia is an obstetrics emergency that occurs when, after the delivery of the fetal head, the baby's anterior shoulder gets stuck behind mother pubic bone.

Management: is as follow:

Initial maneuver:

- **McRobert's maneuver:** have the mother hyperflex her thighs tightly to her abdomen. This maneuver widens the pelvis and flattens the spine in the lumbar region. It is effective in 42 % of the cases
- **Suprapubic pressure:** apply pressure over the bladder. It decreases fetal shoulder breadth
- **Rubin II maneuver:** place two fingers behind anterior shoulder; apply pressure downward and rotate fetus shoulder
- **Wood-Screw maneuver:** place two fingers behind posterior shoulder; apply pressure upward and rotate fetus shoulder

Last resorts are:

- **Zavanelli's maneuver:** push the fetal head back and perform C-section
- **Intentional fetal clavicular fracture**

INDICATIONS OF C-SECTION

Fetal factors	• Abnormal heart rate • Fetal malposition such as transverse lie, incomplete breech, • Big baby • Cephalopelvic disproportion (head is too large to pass through birth canal)
Maternal factors	• Active genital herpes • IIIV • Previous C-section with classic incision • Uterine surgery • Cervical carcinoma • Large uterine fibroids
Placenta or umbilical cord factors	• Umbilical cord prolapse • Placenta previa • Placenta abruption

POSTPARTUM HEMORRHAGE

Postpartum hemorrhage is defined as a loss of blood > 500 ml during vaginal delivery or > 1,000 ml during C-section. Three common types of postpartum hemorrhages are uterine atony, retained placenta, and uterine inversion. Discussed below

Differential diagnosis of postpartum hemorrhage

Cause	Characteristic	Treatment
Uterine atony	• Is the most common cause if postpartum hemorrhage • Caused by over distention of placenta, prolong labor, oxytocin grand parity	**Uterine message**, if this is ineffective then give oxytocin, carboprost* or methylergonovine*
Retained placenta	• Caused by retained part of the placenta. Inspection of placenta shows missing cotyledon	Manual removal of placenta or D&C
Uterine inversion	• Uterus come vagina " red beefy mass" • Results from pulling too hard on the cord	Manuel replacement of placenta plus oxytocin

*Note: carboprost is contraindicated in asthmatic patients and methylergonovine is contraindicated in patients with HTN

LOCHIA

Lochia is the vaginal discharge, which is seen in a woman **4-6 weeks after giving birth.** It contains blood, mucus, and uterine tissue. For first 3-5 days, it is **red** in color due to blood and uterine tissue, as it thins it gradually turns **brownish pink** and **eventually white or yellowish-white.** It has an **odor similar to that of normal menstrual fluid,** but if it is **foul smelly,** then one should suspect **endometritis.**

ENDOMETRITIS
Endometritis is irritation or inflammation of endometrium of the uterus
Risk factors: miscarriage, childbirth, prolong labor, C-section, PID, D& C
Si/Sx: fever, abdominal distention, pelvic pain
Diagnosis:
- WBC count
- ESR
- Endometrial, vaginal, urine and blood culture

Treatment: Empiric treatment with IV gentamicin and clindamycin or broad-spectrum antibiotics until culture and sensitivity is known
Complication: infertility, peritonitis, abscess, and septicemia

POSTPARTUM MOOD DISORDERS
Postpartum mood disorders are mental health disorder that affects women within first year after giving birth

Disorder	Characteristic	Treatment
Postpartum blue	Mother is tearful, but she **continues to take care** of herself and her child	None
Postpartum depression	Mother is tearful, and she **does not take care** of herself and her child	SSRIs
Postpartum psychosis	Mother experience **delusions, hallucinations**, and may have thought about hurting her child	Hospitalization and separate her from her child until she is better

POST TERM PREGNANCY
Post term pregnancy is defined as pregnancy that continues more than 42 weeks of gestation
Complication: post term pregnancy increases the risk of perinatal morbidity and mortality
Diagnosis:
- Clinical diagnosis
- Ultrasound is usually done to confirm the dates

Management:
- If dates are sure and cervix is favorable, then induce the labor with IV oxytocin and artificial rupture of membrane
- If dates are sure, but the cervix is unfavorable, then labor can be induced by prostaglandin E2, followed by IV oxytocin. Other option is to do twice-weekly NSTs and AFIs to ensure fetal well-being
- If dates are unsure preform twice-weekly NSTs and AFIs. If fetal is not doing well any time during the exam, then deliver the baby

Rh INCOMPATIBILITY
Rh incompatibility (also known as rhesus isoimmunization) causes hemolytic anemia in newborn. It is usually seen in second or subsequent pregnancy

Cause: Rh-negative mother and Rh-positive father have a Rh-positive baby. During the first pregnancy mother may get exposed to fetus' blood, and forms antibodies against Rh-positive blood. As a result this reaction is seen second or subsequent pregnancy

Diagnosis:
- Kleihauer-Batke test, this test measures the amount of fetal hemoglobin in mother's blood
- PUBS, it directly measures fetal hematocrit and degree of anemia
- Ultrasound doppler to measure the blood flow through the fetal middle cerebral artery

Treatment: if fetal has severe anemia and is < 34 weeks gestation, then perform intrauterine intravascular transfusion. However, if a fetus with severe anemia is > 34 weeks of gestation, then delivery is usually performed.

Prevention
- Rh-negative mother should receive RhoGAM at 28 weeks of gestation and within 72 hours of **delivery, miscarriage, elective or spontaneous abortion, amniocentesis, placenta abruption, placenta previa or vaginal bleeding**

Note: If both of the parents are Rh-negative, or if the mother is Rh-positive and father is Rh-negative, then there is no need to give RhoGAM

HUMAN IMMUNODEFICIENCY VIRUS

HUMAN IMMUNODEFICIENCY VIRUS (HIV)

HIV is a slow replicating retrovirus that targets and destroys CD4 T cell. As CD 4 T cell declines below a critical level, cell-mediated immunity is lost and body becomes susceptible to opportunistic infection.

Si/Sx: some patients may develop symptoms shortly after the infection. However, it usually **takes years for a person to show symptoms** because a normal person has CD4 count of 600-1000 per μl, and CD 4 count decreases 50-100 per years. Therefore, on the average it takes 5-10 years for CD 4 T cells to decline below critical level and show symptoms

Transmission: blood, semen, pre-seminal fluid, vaginal fluid, anal mucosa, needle stick injury, mother to child during breast milk

Diagnosis:

- Best **initial test is ELISA**; it detects HIV-1 antibodies in the blood, oral fluid or urine. It takes up to 2 weeks for the test result to be available. But sometimes, it may take up to six months for the antibodies to appear after acquiring infection
- If ELISA is positive, then it can be **confirmed** with **western blot**
- **PCR-RNA** test detects the viral genetic material in a person. It is **useful in babies born to HIV positive mothers** because babies' blood can contain their mother's HIV antibodies for several months, but PCR-RNA can determine whether newborns have HIV genetic material in baby's genes. PCR also helps **determine the response and effectiveness of the treatment.**

Treatment: highly active antiretroviral therapy (HAART) is a combination of medicines that slow the rate of HIV virus to make its copies. HAART is started, when:

- Patient has an AIDS defining illness
- CD4< 500, or viral load > 100,000 μl

Any of the following HAART combination can be used:

- **Two nucleosides** combined with **a protease inhibitor** or **Efavirenz**
- **Two nucleosides** combined with **two protease inhibitors**
- **Once–daily** a **combined tablet** of emtricitabine, tenofovir and efavirenz

HAART THERAPY AND ITS SIDE EFFECTS

Type	Medicines	Side effects
Nucleoside reverse transcriptase inhibitors	• Zidovudine • Didanosine • Stavudine • Lamivudine • Abacavir • Emtricitabine • Tenofovir	• All of the nucleoside reverse transcriptase cause lactic acidosis • Zidovudine - **anemia** • Didanosine & stavudine - **pancreatitis and peripheral neuropathy** • Tenofovir – renal insufficiency
Protease inhibitors	• Indinavir • Ritonavir • Tipranavir • Lopinavir	• All protease inhibitor cause hyperglycemia hyperlipidemia, lipodystrophy • Indinavir – **needle shaped kidney stone**
Non-nucleoside reverse transcriptase inhibitors	• Efavirenz • Nevirapine • Efavirenz	

HIV PROPHYLAXIS

HIV prophylaxis medications are given in the following conditions:

1. Anyone exposed to **blood** or have **intercourse** with a **HIV-positive** patient, should receive 3-drug combination for **28 days**

2. Prophylaxis for pneumocystis carinii pneumonia **(PCP) is given** when **CD 4 T cell** counts **fall below 200/mm**. Treatment: Trimethoprim-sulfamethoxazole (TMP-SMX) or dapsone and/or pentamidine.

3. Prophylaxis for mycobacterium avium complex **(MAC)** is given, when CD **4 T cell** counts **fall below 100/mm**. Treatment: daily clarithromycin or weekly azithromycin. It is discontinued when CD 4 T cell goes above 100/mm

HIV-POSITIVE PREGNANT WOMEN MANAGEMENT

Start HAART in pregnant women:
- If CD4 count is <500, then start HAART regardless of gestational age
- If CD4 count is > 500, then start HAART in 2nd trimester

Note: HAART treatment regimen in pregnant women must include ZDV

HAART medicines **contraindicated** in pregnancy are:
- Nevirapine – side effects: fetal hepatotoxicity
- Efavirenz- side effects: neural tube defect
- Didanosine and stavudine – side effects: fetal lactic acidosis

Delivery options for a HIV-positive mothers are following:
- Women should be offered to have a C-section before 38 weeks of gestation, before the rupture of membrane
- Near-term women can have **elective C-section,** if she has high CD 4 T cell count and viral load <1,000 copies/ml
- Near–term pregnant women with **viral loads > 1,000 copies/ml** should have a C-section at 38 weeks gestation, before the rupture of membrane

Notes:

BITES

HUMAN HAND BITE
Human bite is considered a high-grade bite. Patient should be given prophylaxis augmentation (amoxicillin + clavulanate), and then referred to a hand surgeon.

CAT BITE
Cat bite is considered a high-grade bite because their sharp teeth penetrate deeper. Patient should be given prophylaxis augment (amoxicillin + clavulanate)

DOG BITE
Dog bite is considered a low-grade bite, unless the dog is known to have rabies

Treatment: irrigation and proper wound care, observe the dog and treatment is given as follow:

- If the dog **doesn't develop** any symptoms of rabies, then **no vaccination** is needed
- If the dog **develops rabies symptoms** or **known to have rabies,** then give **vaccination** as follow:
  - If the patient **received** human diploid cell vaccine **(HDCV)** in the past, then give **rabies immunoglobulin**
  - If the patient **did not receive HDCV** in the past, then give **HDCV plus rabies immunoglobulin**

BAT BITE
- If the patient **received human diploid cell vaccine (HDCV)** in the past, then give **rabies immunoglobulin**
- If the patient **did not receive HDCV** in the past, then give **HDCV plus rabies immunoglobulin**

Note: there is a high incidence of rabies in the bats and they can spread it by saliva, as well. So if a person is exposed of bat's saliva or bit by a bat, then he should be treated as above. There is no need to locate and watch the bird for rabies symptoms

BLACK WIDOW SPIDER BITE
Symptoms: sharp pain at the site of the bite, deep burning aching pain, vomiting, headache, chest tightness, hypertension and abdominal muscle rigidity.
Treatment: maintain ABCs, tetanus prophylaxis, pain relievers, wound care and nitrate for HTN

BROWN RECLUSE SPIDER BITE
Symptoms: pain and necrosis at the site of bite, fever, chills, arthralgia, myalgia
Treatment: ice compress, oral erythromycin, wound care and plastic surgeons consult

SNAKE BITE
Symptoms: vomiting, diarrhea, restless, dysphagia, muscle weakness, fasciculation
Treatment: Advance cardiac life support (ACLS), tetanus prophylaxis, and type-specific antivenin.

ADULT IMMUNIZATION

Influenza vaccine is given **yearly** to all patients > 65 years of age and those < 65 years of age with the risk factors such as health care workers, pregnant women, immunocompromised, chronic heart disease, diabetes mellitus, and COPD. It should be **avoided** in people with the history of **egg allergy**

Pneumococcal vaccine is given **once** to all patients > 65 years of age and those < 65 years of age with the risk factors (same as influenza). **Revaccination or second dose of pneumococcal vaccine** is only needed, if adults >65 years of age or immunocompromised patient received pneumococcal vaccine more than 5 years ago.

Hepatitis A vaccination is recommended to patients with chronic liver failure, IV drug abuse, chronic liver disease and men who have sex men.

Hepatitis B vaccination is recommended to all young adults and high-risk people such as health care workers, people with recent STD, IV drug abusers

MMR vaccination is recommended to everyone who is born after 1956. Rubella should not be given to pregnant woman. If a childbearing woman receives it, she should avoid for 3 months after the vaccination.

Varicella vaccination is recommended to people with high-risk such as health care workers, teachers, or childcare providers. It should be only given to HIV positive patient if CD 4 T cells are > 500.

Meningococcal vaccination is recommended to college dormitory residents, asplenic, and people with terminal complement deficiency

Tetanus vaccination is recommended to everyone, and then booster dose is given every 10 years. But, there are some other tetanus shot guidelines, which are as follow:

Type wound	Tetanus vaccination
Clean or dirty wound	If the patient received tetanus vaccination **within last 5 years,** then **no vaccination is needed**
Dirty wounds	If the patient received tetanus vaccination within last **5-10 years,** then give **Td booster.** No vaccination is required for clean wounds
Clean and dirty wounds	If the patient received last tetanus vaccination **>10 years ago,** then give **Td booster plus Td immunoglobulin**

TRAVELER PROPHYLAXIS

Malaria
- **Mefloquine or atovaquone-proguanil** is recommended to people traveling to Asia, Africa. Chloroquine is not given to people traveling to these area because of high resistance rate
- **Chloroquine** is to recommended to people traveling to Caribbean, Mexico, and Central America

Typhoid prophylaxis is recommended to people traveling to India, Pakistan, Peru, Chile, and Mexico

Yellow fever prophylaxis is recommended to people traveling to South America and Africa

Meningococcus prophylaxis is recommended to people traveling to sub-Saharan Africa

Hepatitis A vaccination prophylaxis is recommended to all travelers planning to travel after 4 or more weeks, but if patient is planning on traveling within 4 weeks, then give **IVIG**

BIOSTATISTICS

Disease

	(+)	(-)
(+)	A	B
(-)	C	D

Test or Exposure

False positive is defined as a patient without the disease, but has a positive test result

False negative is defined as a patient with the disease, but has a negative test result

Incidence is total number of new cases reported divided by total population

Prevalence is total number of existing cases divided by total population at the given time

Sensitivity is defined as the ability of the test to detect the disease in a patient with a disease. It is calculated, true positive divided by all of the people with the disease. $A/(A+C)$

Specificity is defined as the ability of the test to identify a healthy person in all of the healthy people. It is calculated, true negative divided by all of the people without the disease. $D/(B+D)$

Positive predictive value (PPV), when the test is positive in a patient with the actual disease. It is calculated, true positive divided by all patients tested positive for the disease. $A/(A+B)$

Negative predictive value (NPV), when the test is negative in a patient without the disease. It is calculated, by true negative divided by all of the patients tested negative for the disease. $D/(C+D)$

Relative risk compares the people who are at **risk** of developing disease **when exposed to the risk factor**, to the people at risk of developing a disease **without the risk factors**. It can only be calculated after prospective or experimental studies are done. [A/(A+B)]/ [C/(C+D)]

Odd risk compares the odds of **developing disease** in the people who are **exposed to the risk factor**, to the people with odds of developing disease **without the exposure of risk factors**. It can only be calculated after prospective or experimental studies are done. (A x D) /(B x C)

Attributable risk is the number of cases expected to decrease, if the risk factor is removed. [A/(A+B)] - [C/(C+D)]

Mean is the average numbers
Mode is the most common number.
Median is the middle number
For example: in following numbers 1, 1,2 and 4
- Mean is average of four number: 1+1+2+4 =8/4= 2
- Mode is 1 because it is the most common number
- Median is the middle number, since we don't have a middle number here we can take a average of two middle number (1+2)/2= 1.5

In a **positive skewed** curve, mean >media > mode
In a **negative skewed** curve, mean < median < mode

Types of error
1. **Type I error** occurs when null hypothesis is rejected when in fact it is true
2. **Type II error** occurs when null hypothesis is not rejected when it in fact it is false

TESTS
1. **Chi-squared test** is used to compare percentage
2. **T-test** is used to compare two means
3. **Analysis of variance** (ANOVA) is used to measure three or more means

Correlation coefficient measures the relationship between two variables.

- **Positive 1 correlation means** two variables are positively correlated, which means when one increases so does the other.
- **Negative 1 correlation** means two variables are negatively correlated which means when one goes up, then the other goes down.
- **Zero correlation** means two variables are not related

BIAS

1. **Nonresponse bias** occurs when some subjects choose not to respond to particular questioners

2. **Lead-time bias** occurs when two tests that detect the same disease are compared, but there is no effect in the outcomes of the disease. For example, two tests can screen the cancer, one test finds the cancer at an early age and another test finds the cancer at later age, but patient's life expectancy does not change with the early or late detection.

3. **Admission rate bias** occurs when the hospital's admission criteria influence the outcomes. For example, hospital A has more cases of mortality because they admit only older patients with severe pneumonia. Whereas, hospital B has fewer cases of mortality because they mostly admit young patient with mild pneumonia.

4. **Recall bias** is a risk factor in retrospective studies, it occurs when people cannot accurately recall the exact information. For example, John cannot recall if grandfather died of a heart attack or lung cancer.

5. **Interviewer bias** occurs when an interviewer intentionally or unintentionally makes a decision that affects the study outcome. For example, an interviewer gets incentive to prove certain pain medicine works better than another medicine in arthritis patient. So he only recruits patients with mild or no arthritis pain to prove this medicine works better than another medicine. Blinding can prevent interviewer bias

6. **Unacceptable bias** occurs when people do not admit to some behavior or claim they do more. For example, a person claims that he is cutting down number of cigarettes, but, in fact, he is smoking the same the number of cigarettes.

TYPES OF STUDY

1. **Experimental study** compares two groups; in which one group's variables are intentionally changed and it affects are measured.

2. **Prospective study is** a cohort study, in which group of individuals are chosen and divided into two groups and then followed overtime in the presence and absence of **risk factors.** For example, a study trying to find the incidence of lung cancer, follow the group, in which one group smokes cigarettes and another group does not.

3. **Retrospective study** is a case control study; in which people are chosen based on absence or presence of **disease** and information is collected about risk factors. For example, people with lung cancer are compared without the lung cancer to see if people with lung cancer smoked cigarettes before developing a lung cancer.

4. **Case series study** follows a group of patients with similar disease

5. **Prevalence study** also known as cross-sectional analysis, it looks at the prevalence of a disease and the prevalence of risk-factors

ETHICS

AUTONOMY

An adult patient with a **sound mind** has right to refuse treatment, blood products, or surgery. Frequently asked question in boards, a Jehovah's Witness: who was just involved in a motor vehicle accident and now requires a blood transfusion. However, patient is refusing the blood transfusion. In this case, respect the patient decision; just give him IV fluids, or whatever else is acceptable to the patient.

Pregnant women with a sound mind have right to refuse treatment to **her** and **her unborn child**, regardless of the gestation age. However, once the infant is born, then it becomes physician's responsibility to provide the treatment in newborn's best interest.

Exception: **Incompetent or delirious** patients can be **restrained** or **hospitalized against their will,** if they are a danger to themselves or others.

INFORMED CONSENT

Informed consent is based on patient's autonomy. It can be in **writing or oral**. For the consent to be informed, patient should be informed about **risks, benefits, and alternative treatment or procedures**. It should be in the **language patient can understand** and must be **given for each particular procedure**. Patient should be allowed to make his own decision

DO NOT RESUSCITATE (DNR) ORDER

DNR order is a medical order, which instructs health care providers to not to perform endotracheal intubation and CPR, in the event patient's breathing stops or heart stops beating.

FUTILE CARE

Futile care means that a physician has no obligation to continue providing treatment, if the treatment has no health benefits to the patient.

MEDICAL EMERGENCY PROCEDURES

A competent patient **has right to refuse** any treatment, tests or procedures

If a patient is not capable of making medical decision because of **impaired cognitive function**, then the decision-making process is followed in a following **stepwise manner:**

1. Health care proxy
2. Living will
3. **Previously stated wish** to family, close neighbor or close friends
4. Spouse
5. Patients children who is 18 years of age or older
6. Patient's mother or father
7. Siblings who is 18 years of age or older
8. A close friend, if patient has no family

WITHHOLDING INFORMATION FROM PATIENT

- A patient should always be told about his diagnosis
- If a patient does not want to know the diagnosis, then a physician should ask the patient about the reason for his request and try to resolve the issue. However, if patient is still refusing to know his diagnosis, then have the patient sign the document and withhold the information until patient wants
- If patient's family requests a physician to withhold the diagnosis from the patient, then the physician should first ask the family for the reason of their request. Physician may temporarily hold the information from the patient, but ultimately, patient should always be told about his diagnosis

WITHHOLDING AND WITHDRAWING THE TREATMENT

A competent adult patient has right to withhold and withdraw from any treatment at any time during the treatment

BRAIN DEATH

Brain death is defined as irreversible end of brain activity. The characteristics of brain death are:

- No corneal reflex
- No cortical reflex
- No brain reflex
- **Positive** apnea test

CONFIDENTIALITY

Patient has full right to have his medical information confidential, but **confidentially can be broken in the following situations:**

- Danger to others
- Transmissible disease
- Duty to warn and protect (if patient says that he is going to kill someone, then it is a physician's responsibility to inform the person in danger and the authorities, or both)
- Court mandate
- Suspected child abuse

Frequently test confidentially question

Q. A 25 years old male just been diagnosed with HIV. He is very upset and requests that you do not disclose his HIV status to his wife. What is the next step in management?

A. Encourage the patient to talk to his wife

DOCTOR-PATIENT RELATIONSHIP

A Physician has **no obligation to accept** a patient. However, **once** physician **accepts** the patient, and then physician **cannot abandon** the patient, **until a substitute** physician is found

Physician has right to refuse treatment to a HIV positive patient

SEXUAL CONTACT WITH PATIENT

Sexual contact between a **psychiatrist and patient** is **never acceptable.** However, sexual contact between **other physicians and patient** is **acceptable,** but only after they **end their doctor-patient relationship**

GIFTS
Small gifts that are **not given with the intensions of specific** treatment, procedures or tests, are **acceptable**. Any gift tied to a **specific treatment, procedure or test, is not acceptable**

PHYSICIAN ASSISTED SUICIDE
Physician assisted suicide is always wrong. However, physician may give a pain reliever with **the primary goal to reduce the pain,** which may also shorten the patient's life span.

ORGAN DONATION
Even if person's driver license says that he is an organ donor, a physician is still required to get that person's family or health care proxy's approval for organ donation

IMPAIRED PHYSICIAN
Impaired physician should be reported to a higher authority. Impaired physician means, that a physician, who is a danger to the medical care. A physician drinking, getting in fights or stealing outside his hospital, is not considered impaired physician and is not reportable. Impaired physician can be reported to the following authorities:
- **Residents or physician in training** should be reported to the program **director** or department **chair**
- **Faculty** should be reported to the **dean** or department **chair**
- **A physician in practice should be** reported to the **state medical board**

REPORTING ABUSE
All health care providers are **obligated to report child abuse and elderly** abuse. Even if the claim is found to be false, health care provider **has immunity by the court,** as long as, the report was made in good faith.

Health care providers **cannot report** domestic violence or spousal abuse without **patient's wish.**

PATIENT'S MEDICAL RECORDS
A physician cannot release patient's medical records to anyone without patient's consent. However, physician can release patient's medical records without patient's consent, if court orders or subpoena

A physician cannot obtain patient's medical records from patient's previous physician or other current physicians without patient's consent

MINORS
Patients under 18 years of age do not have capacity to understand their medical condition; they need parents or guardian to make their medical decisions

Exception: In a life-threatening situation, physician can ignore parent or guardian refusal of intervention and proceed to treat a minor. For example, if Jehovah's Witness parents or guardian is refusing lifesaving blood transfusion to the **minor, then physician can overrule their wish** and proceed to blood transfusion

EMANCIPATED MINOR
Emancipated minor is a legal term by which minor who is < 18 years of age is free from control of his or her parents or guardian, moreover, parents or guardian are also free from any obligation towards that minor. Minors are considered emancipated minors, if they are:
- Married
- Living independently and financially independent
- Serving in the military
- Raising their own children

Partial emancipation is a legal term in which minors are emancipated for particular purpose such as:
- Obtaining OCPs
- STD treatment
- Seeking treatment or intervention for substance abuse
- Seeking treatment for psychiatric illness

Notes:

DERMATOLOGY

YEAST SKIN INFECTION

TINEA

Tinea is a superficial skin infection caused by fungus. It is common in children, and thrives in warm moist areas

Specific name depends on the body area it affects:

- Tinea **corporis** affects the skin of the body. It appears **red-colored, raised** border that **clears centrally as it expands**
- Tinea **versicolor** is chronic fungal infection of the skin caused by Pityrosporum (also known as Malassezia furfur). Patient usually present with hypopigmented macules on face and trunk in summers
- Onychomycosis affects the nail, and causes **brittle and yellow discolored nails**
- Tinea **cruris** affects **groins area**
- Tinea **capitis** affects the **head**
- **Tinea pedis** affects the **feet**

Diagnosis:

- Best initial test is KOH prep
- **Note:** KOH prep of tenia versicolor shows classic spaghetti-meatballs appearance
- Most accurate test is fungus culture

Treatment: most of the tinea infections are treated with **topical azoles** such as ketoconazole, clotrimazole, with the exception of followings:

- Tinea versicolor is treated with **selenium sulfide, ketoconazole is the 2nd choice**
- **Nail infection** is treated with **oral itraconazole or terbinafine**
- Tinea capitis **is treated with griseofulvin**

BACTERIAL SKIN INFECTION

1.   IMPETIGO
Impetigo is a superficial skin infection caused **by Staphylococcus aureus** (most common cause) **and Streptococcus pyogenes**. It spreads either by direct contact with skin-to-skin either or auto-inoculates in nose or mouth
Si/S: Red sores, which breaks **open, oozes fluid, and honey colored crusts**
Diagnosis: clinical diagnosis
Treatment:
- **Local** skin infection is treated with **topical mupirocin**
- **Bullous or extensive** disease is treated with **oral** dicloxacillin, or cephalexin

2.   ERYSIPELAS
Erysipelas is a dermis and epidermis infection caused by **group A-beta-hemolytic streptococcus** (Pyogenes)
Si/Sx: bright red appearance of face, high fever, chills, vomiting, and headaches, which starts within 48 hours of infection
Diagnosis: clinical diagnosis
Treatment:
- **Stable patient** is treated with **oral** dicloxacillin or cephalexin
- **Serve disease** or **unstable** patient is treated empirically with IV Nafcillin or oxacillin, until the sensitivity is known.

3.   CELLULITIS
Cellulitis is a severe inflammation of **dermis** and **subcutaneous tissues** caused by **staphylococcus aureus or streptococcus pyogenes**
Diagnosis: clinical diagnosis
Treatment:
- **Stable patient** is treated with **oral** dicloxacillin, or cephalexin
- **Serve disease** or **unstable** patient is treated empirically with IV Nafcillin or oxacillin, until the sensitivity is known

4.   NECROTIZING FASCIITIS
Necrotizing fasciitis is a life-threatening condition, which begins with a traumatic injury to the skin, and then quickly spreads into the fascial planes of the skin.

Cause: **Staphylococcus aureus, clostridium perfringens**
Si/Sx: high fever, pain out of proportion, crepitus, local inflammation may be absent
Diagnosis: X-ray, MRI or CT shows air in tissues
Treatment: Immediate surgical debridement plus antibiotics clindamycin and penicillin to keep the infection from spreading

HAIR FOLLICLE INFECTION
Three most common hair follicle infections are folliculitis, furuncles and carbuncles. Folliculitis leads to furuncle that further leads to carbuncles
Cause:
- Most common cause is **Staph. Aureus**
- Hot tub folliculitis caused by **Pseudomonas aeruginosa**

1. FOLLICULITIS
Folliculitis is inflammation and infection of the hair follicles of the skin. Folliculitis may look like a red pimple with pus in it
Treatment: warm compress or topical mupirocin (2nd choice)

2. FURUNCLES
Furuncle is a **deep folliculitis** that causes painful swollen area. It is full of pus and dead tissue
Treatment: Warm compression, incision and drainage, oral dicloxacillin or cephalexin

3. CARBUNCLES
Carbuncles is a **cluster of furuncles** that fused to become a single lesion
Treatment: Incision and drainage, oral dicloxacillin or cephalexin

AUTOIMMUNE SKIN DISEASE

1. BULLOUS PEMPHIGOID
Bullous pemphigoid is an autoimmune skin disease that causes the formation of bullae between dermis and epidermis
Si/Sx: **thick walled bullae** that **do not rupture easily**
Diagnosis: **Biopsy** with **immunofluorescent antibody** shows IgG **antibodies** and **complement deposit along the basement membrane**
Treatment: Oral corticosteroids

2.   PEMPHIGUS VULGARIS

Pemphigus is an autoimmune disease that causes the formation of **blisters on the skin** and **oral mucosa.**

Si/Sx: **thin** and **fragile** blisters, **painful oral ulcers, Nikolsky sign**

Diagnosis: Most accurate test is **biopsy**

Treatment: **Oral corticosteroids.** If corticosteroids are ineffective, then give cyclophosphamide, azathioprine or IVIG

MALIGNANT AND PREMALIGNANT LESIONS

1.   SEBORRHEIC KERATOSIS

Seborrheic keratosis usually appears as a **greasy hyperpigmented crusty lesions** that appear to be **stuck onto skin** surface. It is commonly seen in elderly

Diagnosis: shave biopsy

Treatment: liquid nitrogen or excision

2.   ACTINIC KERATOSIS

Actinic keratosis is a **non-tender** erythematous macule that develops on the **sun-exposed areas.** It is a premalignant skin condition that can progress to squamous cell carcinoma

Diagnosis: local **excision**

Treatment: cryotherapy, topical 5-fluorouracil

3.   SQUAMOUS CELL CARCINOMA

Squamous cell carcinoma of the skin appears **as an ulcerated nodular mass** that develops on the **sun-exposed** areas such as lips, ears, neck, arm or hands.

Diagnosis: biopsy

Treatment: surgical excision

4.   BASAL CELL CARCINOMA

Basal cell carcinoma is the most common form of cancer in the US. It develops on sun-exposed areas. It looks like **pearly papules** on the skin

Diagnosis: shaves or **punch biopsy**

Treatment: Moh's surgery

5.   MALIGNANT MELANOMA

Malignant melanoma is the leading cause of death from skin disease. It usually starts as a simple mole, which later **develops** into cancer.

Common **characteristics** of melanoma are: Mnemonic **ABCDE**

- **A**symmetric
- **I**rregular Border
- **C**hange in colors
- **D**iameter > 6 mm
- **E**nlarging or growing

Diagnosis: Full thickness biopsy

Management: Excision and Interferon. Interferon appears to reduce the recurrence

Prognosis depends on the depth of melanoma

6.   KAPOSI'S SARCOMA

Kaposi's sarcoma is caused by **human herpesvirus 8.** It is common in immunocompromised patients or **HIV positive** patient with **CD 4 counts < 100.** Patients have **purplish lesion on the skin**

Treatment:

- Best initial treatment for HIV-related Kaposi's sarcoma is HAART treatment, which can help raise CD4 count. Patients usually show complete resolution of the skin lesions while on HAART.
- Specific treatment for Kaposi's sarcoma is liposomal Adriamycin and vinblastine

SEBORRHEIC DERMATITIS

Seborrheic dermatitis **is an erythematous greasy patch** with white flaking **(dandruff).** It is usually found around eyebrows, nasolabial folds, or scalp

Treatment: Topical **ketoconazole or selenium sulfide**

CONTACT DERMATITIS

Contact dermatitis is a **linear pruritic rash** that appears at the site of contact with irritant such as belt buckle site, wristwatch area, or a body part that came in contact with poison ivy

Diagnosis: Definitive diagnosis is **skin patch testing**

Treatment:

- Identifying and remove the source
- **Mild** contact dermatitis is treated with **topical steroids**

- Extensive contact dermatitis is treated with high dose **oral steroids for 2-3 weeks, and then steroids are gradually tapered** to prevent the relapse

PITYRIASIS ROSEA

Pityriasis Rosea is a pruritic skin eruption **that starts as a herald patch, and** then **spreads in a " Christmas tree distribution"**, but **palms and soles are spared**
Treatment: **no treatment is required, it usually resolves** in 1-3 months

ROSACEA

Rosacea is a chronic skin condition characterized by **flushing and redness** on **nose, cheeks, chin, and forehead. It exacerbates** with food, exercise, sun exposure, hot weather, stress, spicy foods, alcohol, or hot baths. It usually coexists with **blepharitis**
Treatment: Topical metronidazole, but If eyes are involved, then treat it with **oral doxycycline**

ATOPIC DERMATITIS

Itchy inflammatory skin condition that affects the flexor surface of the skin
Treatment:
- **Avoid hot water, drying soaps and other irritants**
- **Keep the skin moist** with creams or emollients

PSORIASIS

Psoriasis is a chronic remitting immune–mediated skin disease. It is characterized by red skin with flaky **silvery scales on the extensor surface**, other symptoms: fingernail pitting, **Auspitz sign** (pinpoint bleeding after removal of overlying scales) and **Köbner's phenomenon** (lesions appear at the site of skin injury)
Treatment:
- Mild disease: **topical salicylic** acid is used initially to remove the collection of scaly material, and then **emollient**
- Moderate disease -**Topical vitamin D derivative** (calcipotriene) **vitamin A** (tazarotene)
- If >30% body is involved - **UV light therapy**
- Systemic disease - **DMARDS** (Methotrexate, cyclosporine)

HERPES ZOSTER

Herpes zoster **is also known, as shingles is the** reactivation of chicken pox virus in **sensory nerve ganglion**, which causes painful skin rash with blisters and burning sensation over the affected dermatomes. It is often seen in elderly and immunocompromised patients

Diagnosis:
- Clinical diagnosis
- Most accurate test is Tzanck test, but it is rarely needed

Treatment:
- Steroid
- Most effective treatment is oral acyclovir or famciclovir
- **Gabapentin** is used to control pain in post-herpetic neuralgia. But, if gabapentin is ineffective, then use **TCAs (amitriptyline or Nortriptyline) or topical capsaicin**

SCABIES

Scabies is a contagious skin condition caused by mites. It usually causes **intense pruritus and burrows** between the fingers and toe, genital area or breast creases

Diagnosis: scrape test: apply mineral oil to burrow, and then scrape the organism out

Treatment: Topical permethrin cream, but if topical permethrin cream is ineffective, then give single dose of oral ivermectin

PEDICULOSIS

Pediculosis is an infection caused by lice. It is easily transmitted from person-to-person during the direct contact

Types: two common types of pediculosis are:
- Pediculosis capitis, which infests head hair
- Pediculosis pubis (crabs), which infests pubic hair

Si/Sx: most common symptom is pruritus

Diagnosis: direct visual inspection with fine-toothed comb

Treatment: Topical permethrin cream, but if topical permethrin cream is ineffective, then give single dose of oral ivermectin

ERYTHEMA NODOSUM

Erythema nodosum is **inflammatory condition of the fat cells,** under the skin that results in **painful, tender nodules.** It is usually seen on anterior surface of the lower legs with smooth and shinny appearance

Cause:

- OCP
- IBD
- Pregnancy
- Sarcoidosis, streptococcal infection, sarcoidosis, syphilis
- Hepatitis, histoplasmosis

Treatment: treat underlying cause and NSAIDs

ERYTHEMA MULTIFORME

Erythema multiforme is a hypersensitive reaction in response to an infection or medicine

Si/Sx: "target" or "iris" like lesions on **palms and soles,** itching, fever, joint aches

Cause:

- HSV or Mycoplasma
- Penicillin, Phenytoin
- Sulfa drugs
- NSAIDs

Treatment: **Antihistamine and treat underlying cause**

MORIBILLIFORM RASH

Moribilliform rash **is a hypersensitive drug reaction that looks like measles** (rash first appears on the trunk, and then spreads to the limbs and neck) and **blanches with pressure.** It may develop few days after starting the medicine or after completing the course of the medicine

Treatment: **Stop offending** medicine **and topical or oral antihistamines**

STEVEN –JOHNSON SYNDROME

Steven –Johnson syndrome is a life-threatening hypersensitivity drug reaction that involves the **skin (<10-15%)** and **mucous membrane**

Cause:

- Penicillin, phenobarbital, phenytoin,
- Sulfa drugs
- NSAIDs

Si/Sx: symptoms begin as flu-like symptoms, then painful red or purplish lesions appears that spreads and blisters, and eventually epidermis layer separates from dermis and sheds

Diagnosis: Skin biopsy

Treatment:

- Stop the offending drug
- IVIG and analgesics
- **Intubate the patient**, if respiratory tract is involved
- Transfer the patient in **ICU or burn unit** care

Complication: Most common cause of death is combination of infection, dehydration and malnutrition

TOXIC EPIDERMAL NECROLYSIS (TEN)

Toxic epidermal necrolysis is a life-threatening hypersensitivity drug reaction. It is a severe form of Steven –Johnson syndrome, involving **> 30% body surface area.** Other characteristic feature of TEN is Nikolsky's sign (top layers of the skin sloughs off with gentle rub)

Cause:

- Phenobarbital, phenytoin,
- NSAIDs
- Allopurinol

Diagnosis: skin biopsy

Management:

- Stop the offending drug
- Transfer the patient in **burn unit care or ICU unit, supportive management and nutritional support**

Complication: Most common cause of **death** is **sepsis**

ACNE

Acne is a skin condition that starts with blockage of the hair follicle, filled with keratin and sebum material, followed by infection of lipophilic bacteria *Propionibacterium acnes,* which breaks down the sebum and causing inflammatory reaction and rupture the cysts

Open comedones are called blackheads and closed comedones are called whiteheads

Diagnosis: clinical diagnosis

Treatment:

- **Mild** acne is treated with **topical benzoyl peroxide.** If benzoyl peroxide is ineffective, then **add topical erythromycin or clindamycin**
- **Moderate** acne is treated with **topical antibiotics** (topical benzyl peroxide or topical erythromycin or clindamycin) and **topical tretinoin**
- **Severe** acne is treated with **oral tetracycline.** If tetracycline is ineffective, then give **oral isotretinoin**

NOTE: oral isotretinoin is teratogenic, **a reproductive age woman** must have **pregnancy test** before starting oral isotretinoin, and then she should be put on **2 forms of contraception's:** one barrier method and an another form of contraceptive

PORPHYRIA CUTANEA TARDA

Porphyria cutanea tarda is autosomal dominant defect in heme synthesis (low activity (<50%) of uroporphyrinogen decarboxylase enzyme in RBC and liver)

Si/Sx: non-healing blisters on sun exposed area, hyperpigmentation of skin, and increased hair growth

Exacerbating factors:

- Alcoholism
- Liver disease, hepatitis C
- **Estrogen containing** oral contraceptives
- Iron overload and diabetes

Diagnosis: Wood lamp urine test of urinary uroporphyrin

Treatment: best initial treatment is phlebotomy. If phlebotomy is not possible, then give deferoxamine

Prevention: stop drinking alcohol, stop estrogen use and sun protection barriers

TOXIC SHOCK SYNDROME

Toxic shock syndrome is a life-threatening condition caused by Staphylococcus aureus

Risk factors: tampons use in menstruating women, surgical wounds, nasal packing

Si/Sx: Low blood pressure, fever, confusion, muscle aches, vomiting, rash resembling sunburn

Treatment:
- Remove foreign objects
- Aggressive hydration + vasopressor (dopamine)
- IV Nafcillin, oxacillin or cefazolin
- Vancomycin or linezolid, if MRSA is suspected

LYME DISEASE

Lyme disease is a bacterial infection caused by *Borrelia burgdorferi*, which is transmitted by a tick infected with *Borrelia burgdorferi*

Si/S: Classic sign of Lyme infection is **erythema chronicum migrans** (circular rash with central clearing, that is often described as " bull's eye); other symptoms may include fatigue, myalgia, headache, arthritis, neurologic abnormalities, myocarditis

Diagnosis:
- Best Initial diagnostic test is **ELISA**
- Confirmatory test is **Western blot**

Treatment:
- Oral doxycycline
- Pregnant women are usually treated with amoxicillin
- If a patients has neurologic abnormalities or 3rd degree heart block, then use **IV ceftriaxone**

ROCKY MOUNTAIN SPOTTED FEVER

Rocky Mountain spotted fever is bacterial infection caused by bacterium *Rickettsia rickettsii,* which is transmitted by a tick infected with bacterium *Rickettsia rickettsii*

Si/Sx: fever, chills, headache or malaise, followed by **centripetal rash** appears, which starts at wrist and ankle, and then spreads to trunk and face

Diagnosis: Serology

Treatment: Doxycycline, pregnant women are treated with chloramphenicol

CAT SCRATCH DISEASE

Cat scratch disease is a bacterial infection caused by Bartonella bacteria, which is transmitted by cat scratch or bite

Si/Sx: lymphadenopathy next to the site of scratch or bite, fever, fatigue, headache, sore throat

Treatment: usually no treatment is required, but in severe cases azithromycin may be helpful

OPHTHALMOLOGY

OPEN-ANGLE GLAUCOMA

Open-angle glaucoma accounts for more than 90% of glaucoma. It is caused by slow clogging of drainage canals. It is called open-angle glaucoma because the angle because angle where between the iris and cornea is wide and open.

Si/Sx: painless gradual peripheral vision loss (also known as tunnel vision), increased cup-to disc ratio on fundoscopy exam, increased intraocular pressure (20-30 mmHg),

Treatment:

- **Topical beta-blockers** (timolol, betaxolol), **prostaglandins** (latanoprost) **carbonic anhydrase inhibitors** (dorzolamide, brinzolamide) or pilocarpine.
- If medicines is ineffective or patients can't tolerate them, then surgery (laser trabeculoplasty) may be performed

ANGLE-CLOSURE GLAUCOMA

Angle-closure glaucoma is a less common form of glaucoma. It is caused by slow clogging of drainage canals. It is called angle-closure glaucoma because the angle because angle where between the iris and cornea is closed. It develops fast and requires immediate medical attention

Si/Sx: painful, sudden vision change, seeing **halos around light, fixed dilated** pupils, increased intraocular pressure >30 mmHg leads to Treatment:

- **Immediate** treatment with **pilocarpine** to constrict the pupils, plus **topical timolol** and IV **acetazolamide**
- Definitive therapy is **laser iridotomy**

RETINAL DETACHMENT

Retinal detachment is condition in which retina gets separated from its underlying supporting layers

Si/Sx: sudden painless unilateral vision loss, **floater and flashes** of light, and blinding in a part of visual filed, which is often described by patient as **curtain falling down** in front of the eyes

Treatment: Immediate retinal reattachment or surgery

RETINAL ARTERY OCCLUSION

Retinal artery occlusion is a blockage of one of the small arteries that supply blood to the retina. It is common in temporal arteritis, emboli, and atherosclerosis

Si/Sx: sudden, acute and painless unilateral vision loss

Diagnosis: Funduscopy shows "**cherry red spot**" with surrounding pale retina

Treatment: Acetazolamide or paracentesis of anterior chamber

RETINAL VEIN OCCLUSION

Retinal vein occlusion is a blockage of small veins that take blood away from the retina. It is common in diabetes, glaucoma, HTN, atherosclerosis

Si/Sx: sudden, acute and painless unilateral vision loss

Diagnosis: Funduscopy shows tortuous retinal veins, **retinal hemorrhage**

Treatment: No specific treatment, treat the underlying cause

CATARACT

A cataract is a clouding of normal clear lens inside the eye that leads to painless vision loss.

Diagnose: opacification of the lens on slit-lamp exam. In advance stages red eye reflex become black

Treatment: Surgical removal of lens

MACULAR DEGENERATION

Macular degeneration is also known as age related macular degeneration is a painless vision loss in the center of the visual field due to damage of the retina

Type: two main types of macular degeneration are:

- **Dry (nonexudative) type** is caused by build up of drusen (cellular debris) between the retina and the choroid
- **Wet (exudative) type** is caused by neovascularization in choroid

Diagnosis:

- Dry type: Funduscopy exam shows **yellow white deposit** (drusen) in and around **macula**
- Wet type is diagnosed with fluorescein angiography

Treatment:
- **Dry type** is treated with laser photocoagulation
- **Wet type** is treated with injection of vascular endothelial growth factor inhibitors or thermal laser photocoagulation

DIABETIC RETINOPATHY
Diabetic retinopathy is a complication of diabetes, it usually occurs approximately 10 years after diabetes
Types: two main types of diabetic retinopathy are:
- **Nonproliferative** or background type is asymptomatic. It can only be detected by **fundoscopy exam**, which usually shows **microaneurysms, cotton wool spots, flame hemorrhages** on the retina.
- **Proliferative** type caused by **neovascularization** at the back of the eyes that can cause vitreous hemorrhages, which cause sudden vision loss, blurred vision floaters in the visual field. It is diagnosed with **fluorescein angiography**

Treatment
- **Dry type: strict glucose and HTN** control
- Wet type is treated with injection of **vascular endothelial growth factor inhibitors** in the eyes to control neovascularization

UVEITIS
Uveitis is an inflammation of uvea. It is associated with **autoimmune disease** (rheumatoid arthritis, reactive arthritis), **infections** (CMV, toxoplasmosis, syphilis), **ulcerative colitis**
Si/Sx: photophobia, blurry vision
Diagnosis: Slit lamp examination shows flare and cells in aqueous humor
Treatment: topical steroids and treat the underlying cause

CORNEAL ABRASION
Corneal abrasion is the most common eye injury from scratching or cutting
Si/Sx: pain, photophobia, foreign-body sensation, watery discharge
Diagnosis: Fluorescein satin with **wood lamp**
Treatment: No specific treatment

KERATITIS
Keratitis is an inflammation of the cornea. It is associated with multiple causes, but herpes simplex virus is most commonly asked on the boards
Si/Sx: pain, photophobia, tearing, decreased vision
Diagnosis: fluorescein stain shows dendritic branching
Treatment: oral acyclovir, famciclovir or valacyclovir
Note: Steroids are **contraindicated in herpes keratitis** because they can worsen the condition

CONJUNCTIVITIS

Condition	Bacterial conjunctivitis	Viral conjunctivitis	Allergic conjunctivitis
Si/Sx	• **Unilateral** • **Purulent discharge** • Rarely preauricular adenopathy (only in Neisseria gonorrhea) • Minimal pain • No vision change or pupillary change	• **Bilateral** • **Watery discharge** • Often preauricular adenopathy • Minimal pain • No vision change or pupillary change	• Bilateral • **Watery discharge** • **Marked pruritus** • No pain, vision change or pupillary change
Treatment	Topical antibiotics	Supportive	Antihistamine or steroid drops

PALPERBRAL INFLAMMATION

1. CHALAZION
Chalazion is a cyst in the eyelid that is caused by blockage and inflammation of internal meibomian gland
Si/Sx: Painless tender lump **away from the eyelid margin**
Treatment: Warm compression

2.   HORDEOLUM

Hordeolum is a common disorder of eyelids, involving sebaceous glands of Ziess or sweat gland of Moll
Si/Sx: painful red tender lump **near the eyelid margin**
Treatment: Warm compression

3.   BLEPHARITIS

Blepharitis is inflammation of the eyelids and eyelashes from infection (S. aureus) or secondary to seborrhea
Si/Sx: red and swollen eyelids dry flaking on lids
Treatment: daily washing eyelids margin

4.   ORBITAL CELLULITIS

Orbital cellulitis is an infection of the tissue-surrounding eye including eyelids
Cause: Staphylococcus aureus, streptococcus pneumonia and H. influenza type b
Si/Sx: red or purple eyelid, painful swelling of upper and lower eyelids, eye pain, painful eye movement, limited eye movement
Treatment: Orbital cellulitis is medical emergency patient should be immediately started on IV Vancomycin plus cefotaxime

5.   PERIORBITAL CELLULITIS

Periorbital cellulitis is an inflammation of eyelid and skin around the eyes. This condition can easily be **confused with orbital cellulitis**. The key difference is in the symptoms; patient with periorbital cellulitis **do not have pain with cye movement, vision change, and limited eye movement.**
Treatment: warm to hot compress to reduce pain and inflammation, and oral antibiotics

VISUAL FILED DEFECTS

Visual field defect	Location of lesion
Bitemporal hemianopsia	Optic chiasm
Right anopsia	Right optic nerve
Right homonymous hemianopsia	Left optic tract
Right upper quadrant anopsia	Optic radiation in **left temporal** lobe
Right lower quadrant anopsia	Optic radiation in **left parietal lobe**
Right homonymous hemianopsia with macular sparing	Left occipital lobe

TOXICOLOGY

1. ANTICHOLINERGIC TOXICITY
Si/Sx

- Mydriasis
- Flushed skin
- Dry mouth
- Constipation

Diagnosis: Clinical
Treatment: Physostigmine

2. ORGANOPHOSPHATE POISONING
Si/Sx:

- Miosis
- Salivation
- Diarrhea
- Lacrimation
- Wheezing

Physiology: Organophosphate inhibits the metabolism of acetylcholine by inhibiting the acetylcholinesterase

Diagnosis:

- Clinical diagnosis
- Specific test is RBC cholinesterase level

Management:

- Respiratory support
- Atropine is the best initial treatment, and pralidoxime is the second choice

Note: Patient may have toxin on his or her clothes, so it is better to remove and wash all the patient's clothes to prevent further exposure of the toxin

3.   ASPIRIN/ SALICYLATE OVERDOSE

Si/Sx: Tinnitus, nausea, vomiting, confusion that can progress to seizure
and coma

Diagnosis:

- Labs show: Respiratory alkalosis with elevated anion gap channel
  acidosis, increased PTT and low glucose level
- **Most specific** test is **aspirin level**

Management:

- **Charcoal** to block absorption and alkalinization of urine with
  D5W + 3amps bicarbonate
- **Dialysis** is for severe cases

4.   CARBON MONOXIDE POISONING

Si/Sx: **fatigue, headaches,** shortness of breath, disorientation, **cherry-red
color skin or lips,**

Diagnosis: **Co-oximetry**

Treatment: **100% oxygen,** severe cases are treated with **hyperbaric oxygen**

5.   METHEMOGLOBINEMIA

Si/Sx: cyanosis, shortness of breath, confusion or seizure, after recent
exposure of nitrate, dapsone, or anesthetics

Diagnosis: **Metahemoglobin level**

Treatment: **100% oxygen and methylene blue** to restore hemoglobin

6.   ACETAMINOPHEN TOXICITY

Si/Sx: nausea and vomiting starts within 2 hours of exposure, which
usually resolves after first 24 hours and then hepatic failure develops

Diagnosis: Acetaminophen level

Treatment: **Charcoal and N-acetyl cysteine** within 8-10 hours

7.   DIGOXIN TOXICITY

Si/Sx: GI disturbance, yellow " halos" around objects, paroxysmal atrial
tachycardia

Diagnosis: blood level

Treatment: **Digoxin-binding antibodies**

8. ETHYLENE GLYCOL

Si/Sx: **Calcium oxalate urine crystals**, high anion gap metabolic acidosis
Dx: Urinalysis shows **envelope crystals**
Treatment: Fomepizole followed by dialysis

9. METHANOL

Si/Sx: **vision disturbance**, high anion gap metabolic acidosis
Diagnosis: blood level
Treatment: Fomepizole followed by dialysis

10. ALKALI BURN

Alkali burn are caused by ingestion dishwasher, detergent, drain cleaners, that can cause musical burn and respiratory compromise
Diagnosis: clinical
Treatment: Milk or water and NPO

Notes:

VITAMINS

Vitamin	Deficiency	Toxicity
Vitamin A	• Night blindness • Dry skin • Metaplasia of respiratory epithelium	• Pseudotumor cerebri • Hyperparathyroidism
Vitamin D	• Rickets in children • Osteomalacia in adults	• Kidney stones • Dementia • Abdominal pain • Depression
Vitamin K	• Clotting factor deficiency that leads to increased PT/INR	• Toxicity is rare
Vitamin B 1 (Thiamine)	• Wet beriberi (high cardiac output, cardiomyopathy) • Dry beriberi (neuropathy)	None
Vitamin B 2 (Riboflavin)	• Angular cheilosis • Stomatitis • Glossitis	None
Vitamin B 3 (Niacin)	• Pellagra (diarrhea, dementia and dermatitis)	None
Vitamin B 5 (Pantothenate)	• Dermatitis, enteritis	None
Vitamin B 6 (Pyridoxine)	• Peripheral neuropathy	None
Vitamin B 12 (Cyanocobalamin)	• Megalobalstic anemia • Peripheral neuropathy	None
Folic acid	• Megalobalstic anemia	None
Vitamin C	• Scurvy: bruising, anemia, poor wound healing, bone pain (seen in people on "tea and toast" or "hot dogs and soda" diet)	None

Notes:

INDEX

11-beta-hydroxylase CAH, 270
17-alpha-hydroxylase CAH, 270
21-hydroxylase CAH, 270

A
Abdominal aorta aneurysm, 26
Abdominal trauma, 162
Abortion, 319
Abruptio placenta, 322
Absence seizure, 200, 262
Acetaminophen toxicity, 372
Achalasia, 133
Achilles tendon rupture, 184
Acid-base disorder, 107
Acne, 362
Acromegaly, 29, 96
Actinic keratosis, 356
Actinomyces, 74
Active tuberculosis, 76,77
Acute adrenal crisis, 92
Acute allergic interstitial
nephropathy, 112
Acute coronary syndrome, 5
Acute dystonia, 219
Acute epidural hematoma, 213
Acute hemolytic reaction, 56
Acute hepatitis B
Acute lymphoblastic leukemia
(ALL), 46
Acute mesenteric ischemia, 161
Acute myelogenous leukemia
(AML), 46, 47
Acute pancreatitis, 157
Acute pharyngitis, 59
Acute rejection, 57
Acute Renal failure, 109
Acute stress disorder, 224
Acute tubular necrosis, 111
Adenocarcinoma, 71
Adenomyosis, 300

Adjustment disorder, 226
Admission rate bias, 345
Adrenal tumor or hyperplasia, 95
Adrenal tumor, 293
Adult respiratory distress
syndrome, 69
Akathisia, 219
Alcohol hallucinosis, 231
Alcohol hepatitis, 155
Alcohol intoxication, 231
Alcohol liver disease, 155
Alcohol screening, 231
Alcohol tremor, 231
Alcohol withdrawal seizure, 231
Alcohol withdrawals, 231
Alkali burn, 373
Allergic anaphylaxis, 57
Allergic conjunctivitis, 368
Allergic reaction, 56
Allergic rhinitis, 61
Alpha-thalassemia, 36
Alport syndrome, 116
Alzheimer disease, 193
Amniocenteses, 315
Amoebic liver abscess, 160
Amphetamine intoxication, 230
Amphetamine withdrawal, 230
Amyotrophic lateral sclerosis,
198
Anaerobes, 73
Analysis of variance, 344
Anaphylaxis, 106
Anaplastic carcinoma, 90
Androgen insensitivity
syndrome, 295
Anemia of chronic disease, 34, 35
Anemia, 33
Angelman syndrome, 275
Angle-closure glaucoma, 365
Ankylosing spondylitis, 167
Anorexia, 229
Anterior cruciate ligament 183
Anterior shoulder dislocation,
179

Anterior spinal artery syndrome, 204
Anticholinergic toxicity, 371
Antisocial PD, 229
Anxiety disorders, 224
Aortic dissection, 1
Aortic regurgitation, 16
Aortic stenosis, 16
Aortoiliac disease, 27
APGAR score, 239
Aplastic anemia, 45
Appendicitis, 161
Arrest disorder, 329
Arterial ulcers, 28
Asbestos, 67
Ascending cholangitis, 159
Ascites, 151
Asherman syndrome, 297
Asperger syndrome, 235
Aspergillus, 76
Aspirin/ salicylate overdose, 372
Asthma exacerbation, 64
Asthma, 62
Astrocytoma, 202
Asymptomatic bacteriuria, 129
Atonic seizures, 200
Atopic dermatitis, 358
Atrial fibrillation, 12
Atrial flutter, 13
Atrial septal defect, 244
Attention deficit hyperactivity disorder (ADHD), 235
Attributable risk, 344
Atypical depression, 222
Atypical pneumonia, 73
Autism, 235
Autoimmune hepatitis, 154
Autonomy, 347
Avoidant PD, 228

B
Back pain, 185
Back sprain, 203
Bacterial conjunctivitis, 368

Bacterial pneumonia, 256
Bacterial prostatitis, 129
Bacterial tracheitis, 253
Bacterial vaginosis, 285
Bacteriemia, 215
Barrett's esophagus, 139
Basal cell carcinoma, 356
Bat bite, 339
Beat-thalassemia, 36
Benign essential tremor, 190
Benign positional vertigo (BPV), 196
Benign prostate hypertrophy, 123
Benzodiazepine intoxication, 230
Benzodiazepine withdrawal, 230
Bereavement, 222
Berylliosis, 67
Biliary colic, 159
Biophysical profile, 316
Bipolar disorder type I, 223
Bipolar disorder type II, 223
Bipolar disorder, 223
Bitemporal hemianopsia, 370
Black widow spider bite, 340
Bladder cancer, 131
Blastomycosis, 76
Blepharitis, 369
Blunt abdominal trauma, 162
Body dysmorphic disorder, 227
Boerhaave syndrome, 137
Borderline PD, 229
Brain abscess, 211
Brain death, 349
Brain lesion, 199
Brain tumors, 202
Breast cancer, 304
Breast milk jaundice, 272
Breastfeeding jaundice, 272
Breech presentation, 330
Brief psychotic disorder, 220
Broca's aphasia, 199
Bronchiectasis, 64
Bronchiolitis, 254
Bronchoalveolar

Brown recluse spider bite, 340
Brown-séquard syndrome, 204
Bulimia, 229
Bullous pemphigoid, 355
Burton agammaglobulinemia, 267
Bypass fistula, 287, 288

C
Calcium oxalate stones, 121
Calcium phosphate stones, 121
Campylobacter, 146
Candida diaper dermatitis, 241
Candidiasis, 285
Caplan syndrome, 167
Caput Succedaneum, 261
Carbon monoxide poisoning, 372
Carbuncles, 355
Carcinoid syndrome, 147
Cardiogenic shock, 105, 106
Cardiomyopathy, 20
Carpel tunnel syndrome, 180
Case series study, 346
Cat bite, 339
Cat scratch disease, 364
Cataract, 366
Cauda equina syndrome, 185, 204
Celiac disease, 148
Cellulitis, 354
Central diabetes, 98
Cephalohematoma, 261
Cerebellar tremors, 190
Cervical cancer, 289
Cervicitis, 286
Chalazion, 368
Chancroid, 130
CHARGE syndrome, 251
Chediak- Higashi syndrome, 267
Chemical conjunctivitis, 240
Chi-squared test, 344
Childhood disintegrative disorder, 235
Chlamydia conjunctivitis, 240

Chlamydia pneumonia, 74
Chlamydia Psittaci, 74
Chlamydia trachomatis, 255
Choanal atresia, 251
Cholecystitis, 159
Choledocholithiasis, 160
Chorioamnionitis, 328
Choriocarcinoma, 291
Choriocarcinoma, 292
Chorionic villus sampling, 315
Chronic bronchitis, 64
Chronic granulomatosis disease, 267
Chronic hypertension, 325
Chronic lymphoblastic leukemia (CLL), 46, 47
Chronic myelogenous leukemia (CML), 46, 48
Chronic obstructive pulmonary disease, 64
Chronic pancreatitis, 148, 157
Chronic rejection, 57
Cirrhosis, 151
Clavicular fracture, 179, 257
Cleft lip, 257
Cleft palate, 257
Clonic seizures, 200
Clostridium difficile, 146
Cluster headache, 195
Coal miner's lung disease, 67
Coarctation of aorta, 29, 245
Cocaine abuse, 1
Cocaine intoxication, 230
Cocaine withdrawal, 230
Coccidioides immitis, 76
Cold-agglutinin hemolysis, 40
Colles fracture, 181
Colon cancer screening, 145
Compartment syndrome, 186
Complete abortion, 320
Complete breech, 330
Complete isosexual precocious puberty, 298
Complex partial seizure, 200

Conduct disorder, 236
Confidentiality, 349
Congenital adrenal hyperplasia, 270, 293
Congenital hip dysplasia, 258
Congenital hypothyroidism, 270
Congestive heart failure, 19
Conjunctivitis, 368
Conn syndrome, 29
Constrictive pericarditis, 22
Contact dermatitis, 358
Contraception, 306
Contraction stress test, 316
Conversion disorder, 227
Corneal abrasion, 367
Costochondritis, 1
Coxiella burnetii, 74
CREST syndrome, 171
Creutzfeldt-Jakob disease, 194
Crohn's disease, 143
Croup, 252
Cryptorchidism, 264
Cryptosporidium, 146
Cushing's disease, 95
Cushing's syndrome, 94
Cutis marmorata, 241
Cyanotic congenital heart disease, 243
Cyclothymia, 223
Cystic fibrosis, 254
Cystine stones, 121
Cystitis, 127
Cystocele, 303
Cytomegalovirus, 278

D
D-xylose test, 149
Dawn phenomenon, 82
De Quervain tenosynovitis, 182
Deep vein thrombosis, 215
Delirium tremens, 231
Delusional disorder, 224
Dementia, 193
Dependent PD, 228

Depo-Provera, 306
Dermatomyositis, 172
Development miles stones, 242
Diabetes insipidus, 98
Diabetes, 81
Diabetic ketoacidosis, 82
Diabetic nephropathy, 117
Diabetic retinopathy, 367
Diaper rash, 241
Diffuse esophageal spasm, 135
Diffuse scleroderma, 170
DiGeorge's syndrome, 267
Digoxin toxicity, 372
Dilated cardiomyopathy, 21
Direct inguinal hernia, 163
Disk herniation, 185
Diverticulitis, 161
Diverticulosis, 161
Do not resuscitate (DNR) order, 347
Doctor-patient relationship, 349
Dog bite, 339
Double Y males, 274
Down syndrome, 274
Drug hepatitis, 155
Drug-induced lupus, 170
Ductal carcinoma in situ, 304
Dumping syndrome, 143
Duodenal atresia, 247
Duodenal ulcer, 140
Dupuytren contracture, 182
Dysfunctional uterine bleeding, 301
Dysgerminoma, 291
Dysthymia, 222

E
Early decelerations, 321
Ebstein anomaly, 223
Eclampsia, 325
Ectopic pregnancy, 321
Edwards' syndrome, 274
Ehlers-Danlos syndrome, 274
Electrolytes, 99

Emancipated minor, 351
Emphysema, 65
Encephalitis, 210
End-stage renal failure, 119
Endocarditis, 24
Endometrial cancer, 288
Endometriosis, 299
Endometritis, 333
Entamoeba histolytica, 146
Entero- hemorrhagic E.coli
(0517:H7), 146
Enterocele, 303
Ependymomas, 202
Epididymitis, 129, 266
Epiglottitis, 252
Epispadias, 264
Epithelial cell tumors, 290
Erb-Duchenne palsy, 257
Erectile dysfunction, 123
Erysipelas, 354
Erythema infectiosum, 268
Erythema multiforme, 360
Erythema nodosum, 360
Erythema toxicum, 241
Esophageal cancer, 139
Esophageal scleroderma, 134
Esophageal spasm, 1
Esophageal varices, 137
Esophagitis, 136
Essential thrombocythemia, 44
Estrogen progesterone challenge
test, 297
Estrogen- progesterone
combined contraceptives, 306
Ethics, 347
Ethylene glycol, 373
Ewing sarcoma, 176
Exhibitionism, 232
Exogenous thyroid hormone
abuse, 86, 87
Experimental study, 346
Extrapulmonary diseases, 68
Exudative diarrhea, 147

F
Fabry's syndrome, 273
Factious disorder, 227
Factitious disorder by proxy, 227
Failure to thrive, 275
False negative, 343
False positive, 343
Febrile nonhemolytic reaction, 56
Febrile seizure, 262
Felty syndrome, 167
Female diaphragm, 306
Femoral hernia, 163
Femoral shaft fracture, 183
Femoropopliteal disease, 27
Fetal heart rate, 321
Fetishism, 232
Fibroadenoma, 304
Fibrocystic breast disease, 303
Fibromyalgia, 173
Fibronectin test, 327
First-degree heart block, 10
Focal segmental
glomerulosclerosis, 116
Folate deficiency, 38
Folic acid deficiency, 375
Follicular carcinoma, 90
Folliculitis, 355
Footling or incomplete breech,
330
Foreign body aspiration, 253
Fragile X syndrome, 273
Frank breech, 330
Frotteurism, 232
Fungal meningitis, 209
Furuncle, 355
Futile care, 347

G
Galactosemia, 275
Galeazzi fracture, 181
Gardner's syndrome, 145
Gastric ulcer, 140
Gastritis, 140
Gastroparesis, 84, 142

Gastroschisis, 249
Gaucher disease, 273
Gender identity disorder, 232
Gender identity, 232
Gender role, 232
Generalized anxiety disorder, 225
GERD, 1, 138
Germ cell tumors, 290
Gestational diabetes, 312, 313
Gestational hypertension, 325
Gestational trophoblastic tumor, 292
GI bleeding, 150
Giant cell tumor, 176
Giardia, 146
Gifts, 350
Glucose-6-phosphate dehydrogenase (g6pd) deficiency, 42
Golfer Elbow, 180
Gonadal failure, 298
Gonococcal arthritis, 177
Gonococcal conjunctivitis, 240
Gonococcal urethritis, 130
Goodpasture syndrome, 114
Gout, 173
Granuloma inguinale, 130
Granulosa cell tumor, 299
Grave's disease, 86, 87
Gravida, 309
Group b beta-hemolytic streptococci screening, 314
Guillain-barré syndrome, 197

H
Hairy cell leukemia, 49
Hallucinogens intoxication, 230
Hashimoto's disease, 88
Headache, 194
Healthcare associated pneumonia, 75
Heat cramps, 104
Heat exhaustion, 104

Heat stroke, 104
HELLP syndrome, 326
Hemangioma, 240
Hemineglect, 199
Hemochromatosis, 154
Hemolytic uremic syndrome (HUS), 43
Disseminated intravascular coagulation (DIC), 43
Hemophilia A, 55
Hemophilia B, 55
Hemorrhagic stroke, 187
Hemorrhoids, 150
Hemothorax, 79
Henoch-Schönlein purpura, 260
Hepatic adenoma, 160
Hepatitis A prophylaxis, 342
Hepatitis A vaccination, 341
Hepatitis A, 155
Hepatitis B vaccination, 341
Hepatitis B, 156
Hepatitis C, 156
Hereditary angioedema, 266
Hereditary spherocytosis, 40
Herpes simplex encephalitis, 210
Herpes symplex virus, 278
Herpes zoster, 359
High anion gap metabolic acidosis, 125
Hip dislocation, 183
Hip fracture, 183
Hirschsprung disease, 247
Hirsutism, 293
Histoplasmosis, 76
HIV-positive pregnant women management, 337
Hodgkin's lymphoma, 50
Hordeolum, 369
Hospital acquired pneumonia, 75
HSV, 130
Human bite, 339
Human immunodeficiency virus (HIV), 335
Hunter's syndrome, 273

Huntington disease, 191
Hurler's syndrome, 273
Hydatiform mole, 292
Hydrocele, 264
Hyperacute rejection, 57
Hyperaldosteronism, 92
Hypercalcemia, 102
Hyperkalemia, 100
Hypermagnesemia, 103
Hypernatremia, 99
Hyperosmolar diabetic coma, 84
Hyperparathyroidism, 91
Hypertension, 29, 325
Hypertensive emergency, 32
Hypertensive urgency, 31
Hyperthyroidism, 29, 86
Hypertrophic obstructive
cardiomyopathy, 21
Hypoadrenalism, 91
Hypocalcemia, 102
Hypochondriasis, 227
Hypoglycemia, 85
Hypokalemia, 101
Hypomagnesemia, 103
Hypomania, 223
Hyponatremia, 99
Hypospadias, 264
Hypothalamic-pituitary failure,
296
Hypothalamus-pituitary
dysfunction, 298
Hypothermia, 104
Hypothyroidism, 86,88, 297
Hypovolemic shock, 105, 106

I
Idiopathic thrombocytopenic
purpura, 53
IgA deficiency, 267
IgA nephropathy, 114
Impaired physician, 350
Imperforate anus, 247
Imperforated hymen, 295
Impetigo, 354

Impulse control disorder, 228
Incidence, 343
Incomplete abortion, 320
Incomplete isosexual precocious
puberty, 298
Indications of C-section, 331
Indirect inguinal hernia, 163
Inevitable abortion, 320
Infectious diarrhea, 146
Infertility, 301
Inflammatory bowel disease, 143,
304
Influenza vaccine, 341
Influenza, 61
Informed consent, 347
Inhalants intoxication, 230
Intermittent explosive disorder,
228
Interstitial lung disease, 67
Interviewer bias, 345
Intestinal malrotation, 248
Intrarenal failure, 109, 110
Intrauterine device (IUD), 306,
307
Intrauterine growth retardation
(IUGR), 317
Intussusception, 247
Iron deficiency anemia, 34
Irritable bowel syndrome, 149
Irritant diaper dermatitis, 241
Ischemic stroke, 187

J
Jersey finger, 182
Juvenile rheumatoid arthritis,
259

K
Kallmann syndrome, 296
Kaposi's sarcoma, 357
Kawasaki disease, 260
Keratitis, 368
Klebsiella, 73
Kleptomania, 228

Klinefelter syndrome, 274
Klumpke paralysis, 257
Knee injury, 183
Krabbe's disease, 273

L
Labor, 327, 329
Labyrinthitis, 196
Lambert-Eaton syndrome, 192
Large bowel obstruction, 163
Large cell carcinoma, 71
Late decelerations, 322
Latent tuberculosis, 76, 77
Lead poisoning, 263
Lead-time bias, 345
Legg-cavlé-perthes, 258
Legionella, 74
Leukemia, 46
Liver disease, 55
Lobular carcinoma in situ, 304
Lochia, 332
Lower GI bleeding, 150
LSD intoxication, 230
Lung cancer, 70, 71
Lyme disease, 363
Lymphogranuloma venereum, 130
Lymphoma, 50

M
Macrocytic anemia, 34, 38
Macular degeneration, 366
Major depression disorder, 220
Malabsorption diarrhea, 148
Malaria, 342
Male condoms, 306
Malignant hyperthermia, 215
Malignant melanoma, 357
Malingering disorder, 228
Mallet finger, 182
Mallory-Weiss syndrome, 137
Mania, 223
Marfan syndrome, 274
Marijuana intoxication, 230

Masochism, 232
Mastitis, 304
McCune-Albert syndrome, 298
Mean, 344
Measles, 268
Meckel's diverticulum, 249
Meconium ilium, 246
Median, 344
Medical emergency procedures, 348
Medullary carcinoma, 90
Medulloblastoma, 202
Membranoproliferative glomerulonephritis, 117
Membranous glomerulonephritis, 117
MEN Type 1 (Wermer's syndrome), 90
MEN Type IIa (Sipple syndrome), 90
MEN Type IIb, 90
Meniere's disease, 196
Meningioma, 202
Meningitis, 207
Meningocele, 261
Meningococcal vaccination, 341
Meningococcus, 342
Meniscal tear, 184
Menopause, 307
Mental retardation, 236
Metabolic acidosis, 107
Metabolic alkalosis, 107
Metachromatic leukodystrophy, 273
Metastatic malignancy of spine, 185
Methanol, 373
Methemoglobinemia, 372
Microangiopathic hemolytic anemia, 43
Microcytic anemia, 34
Migraine headache, 194
Mild pre-eclampsia, 325
Milia, 241

Minimal change disease, 116
Missed abortion, 320
Mitral regurgitation, 17
Mitral stenosis, 17
Mitral valve prolapse, 18
Mixed acid-base disorders, 108
MMR vaccination, 341
Mode, 344
Molar pregnancy, 292
Mongolian spots, 241
Monteggia fracture, 181
Moribilliform rash, 360
Morton neuroma, 175
Müllerian agenesis, 295
Multifocal atrial tachycardia, 14
Multiple endocrine neoplasia
syndromes (MEN), 90
Multiple myeloma, 52
Multiple sclerosis, 197
Mumps, 268
Myasthenia gravis, 191
Mycobacterium avium complex,
336
Mycoplasma pneumonia, 256
Mycoplasma, 74
Myelodysplastic syndrome, 48
Myelofibrosis, 45
Myelomeningocele, 261
Myoclonic seizures, 200
Myxedema coma, 88

N
Nagele rule, 309
Narcissistic PD, 229
Narcolepsy, 233
Necrotizing enterocolitis, 246
Necrotizing fasciitis, 354
Negative 1 correlation, 345
Negative predictive value, 343
Negative skewed curve, 344
Neisseria meningitis, 208
Neonate acne, 241
Nephritis syndrome, 113
Nephrogenic diabetes, 98

Nephrolithiasis, 120
Nephrotic syndrome, 113, 116
Neuroblastoma, 265
Neurocysticercosis, 211
Neurofibromatosis, 262
Neurogenic shock, 105, 106
Neuroleptic malignant
syndrome, 219
Newborn jaundice, 271
Newborn screening, 239
Niemann-Pick disease, 273
Night terrors, 233
Nightmares, 233
Nightstick fracture, 181
Nocardia, 74
Non-gonococcal arthritis, 177
Non-Gonococcal urethritis, 130
Non-Hodgkin's lymphoma, 51
Non-ST-segment elevation MI, 5
Non-stress test, 315
Nonalcoholic steatohepatitis, 155
Nonresponse bias, 345
Normocytic anemia, 34

O
Obsessive-compulsive disorder,
226
Obsessive-compulsive
personality disorder (OCPD),
226, 229
Obstructive lung disease, 62
Odd risk, 344
Oligohydromona, 316
Omphalocele, 249
Onychomycosis, 353
Open pneumothorax, 79
Open-angle glaucoma, 365
Opiate intoxication, 230
Opiate withdrawal, 230
Oppositional defiant disorder,
236
Oral glucose tolerance test, 312
Orbital cellulitis, 369
Organ donation, 350

Organophosphate poisoning, 371
Osmotic diarrhea, 147
Osteoarthritis, 165
Osteochondroma, 176
Osteogenic sarcoma
(osteosarcoma), 176
Osteomyelitis, 178
Osteoporosis, 308
Otitis Externa, 269
Otitis Media, 269
Ovarian cancer, 293
Ovarian cysts, 291
Ovarian tumors, 290
Overflow incontinence, 287, 288

P
Paget disease of bones, 175
Paget disease of breast, 305
Pain disorder, 227
Pancreatic abscess, 158
Pancreatic cancer, 158
Pancreatic pseudocyst, 158
Panic attacks, 1
Panic disorder, 225
Papillary carcinoma, 89
Paranoid PD, 228
Parenchymal hemorrhage, 213
Parity, 309
Parkinson's disease, 189
Parkinsonism, 219
Paroxysmal nocturnal
hemoglobinuria, 42
Partial emancipation, 351
Patau's syndrome, 274
Patent ductus arteriosus, 245
Pathologic jaundice, 271
Patient's medical records, 351
PCP intoxication, 230
Pediculosis, 359
Pedophilia, 232
Pelvic inflammatory disease, 286
Pelvic organ prolapse, 302
Pemphigus, 356
Peptic stricture, 135

Peptic ulcer, 140
Percutaneous umbilical blood
sampling, 315
Pericardial tamponade, 24
Pericarditis, 1
Pericarditis, 24
Periorbital cellulitis, 369
Peripheral vascular disease, 27
Permanent sterilization, 307
Personality disorder
Pertussis, 251
Pervasive development
disorders, 235
Phenylketonuria, 274
Pheochromocytoma, 29, 94
Phobia, 225
Physician assisted suicide, 350
Physiologic jaundice, 271
Picks disease, 193
Pituitary tumor, 86, 87
Pityriasis rosea, 358
Placenta previa, 323
Plantar fasciitis, 175
Pleural effusion, 68
Plummer-Vinson syndrome, 135
Plummer's disease (Toxic
multinodular goiter), 86, 87
Pneumococcal vaccine, 341
Pneumoconiosis, 67
Pneumocystis carinii, 76, 336
Pneumonia, 73
Pneumothorax, 1
Polyarteritis nodosa, 115
Polycystic kidney disease, 122
Polycystic ovarian syndrome, 293
Polycythemia Vera, 44
Polyhydramnios, 316
Polymyalgia rheumatica, 172
Polymyositis, 172
Porphyria cutanea tarda, 362
Port–wine stain, 240
Positive 1 correlation, 345
Positive predictive value, 343
Positive skewed curve, 344

Post term pregnancy, 333
Post-traumatic stress disorder
(PTSD), 224
Posterior cruciate ligament, 184
Posterior shoulder dislocation,
179
Postoperative fever, 215
Postpartum blue, 333
Postpartum depression, 333
Postpartum hemorrhage, 332
Postpartum mood disorders, 333
Postpartum psychosis, 333
Postrenal failure, 109, 110
Poststreptococcal
glomerulonephritis, 113
Prader-Willi syndrome, 275
Pre-eclampsia, 325
Precocious puberty, 298
Premature delivery, 309
Premature rupture of membrane,
328
Prerenal failure, 109
Preterm delivery, 309
Preterm labor, 327
Prevalence study, 346
Prevalence, 343
Primary amenorrhea, 294
Primary biliary cirrhosis, 153
Primary dysmenorrhea, 299
Primary hyperaldosteronism, 92
Primary hyperparathyroidism,
91
Primary hypertension, 29
Primary sclerosis cholangitis, 153
Primary syphilis, 130
Prinzmetal angina, 9
Progesterone challenge test, 297
Progestin only contraceptives,
306
Prolactinoma, 95
Prospective study, 346
Prostate cancer, 131
Protracted disorder, 329
Pseudogout, 174

Pseudohyperkalemia, 101
Pseudomonas, 73
Pseudotumor cerebri, 195
Psoriasis, 358
Psoriatic arthritis, 167,168
Pulmonary edema, 20
Pulmonary embolism, 69
Pyelonephritis, 128
Pylorus stenosis, 248
Pyogenic liver abscess, 160
Pyromania, 228

R
Rapid cycling bipolar disorder,
223
Reactive arthritis, 167,169
Recall bias, 345
Rectocele, 303
Relative risk, 344
Renal amyloidosis, 118
Renal artery stenosis, 29, 122
Renal cell carcinoma, 131
Renal tubular acidosis, 124, 125
Reporting abuse, 350
Respiratory acidosis, 107
Respiratory alkalosis, 107
Respiratory distress syndrome,
250
Restless leg syndrome, 191
Restrictive cardiomyopathy, 22
Restrictive lung disease, 66
Retained placenta, 332
Retinal artery occlusion, 366
Retinal detachment, 365
Retinal vein occlusion, 366
Retrospective study, 346
Rett syndrome, 235
Rh incompatibility, 334
Rheumatic fever, 279
Rheumatoid arthritis, 165
Right anopsia, 370
Right homonymous hemianopsia
with macular sparing, 370

Right homonymous hemianopsia, 370
Right lower quadrant anopsia, 370
Right upper quadrant anopsia, 370
Rocky Mountain spotted, 364
Rosacea, 358
Roseola, 268
Rotator cuff injury, 179
Rubella, 268
Rubella, 278

S
Sadism, 232
Safe drugs during pregnancy, 318
Salmonella, 146
Sarcoidosis, 67
Scabies, 359
Scaphoid fracture, 181
Scarlet fever, 278
Schatzki's ring, 135
Schizoaffective disorder, 220
Schizoid PD, 228
Schizophrenia, 217
Schizophreniform disorder, 220
Schizotypal PD, 228
Schwannomas, 202
Scleroderma, 170
Seasonal depressive disorder, 222
Seborrheic dermatitis, 357
Seborrheic keratosis, 356
Second-degree type I heart block, 10
Second-degree type II heart block, 11
Secondary amenorrhea, 296
Secondary hyperaldosteronism, 93
Secondary hyperparathyroidism, 91
Secondary hypertension, 29
Secondary syphilis, 130

Secretin stimulation test, 149
Secretory diarrhea, 147
Seizures, 199
Sensitivity, 343
Septic arthritis, 177
Septic shock, 105, 106
Seronegative arthropathies, 167
Serotonin syndrome, 222
Sertoli-Leydig tumor, 291
Severe combined immune deficiency, 267
Severe pre-eclampsia, 325
Sexual contact with patient, 349
Sexual identity, 232
Sexual orientation, 232
Sexual paraphilia, 232
Shigella, 146
Shock, 105
Shoulder dystocia, 330
SIADH, 97
Sickle cell anemia, 39
Sideroblastic anemia, 36
Sigmoid volvulus, 162
Silicosis, 67
Simple partial seizure, 200
Sinus bradycardia, 9
Sinusitis, 60
Sleep apnea, 80
Sleep disorders, 233
Sleepwalking, 233
Slipped capital femoral epiphysis, 258
Small bowel obstruction, 163
Small cell cancer, 95
Small cell carcinoma, 71
Smoking cessation, 72
Snakebite, 340
Solitary pulmonary nodule, 70
Somatization disorder, 226
Somatoform disorders, 226
Somogyi effect, 82
Specificity, 343
Spina bifida occulta, 261
Spinal stenosis, 186, 203

Spinal tumor, 204
Splenic rupture, 161
Spontaneous abortion, 320
Spontaneous bacterial peritonitis, 152
Squamous cell carcinoma, 71, 356
ST-segment elevation MI, 5
Stable angina, 2
Stages and duration of labor, 329
Status epilepticus, 201
Steven–Johnson syndrome, 361
Streptococcus pneumonia, 73
Stress incontinence, 287, 288
Stroke, 187
Stromal cell tumors, 291
Struvite stones, 121
Subacute combined degeneration, 204
Subacute thyroiditis, 86, 87
Subarachnoid hemorrhage, 215
Subclavian steal syndrome, 28
Substance abuse, 230
Suicide, 233
Supraventricular tachycardia, 13
Syndrome, 71
Syphilis, 130, 277
Syringomyelia, 203
Systemic lupus erythematosus, 118, 169
Systemic still's disease, 259

T
T-test, 344
Tardive dyskinesia, 219
Tay-Sachs disease, 273
Temporal arteritis, 196
Tennis elbow, 180
Tension headache, 195
Tension pneumothorax, 79
Teratogen drugs, 318
Term delivery, 309
Tertiary syphilis, 130
Testicular cancer, 132
Testicular torsion, 266

Tetanus vaccination, 342
Tetralogy of Fallot, 243
Thalassemia, 36
Third-degree heart block, 11
Thoracic aorta dissection, 26
Threatened abortion, 320
Thrombotic thrombocytopenia purpura (TTP), 43
Thyroid cancer, 89
Thyroid disorder, 86
Thyroid nodule, 89
Thyroid storm, 88
Tibial fracture, 183
Tinea capitis, 353
Tinea corporis, 353
Tinea cruris, 353
Tinea pedis, 353
Tinea versicolor, 353
Tonic seizures, 200
Tonic- clonic seizure, 200
TORCH syndrome, 277
Tourette's syndrome, 236
Toxic epidermal necrolysis, 361
Toxic shock syndrome, 363
Toxicology, 371
Toxoplasmosis encephalitis, 210
Toxoplasmosis, 277
Tracheoesophageal fistula, 250
Transfusion reaction, 56
Transfusion-associated acute lung injury, 56
Transient ischemia, 188
Transient synovitis, 259
Transient tachypnea of newborn, 250
Transplant rejection, 57
Transposition of the great arteries, 243
Transverse vaginal pouch, 295
Traveler prophylaxis, 342
Trichomonas, 285
Trichotillomania, 228
Trigger finger, 182
Trisomy 18, 314

Trisomy 21, 314
Tropical spruce, 148
Tuberculosis meningitis, 209
Tuberculosis, 76
Turcot's syndrome, 145
Turner syndrome, 274
Turner syndrome, 296
Type 1 diabetes, 81
Type 2 diabetes, 83
Type I error, 344
Type II error, 344
Typhoid, 342
Typical pneumonia, 73

U
Ulcerative colitis (UC), 143
Umbilical cord prolapse, 322
Umbilical hernia, 249
Unacceptable bias, 346
Unhappy triad, 184
Unstable angina, 5
Upper GI bleeding, 150
Urethritis, 128
Urge incontinence, 287, 288
Uric acid stones, 121
Urinary tract infection, 127, 215
Urine incontinence, 287
Uterine atony, 332
Uterine inversion, 332
Uterine leiomyoma, 300
Uterine prolapse, 303
Uterine rupture, 323
Uveitis, 367

V
VACTERL syndrome, 251
Vaginitis, 285
Variable decelerations, 322
Varicella vaccination, 341
Varicella-Zoster, 277
Varicella, 268
Varicocele, 264
Vasa previa, 324
Vascular dementia, 193

Vasomotor rhinitis, 61
Venous ulcers, 28
Ventilator associated pneumonia, 75
Ventricular fibrillation, 11
Ventricular septal defect, 244
Ventricular tachycardia, 12
Vertigo, 196
Vestibular neuritis, 196
Viral conjunctivitis, 368
Viral hepatitis, 155
Viral pneumonia, 255
Virilization, 293
Vitamin A deficiency, 375
Vitamin A toxicity, 375
Vitamin B 1 deficiency, 375
Vitamin B 12 deficiency, 375
Vitamin B 2 deficiency, 375
Vitamin B 3 deficiency, 375
Vitamin B 5 deficiency, 375
Vitamin B 6 deficiency, 375
Vitamin B- 12 deficiency, 38
Vitamin C deficiency, 375
Vitamin D deficiency, 375
Vitamin D toxicity, 375
Vitamin K deficiency, 375
Vitamin K deficiency, 55
Vitamin K toxicity, 375
Von Willebrand disease, 54
Vulvar cancer, 290

W
Waldenstrom's
macroglobulinemia, 53
Wandering pacemaker, 14
Warm autoimmune hemolysis, 41
Wegner's granulomatosis, 115
Wernicke's aphasia, 199
Whipple disease, 148
Wilms' tumor, 265
Wilson disease, 154
Wiskott-Aldrich syndrome, 267

Withholding and withdrawing
the treatment, 348
Withholding information from
patient, 348
Wolff–Parkinson–white
syndrome, 14

Y
Yellow fever, 342
Yersinia, 146

Z
Zenker diverticulum, 134
Zero correlation, 345
Zollinger-Ellison syndrome, 142